Essential Psychopharmacology

The Prescriber's Guide

ANTIDEPRESSANTS

New!

In response to the rapid developments in psychopharmacology, this is a spin-off from Stephen Stahl's new, completely revised and updated edition of his much acclaimed *Prescriber's Guide*. It covers the most important drugs in use today for treating depression.

In full color throughout, and with four or more pages for each antidepressant, Stephen Stahl distills his great expertise into a pragmatic formulary that gives all the information a prescriber needs to treat patients effectively. Each drug is covered in five categories: • *general therapeutics,* • *dosing and use,* • *side effects,* • *special populations,* and • *pearls.*

Target icons appear next to key categories for each drug so that the prescriber can go easily and instantly to the information needed. Two indexes are included, listing drugs by name (generic and international) and use. In addition Dr. Stahl indicates which drugs have FDA approval, and also gives the FDA Use-in-Pregnancy Ratings.

Stephen M. Stahl is Adjunct Professor of Psychiatry at the University of California, San Diego. He has conducted numerous research projects awarded by the National Institute of Mental Health, the Veteran's Administration, and the pharmaceutical industry. The author of more than 300 articles and chapters, Stephen Stahl is an internationally recognized clinician, researcher, and teacher in psychiatry with subspecialty expertise in psychopharmacology.

From reviews of the first *Prescriber's Guide:*

". . . instead of a laundry list, Dr. Stahl presents what the clinician ought to be looking for – this is not your father's PDR (*Physician's Desk Reference*)! The clinical tips and pearls that are found in each entry are invaluable – not only are dosing guidelines provided, but also the author's educated and respected opinion regarding potential advantages and disadvantages of each drug . . . a real bargain. . . . The book's major strength is its readability and user friendliness. The art of psychopharmacology is finally given the space it deserves. . . . This guidebook is an excellent source of information for the art of prescribing psychotropic medications and belongs in every clinician's library."
The Annals of Pharmacotherapy

"I think that this manual has all the characteristics of a true bestseller. The format is very attractive, the information is complete, the consultation is easy. In no other recent text will a clinician find so much information in such a concise and user-friendly format."
Acta Psychiatrica Scandinavica, reviewer Mario Maj

Essential Psychopharmacology
The Prescriber's Guide
ANTIDEPRESSANTS

Stephen M. Stahl, M.D., Ph.D.

Adjunct Professor of Psychiatry
University of California at San Diego

Editorial assistant
Meghan M. Grady

With illustrations by
Nancy Muntner

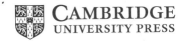
CAMBRIDGE
UNIVERSITY PRESS

Every effort has been made in preparing this book to provide accurate and up-to-date information that is in accord with accepted standards and practice at the time of publication. Nevertheless, the author, editors and publisher can make no warranties that the information contained herein is totally free from error, not least because clinical standards are constantly changing through research and regulation. The authors, editors and publisher therefore disclaim all liability for direct or consequential damages resulting from the use of material contained in this book. Readers are strongly advised to pay careful attention to information provided by the manufacturer of any drugs or equipment that they plan to use.

PUBLISHED BY CAMBRIDGE UNIVERSITY PRESS
Cambridge, New York, Melbourne, Madrid, Cape Town, Singapore, São Paulo

CAMBRIDGE UNIVERSITY PRESS
20 West 20th Street, New York NY, 10011-4211 USA
www.cambridge.org

Information on this title: www.cambridge.org/9780521616348

First published 2006

Printed in Canada by Friesens

*A catalog record for this book is available from
the British Library*

Library of Congress Cataloging-in-Publication Data
Stahl, S. M.
    Essential psychopharmacology : the prescriber's guide : antidepressants
    / Stephen M. Stahl ; editorial assistant, Meghan M. Grady ; with illustra-
    tions by Nancy Muntner.
        p. ; cm.
    Includes bibliographical references and index.
    ISBN-13: 978-0-521-61634-8 (pbk.)
    ISBN-10: 0-521-61634-4 (pbk.)
    1. Antidepressants--Handbooks, manuals, etc.   I. Title. II. Title:
    Prescriber's guide. III. Title: Antidepressants.
    [DNLM: 1. Antidepressive Agents--therapeutic use--Handbooks.
    QV 39 S781eb 2006]
    RM332.S73 2006
    615'.78--dc22
    2006007301

To members of the Neuroscience Education Institute and prescribers of psychopharmacologic agents everywhere. Your relentless determination to find the best portfolio of treatments for each individual patient within your practice is my inspiration.

Table of contents

Introduction   ix

List of icons   xi

1. amitriptyline   1
2. amoxapine   9
3. atomoxetine   17
4. bupropion   23
5. citalopram   29
6. clomipramine   35
7. desipramine   43
8. dothiepin   51
9. doxepin   57
10. duloxetine   65
11. escitalopram   71
12. fluoxetine   77
13. fluvoxamine   83
14. imipramine   89
15. isocarboxazid   95
16. lofepramine   101
17. maprotiline   107
18. milnacipran   113
19. mirtazapine   119
20. moclobemide   125
21. nefazodone   131
22. nortriptyline   137
23. paroxetine   145
24. phenelzine   153
25. protriptyline   159
26. reboxetine   165
27. selegiline   171
28. sertraline   179
29. tianeptine   185
30. tranylcypromine   189
31. trazodone   195
32. trimipramine   201
33. venlafaxine   207

Index by drug name   213
  (generic and international trade names)
Index by use   217

Abbreviations   219

(FDA) Use-In-Pregnancy Ratings   221

Introduction

This *Guide* is intended to complement *Essential Psychopharmacology*. *Essential Psychopharmacology* emphasizes mechanisms of action and how psychotropic drugs work upon receptors and enzymes in the brain. This *Guide* gives practical information on how to use antidepressants in clinical practice.

It would be impossible to include all available information about any antidepressant in a single work and no attempt is made here to be comprehensive. The purpose of this *Guide* is instead to integrate the art of clinical practice with the science of psychopharmacology. That means including only essential facts in order to keep things short. Unfortunately that also means excluding less critical facts as well as extraneous information, which may nevertheless be useful to the reader but would make the book too long and dilute the most important information. In deciding what to include and what to omit, the author has drawn upon common sense and 30 years of clinical experience with patients. He has also consulted with many experienced clinicians and analysed the evidence from controlled clinical trials and regulatory filings with government agencies.

In order to meet the needs of the clinician and to facilitate future updates of this *Guide*, the opinions of readers are sincerely solicited. Feedback can be emailed to feedback@neiglobal.com. Specifically, are the best and most essential antidepressant drugs included here? Do you find any factual errors? Are there agreements or disagreements with any of the opinions expressed here? Are there suggestions for any additional tips or pearls for future editions? Any and all suggestions and comments are welcomed.

All of the selected drugs are presented in the same design format in order to facilitate rapid access to information. Specifically, each drug is broken down into five sections, each designated by a unique color background: ■ therapeutics, ■ side effects, ■ dosing and use, ■ special populations, and ■ the art of psychopharmacology, followed by key references.

Therapeutics covers the brand names in major countries; the class of drug; what it is commonly prescribed and approved for by the United States Food and Drug Administration (FDA); how the drug works; how long it takes to work; what to do if it works or if it doesn't work; the best augmenting combinations for partial response or treatment resistance, and the tests (if any) that are required.

Side effects explains how the drug causes side effects; gives a list of notable, life threatening or dangerous side effects; gives a specific rating for weight gain or sedation, and advice about how to handle side effects, including best augmenting agents for side effects.

Dosing and use gives the usual dosing range; dosage forms; how to dose and dosing tips; symptoms of overdose; long-term use; if habit forming, how to stop; pharmacokinetics; drug interactions, when not to use and other warnings or precautions.

Special populations gives specific information about any possible renal, hepatic and cardiac impairments, and any precautions to be taken for treating the elderly, children, adolescents, and pregnant and breast-feeding women.

The art of psychopharmacology gives the author's opinions on issues such as the potential advantages and disadvantages of any one drug, the primary target symptoms, and clinical pearls to get the best out of a drug.

At the back of the *Guide* are two indexes. The first is an index by drug name, giving both generic names (uncapitalized) and trade names (capitalized and followed by the generic name in parentheses). The second is an index of common uses for the generic drugs included in the *Guide* and is organized by disorder/symptom. Agents that are approved by the FDA for a particular use are shown in bold. In addition to these indexes there is a list of abbreviations; FDA definitions for the Pregnancy Categories A, B, C, D and X, and, finally, an index of the icons used in the *Guide*.

Readers are encouraged to consult standard references[1] and comprehensive psychiatry and pharmacology textbooks for more in-depth information. They are also reminded that the art of psychopharmacology section is the author's opinion.

It is strongly advised that readers familiarize themselves with the standard use of these drugs before attempting any of the more exotic uses discussed, such as unusual drug combinations and doses. Reading about both drugs before augmenting one with the other is also strongly recommended. Today's psychopharmacologist should also regularly track blood pressure, weight and body mass index for most of their patients. The dutiful clinician will also check out the drug interactions of non-central-nervous-system (CNS) drugs with those that act in the CNS, including any prescribed by other clinicians.

Certain drugs may be for experts only and might include nefazodone and MAO inhibitors, among others. Off-label uses not approved by the FDA and inadequately studied doses or combinations of drugs may also be for the expert only, who can weigh risks and benefits in the presence of sometimes vague and conflicting evidence. Pregnant or nursing women, or people with two or more psychiatric illnesses, substance abuse, and/or a concomitant medical illness may be suitable patients for the expert only. Use your best judgement as to your level of expertise and realize that we are all learning in this rapidly advancing field. The practice of medicine is often not so much a science as it is an art. It is important to stay within the standards of medical care for the field, and also within your personal comfort zone, while trying to help extremely ill and often difficult patients with medicines that can sometimes transform their lives and relieve their suffering.

Finally, this book is intended to be genuinely helpful for practitioners of psychopharmacology by providing them with the mixture of facts and opinions selected by the author. Ultimately, prescribing choices are the reader's responsibility. Every effort has been made in preparing this book to provide accurate and up-to-date information in accord with accepted standards and practice at the time of publication. Nevertheless, the psychopharmacology field is evolving rapidly and the author and publisher make no warranties that the information contained herein is totally free from error, not least because clinical standards are constantly changing through research and regulation. Furthermore, the author and publisher disclaim any responsibility for the continued currency of this information and disclaim all liability for any and all damages, including direct or consequential damages, resulting from the use of information contained in this book. Doctors recommending and patients using these drugs are strongly advised to pay careful attention to, and consult information provided by the manufacturer.

---

[1] For example, *Physician's Desk Reference* and *Martindale's*

List of icons

 alpha 2 agonist

 anticonvulsant

 antihistamine

 benzodiazepine

 cholinesterase inhibitor

 conventional antipsychotic

 dopamine stabilizer

 lithium

 modafinil (wake-promoter)

 monoamine oxidase inhibitor

 nefazodone (serotonin antagonist/reuptake inhibitor)

 N-methyl-d-aspartate antagonist

 noradrenergic and specific serotonergic antidepressant

norepinephrine and dopamine reuptake inhibitor

 sedative hypnotic

 selective norepinephrine reuptake inhibitor

 selective serotonin reuptake inhibitor

 serotonin-dopamine antagonist

 serotonin and norepinephrine reuptake inhibitor

 serotonin 1A partial agonist

 stimulant

 trazodone (serotonin antagonist/reuptake inhibitor)

 tricyclic/tetracyclic antidepressant

 How the drug works, mechanism of action

 Best augmenting agents to add for partial response or treatment-resistance

 Life-threatening or dangerous side effects

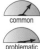   **Weight Gain:** Degrees of weight gain associated with the drug, with unusual signifying that weight gain has been reported but is not expected; not unusual signifying that weight gain occurs in a significant minority; common signifying that many experience weight gain and/or it can be significant in amount; and problematic signifying that weight gain occurs frequently, can be significant in amount, and may be a health problem in some patients

    Sedation: Degrees of sedation associated with the drug, with unusual signifying that sedation has been reported but is not expected; not unusual signifying that sedation occurs in a significant minority; common signifying that many experience sedation and/or it can be significant in amount; and problematic signifying that sedation occurs frequently, can be significant in amount, and may be a health problem in some patients

Tips for dosing based on the clinical expertise of the author

Drug interactions that may occur

Warnings and precautions regarding use of the drug

Dosing and other information specific to children and adolescents

Information regarding use of the drug during pregnancy

Clinical pearls of information based on the clinical expertise of the author

THERAPEUTICS

Brands • Elavil
see index for additional brand names

Generic? Yes

Class

• Tricyclic antidepressant (TCA)
• Serotonin and norepinephrine/noradrenaline reuptake inhibitor

Commonly Prescribed For
(bold for FDA approved)

• **Depression**
• **Endogenous depression**
✳ Neuropathic pain/chronic pain
✳ Fibromyalgia
✳ Headache
✳ Low back pain/neck pain
• Anxiety
• Insomnia
• Treatment-resistant depression

How The Drug Works

• Boosts neurotransmitters serotonin and norepinephrine/noradrenaline
• Blocks serotonin reuptake pump (serotonin transporter), presumably increasing serotonergic neurotransmission
• Blocks norepinephrine reuptake pump (norepinephrine transporter), presumably increasing noradrenergic neurotransmission
• Presumably desensitizes both serotonin 1A receptors and beta adrenergic receptors
• Since dopamine is inactivated by norepinephrine reuptake in frontal cortex, which largely lacks dopamine transporters, amitriptyline can increase dopamine neurotransmission in this part of the brain

How Long Until It Works

• May have immediate effects in treating insomnia or anxiety
• Onset of therapeutic actions usually not immediate, but often delayed 2 to 4 weeks
• If it is not working within 6 to 8 weeks for depression, it may require a dosage increase or it may not work at all
• May continue to work for many years to prevent relapse of symptoms

If It Works

• The goal of treatment of depression is complete remission of current symptoms as well as prevention of future relapses
• The goal of treatment of chronic pain conditions such as neuropathic pain, fibromyalgia, headaches, low back pain, and neck pain is to reduce symptoms as much as possible, especially in combination with other treatments
• Treatment of depression most often reduces or even eliminates symptoms, but not a cure since symptoms can recur after medicine stopped
• Treatment of chronic pain conditions such as neuropathic pain, fibromyalgia, headache, low back pain, and neck pain may reduce symptoms, but rarely eliminates them completely, and is not a cure since symptoms can recur after medicine is stopped
• Continue treatment of depression until all symptoms are gone (remission)
• Once symptoms of depression are gone, continue treating for 1 year for the first episode of depression
• For second and subsequent episodes of depression, treatment may need to be indefinite
• Use in anxiety disorders and chronic pain conditions such as neuropathic pain, fibromyalgia, headache, low back pain, and neck pain may also need to be indefinite, but long-term treatment is not well studied in these conditions

If It Doesn't Work

• Many depressed patients only have a partial response where some symptoms are improved but others persist (especially insomnia, fatigue, and problems concentrating)
• Other depressed patients may be nonresponders, sometimes called treatment-resistant or treatment-refractory
• Consider increasing dose, switching to another agent or adding an appropriate augmenting agent
• Consider psychotherapy
• Consider evaluation for another diagnosis or for a comorbid condition (e.g., medical illness, substance abuse, etc.)
• Some patients may experience apparent lack of consistent efficacy due to activation of latent or underlying bipolar disorder, and

require antidepressant discontinuation and a switch to a mood stabilizer

Best Augmenting Combos for Partial Response or Treatment-Resistance

- Lithium, buspirone, thyroid hormone (for depression)
- Gabapentin, tiagabine, other anticonvulsants, even opiates if done by experts while monitoring carefully in difficult cases (for chronic pain)

Tests

- None for healthy individuals
- * Since tricyclic and tetracyclic antidepressants are frequently associated with weight gain, before starting treatment, weigh all patients and determine if the patient is already overweight (BMI 25.0–29.9) or obese (BMI ≥30)
- Before giving a drug that can cause weight gain to an overweight or obese patient, consider determining whether the patient already has pre-diabetes (fasting plasma glucose 100–125 mg/dl), diabetes (fasting plasma glucose >126 mg/dl), or dyslipidemia (increased total cholesterol, LDL cholesterol and triglycerides; decreased HDL cholesterol), and treat or refer such patients for treatment, including nutrition and weight management, physical activity counseling, smoking cessation, and medical management
- * Monitor weight and BMI during treatment
- * While giving a drug to a patient who has gained >5% of initial weight, consider evaluating for the presence of pre-diabetes, diabetes, or dyslipidemia, or consider switching to a different antidepressant
- EKGs may be useful for selected patients (e.g., those with personal or family history of QTc prolongation; cardiac arrhythmia; recent myocardial infarction; uncompensated heart failure; or taking agents that prolong QTc interval such as pimozide, thioridazine, selected antiarrhythmics, moxifloxacin, sparfloxacin, etc.)
- Patients at risk for electrolyte disturbances (e.g., patients on diuretic therapy) should have baseline and periodic serum potassium and magnesium measurements

avoid other anticholinergics

SIDE EFFECTS

How Drug Causes Side Effects

- Anticholinergic activity may explain sedative effects, dry mouth, constipation, and blurred vision
- Sedative effects and weight gain may be due to antihistamine properties
- Blockade of alpha adrenergic 1 receptors may explain dizziness, sedation, and hypotension
- Cardiac arrhythmias and seizures, especially in overdose, may be caused by blockade of ion channels

Notable Side Effects

- Blurred vision, constipation, urinary retention, increased appetite, dry mouth, nausea, diarrhea, heartburn, unusual taste in mouth, weight gain
- Fatigue, weakness, dizziness, sedation, headache, anxiety, nervousness, restlessness
- Sexual dysfunction (impotence, change in libido)
- Sweating, rash, itching

Life Threatening or Dangerous Side Effects

- Paralytic ileus, hyperthermia (TCAs + anticholinergic agents)
- Lowered seizure threshold and rare seizures
- Orthostatic hypotension, sudden death, arrhythmias, tachycardia
- QTc prolongation
- Hepatic failure, extrapyramidal symptoms
- Increased intraocular pressure
- Rare induction of mania
- Rare activation of suicidal ideation and behavior (suicidality)

Weight Gain

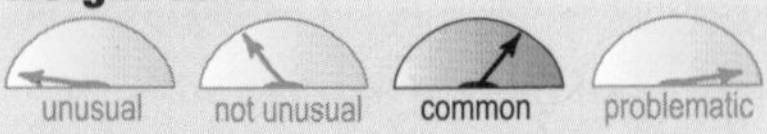
unusual
not unusual
common
problematic

- Many experience and/or can be significant in amount
- Can increase appetite and carbohydrate craving

Sedation

unusual   not unusual   **common**   problematic

- Many experience and/or can be significant in amount
- Tolerance to sedative effects may develop with long-term use

What To Do About Side Effects

- Wait
- Wait
- Wait
- Lower the dose
- Switch to an SSRI or newer antidepressant

Best Augmenting Agents for Side Effects

- Many side effects cannot be improved with an augmenting agent

DOSING AND USE

Usual Dosage Range

- 50–150 mg/day

Dosage Forms

- Capsule 25 mg, 50 mg, 100 mg

How to Dose

- Initial 25 mg/day at bedtime; increase by 25 mg every 3–7 days
- 75 mg/day in divided doses; increase to 150 mg/day; maximum 300 mg/day

 Dosing Tips

- If given in a single dose, should generally be administered at bedtime because of its sedative properties
- If given in split doses, largest dose should generally be given at bedtime because of its sedative properties
- If patients experience nightmares, split dose and do not give large dose at bedtime
- Patients treated for chronic pain may only require lower doses
- If intolerable anxiety, insomnia, agitation, akathisia, or activation occur either upon dosing initiation or discontinuation, consider the possibility of activated bipolar disorder, and switch to a mood stabilizer or an atypical antipsychotic

Overdose

- Death may occur; CNS depression, convulsions, cardiac dysrhythmias, severe hypotension, ECG changes, coma

Long-Term Use

- Safe

Habit Forming

- No

How to Stop

- Taper to avoid withdrawal effects
- Even with gradual dose reduction, some withdrawal symptoms may appear within the first 2 weeks
- Many patients tolerate 50% dose reduction for 3 days, then another 50% reduction for 3 days, then discontinuation
- If withdrawal symptoms emerge during discontinuation, raise dose to stop symptoms and then restart withdrawal much more slowly

Pharmacokinetics

- Substrate for CYP450 2D6 and 1A2
- Plasma half-life 10–28 hours
- Metabolized to an active metabolite, nortriptyline, which is predominantly a norepinephrine reuptake inhibitor, by demethylation via CYP450 1A2

 Drug Interactions

- Tramadol increases the risk of seizures in patients taking TCAs
- Use of TCAs with anticholinergic drugs may result in paralytic ileus or hyperthermia
- Fluoxetine, paroxetine, bupropion, duloxetine, and other CYP450 2D6 inhibitors may increase TCA concentrations
- Fluvoxamine, a CYP450 1A2 inhibitor, can decrease the conversion of amitriptyline to nortriptyline and increase amitriptyline plasma concentrations
- Cimetidine may increase plasma concentrations of TCAs and cause anticholinergic symptoms
- Phenothiazines or haloperidol may raise TCA blood concentrations
- May alter effects of antihypertensive drugs; may inhibit hypotensive effects of clonidine
- Use of TCAs with sympathomimetic agents may increase sympathetic activity

- Methylphenidate may inhibit metabolism of TCAs
- Activation and agitation, especially following switching or adding antidepressants, may represent the induction of a bipolar state, especially a mixed dysphoric bipolar II condition sometimes associated with suicidal ideation, and require the addition of lithium, a mood stabilizer or an atypical antipsychotic, and/or discontinuation of amitriptyline

 Other Warnings/ Precautions

- Add or initiate other antidepressants with caution for up to 2 weeks after discontinuing amitriptyline
- Generally, do not use with MAO inhibitors, including 14 days after MAOIs are stopped; do not start an MAOI until 2 weeks after discontinuing amitriptyline, but see Pearls
- Use with caution in patients with history of seizures, urinary retention, narrow angle-closure glaucoma, hyperthyroidism
- TCAs can increase QTc interval, especially at toxic doses, which can be attained not only by overdose but also by combining with drugs that inhibit TCA metabolism via CYP450 2D6, potentially causing torsade de pointes-type arrhythmia or sudden death
- Because TCAs can prolong QTc interval, use with caution in patients who have bradycardia or who are taking drugs that can induce bradycardia (e.g., beta blockers, calcium channel blockers, clonidine, digitalis)
- Because TCAs can prolong QTc interval, use with caution in patients who have hypokalemia and/or hypomagnesemia, or who are taking drugs that can induce hypokalemia and/or magnesemia (e.g., diuretics, stimulant laxatives, intravenous amphotericin B, glucocorticoids, tetracosactide)
- When treating children, carefully weigh the risks and benefits of pharmacological treatment against the risks and benefits of nontreatment with antidepressants and make sure to document this in the patient's chart
- Distribute the brochures provided by the FDA and the drug companies

- Warn patients and their caregivers about the possibility of activating side effects and advise them to report such symptoms immediately
- Monitor patients for activation of suicidal ideation, especially children and adolescents

Do Not Use

- If patient is recovering from myocardial infarction
- If patient is taking agents capable of significantly prolonging QTc interval (e.g., pimozide, thioridazine, selected antiarrhythmics, moxifloxacin, sparfloxacin)
- If there is a history of QTc prolongation or cardiac arrhythmia, recent acute myocardial infarction, uncompensated heart failure
- If patient is taking drugs that inhibit TCA metabolism, including CYP450 2D6 inhibitors, except by an expert
- If there is reduced CYP450 2D6 function, such as patients who are poor 2D6 metabolizers, except by an expert and at low doses
- If there is a proven allergy to amitriptyline or nortriptyline

Renal Impairment

- Use with caution; may need to lower dose

Hepatic Impairment

- Use with caution; may need to lower dose

Cardiac Impairment

- TCAs have been reported to cause arrhythmias, prolongation of conduction time, orthostatic hypotension, sinus tachycardia, and heart failure, especially in the diseased heart
- Myocardial infarction and stroke have been reported with TCAs
- TCAs produce QTc prolongation, which may be enhanced by the existence of bradycardia, hypokalemia, congenital or acquired long QTc interval, which should be evaluated prior to administering amitriptyline
- Use with caution if treating concomitantly with a medication likely to produce

prolonged bradycardia, hypokalemia, slowing of intracardiac conduction, or prolongation of the QTc interval

- Avoid TCAs in patients with a known history of QTc prolongation, recent acute myocardial infarction, and uncompensated heart failure
- TCAs may cause a sustained increase in heart rate in patients with ischemic heart disease and may worsen (decrease) heart rate variability, an independent risk of mortality in cardiac populations
- Since SSRIs may improve (increase) heart rate variability in patients following a myocardial infarct and may improve survival as well as mood in patients with acute angina or following a myocardial infarction, these are more appropriate agents for cardiac population than tricyclic/tetracyclic antidepressants
- *Risk/benefit ratio may not justify use of TCAs in cardiac impairment*

Elderly

- May be more sensitive to anticholinergic, cardiovascular, hypotensive, and sedative effects
- Initial dose 50 mg/day; increase gradually up to 100 mg/day

 ## Children and Adolescents

- Carefully weigh the risks and benefits of pharmacological treatment against the risks and benefits of nontreatment with antidepressants and make sure to document this in the patient's chart
- Use with caution, observing for activation of known or unknown bipolar disorder and/or suicidal ideation, and inform parents or guardian of this risk so they can help observe child or adolescent patients
- Monitor patients face-to-face regularly, particularly during the first several weeks of treatment
- Not generally recommended for use under age 12
- Several studies show lack of efficacy of TCAs for depression
- May be used to treat enuresis or hyperactive/impulsive behaviors
- Some cases of sudden death have occurred in children taking TCAs

- Adolescents: initial dose 50 mg/day; increase gradually up to 100 mg/day

Pregnancy

- Risk Category C [some animal studies show adverse effects, no controlled studies in humans]
- Crosses the placenta
- Adverse effects have been reported in infants whose mothers took a TCA (lethargy, withdrawal symptoms, fetal malformations)
- Must weigh the risk of treatment (first trimester fetal development, third trimester newborn delivery) to the child against the risk of no treatment (recurrence of depression, maternal health, infant bonding) to the mother and child
- For many patients this may mean continuing treatment during pregnancy

Breast Feeding

- Some drug is found in mother's breast milk
- *Recommended either to discontinue drug or bottle feed
- Immediate postpartum period is a high-risk time for depression, especially in women who have had prior depressive episodes, so drug may need to be reinstituted late in the third trimester or shortly after childbirth to prevent a recurrence during the postpartum period
- Must weigh benefits of breast feeding with risks and benefits of antidepressant treatment versus non-treatment to both the infant and the mother
- For many patients this may mean continuing treatment during breast feeding

THE ART OF PSYCHOPHARMACOLOGY

Potential Advantages

- Patients with insomnia
- Severe or treatment-resistant depression
- Patients with a wide variety of chronic pain syndromes

Potential Disadvantages

- Pediatric and geriatric patients
- Patients concerned with weight gain
- Cardiac patients

Primary Target Symptoms

- Depressed mood
- Symptoms of anxiety
- Somatic symptoms
- Chronic pain
- Insomnia

 Pearls

- Was once one of the most widely prescribed agents for depression
- Remains one of the most favored TCAs for treating headache and a wide variety of chronic pain syndromes, including neuropathic pain, fibromyalgia, migraine, neck pain, and low back pain
- ✳ Preference of some prescribers for amitriptyline over other tricyclic/tetracyclic antidepressants for the treatment of chronic pain syndromes is based more upon art and anecdote rather than controlled clinical trials, since many TCAs/tetracylics may be effective for chronic pain syndromes
- Tricyclic antidepressants are no longer generally considered a first-line treatment option for depression because of their side effect profile
- ✳ Amitriptyline has been shown to be effective in primary insomnia
- TCAs may aggravate psychotic symptoms
- Alcohol should be avoided because of additive CNS effects
- Underweight patients may be more susceptible to adverse cardiovascular effects
- Children, patients with inadequate hydration, and patients with cardiac disease may be more susceptible to TCA-induced cardiotoxicity than healthy adults
- For the expert only: although generally prohibited, a heroic but potentially dangerous treatment for severely treatment-resistant patients is to give a tricyclic/tetracyclic antidepressant other than clomipramine simultaneously with an MAO inhibitor for patients who fail to respond to numerous other antidepressants
- If this option is elected, start the MAOI with the tricyclic/tetracyclic antidepressant simultaneously at low doses after appropriate drug washout, then alternately increase doses of these agents every few days to a week as tolerated
- Although very strict dietary and concomitant drug restrictions must be observed to prevent hypertensive crises and serotonin syndrome, the most common side effects of MAOI/tricyclic or tetracyclic combinations may be weight gain and orthostatic hypotension
- Patients on TCAs should be aware that they may experience symptoms such as photosensitivity or blue-green urine
- SSRIs may be more effective than TCAs in women, and TCAs may be more effective than SSRIs in men
- Since tricyclic/tetracyclic antidepressants are substrates for CYP450 2D6, and 7% of the population (especially Caucasians) may have a genetic variant leading to reduced activity of 2D6, such patients may not safely tolerate normal doses of tricyclic/tetracyclic antidepressants and may require dose reduction
- Phenotypic testing may be necessary to detect this genetic variant prior to dosing with a tricyclic/tetracyclic antidepressant, especially in vulnerable populations such as children, elderly, cardiac populations, and those on concomitant medications
- Patients who seem to have extraordinarily severe side effects at normal or low doses may have this phenotypic CYP450 2D6 variant and require low doses or switching to another antidepressant not metabolized by 2D6

Suggested Reading

Anderson IM. Meta-analytical studies on new antidepressants. Br Med Bull 2001; 57:161–178.

Anderson IM. Selective serotonin reuptake inhibitors versus tricyclic antidepressants: a meta-analysis of efficacy and tolerability. J Aff Disorders 2000;58:19–36.

Barbui C, Hotopf M. Amitriptyline v. the rest: still the leading antidepressant after 40 years of randomised controlled trials. Br J Psychiatry 2001;178:129–144.

Bryson HM, Wilde MI. Amitriptyline. A review of its pharmacological properties and therapeutic use in chronic pain states. Drugs Aging 1996;8:459–76.

THERAPEUTICS

Brands
• Asendin
see index for additional brand names

Generic? Yes

Class
• Tricyclic antidepressant (TCA), sometimes classified as a tetracyclic antidepressant
• Norepinephrine/noradrenaline reuptake inhibitor
• Serotonin 2A antagonist
• Parent drug and especially an active metabolite are dopamine 2 antagonists

Commonly Prescribed For
(bold for FDA approved)
• **Neurotic or reactive depressive disorder**
• **Endogenous and psychotic depressions**
• **Depression accompanied by anxiety or agitation**
• Depressive phase of bipolar disorder
• Anxiety
• Insomnia
• Neuropathic pain/chronic pain
• Treatment-resistant depression

How The Drug Works
• Boosts neurotransmitter norepinephrine/noradrenaline
• Blocks norepinephrine reuptake pump (norepinephrine transporter), presumably increasing noradrenergic neurotransmission
• Since dopamine is inactivated by norepinephrine reuptake in frontal cortex, which largely lacks dopamine transporters, amoxapine can thus increase dopamine neurotransmission in this part of the brain
• A more potent inhibitor of norepinephrine reuptake pump than serotonin reuptake pump (serotonin transporter)
• At high doses may also boost neurotransmitter serotonin and presumably increase serotonergic neurotransmission
• Blocks dopamine 2 receptors, reducing positive symptoms of psychosis

How Long Until It Works
• Onset of therapeutic actions usually not immediate, but often delayed 2 to 4 weeks

• If it is not working within 6 to 8 weeks for depression, it may require a dosage increase or it may not work at all
• May continue to work for many years to prevent relapse of symptoms

If It Works
• The goal of treatment is complete remission of current symptoms as well as prevention of future relapses
• Treatment most often reduces or even eliminates symptoms, but not a cure since symptoms can recur after medicine stopped
• Continue treatment until all symptoms are gone (remission)
• Once symptoms gone, continue treating for 1 year for the first episode of depression
• For second and subsequent episodes of depression, treatment may need to be indefinite
• Use in anxiety disorders may also need to be indefinite

If It Doesn't Work
• Many patients only have a partial response where some symptoms are improved but others persist (especially insomnia, fatigue, and problems concentrating)
• Other patients may be nonresponders, sometimes called treatment-resistant or treatment-refractory
• Consider increasing dose, switching to another agent or adding an appropriate augmenting agent
• Consider psychotherapy
• Consider evaluation for another diagnosis or for a comorbid condition (e.g., medical illness, substance abuse, etc.)
• Some patients may experience apparent lack of consistent efficacy due to activation of latent or underlying bipolar disorder, and require antidepressant discontinuation and a switch to a mood stabilizer

Best Augmenting Combos for Partial Response or Treatment-Resistance
• Lithium, buspirone, thyroid hormone

Tests
• None for healthy individuals
✱ Since tricyclic and tetracyclic antidepressants are frequently associated with weight gain, before starting treatment,

weigh all patients and determine if the patient is already overweight (BMI 25.0–29.9) or obese (BMI ≥30)

- Before giving a drug that can cause weight gain to an overweight or obese patient, consider determining whether the patient already has pre-diabetes (fasting plasma glucose 100–125 mg/dl), diabetes (fasting plasma glucose >126 mg/dl), or dyslipidemia (increased total cholesterol, LDL cholesterol and triglycerides; decreased HDL cholesterol), and treat or refer such patients for treatment, including nutrition and weight management, physical activity counseling, smoking cessation, and medical management

 Monitor weight and BMI during treatment

 While giving a drug to a patient who has gained >5% of initial weight, consider evaluating for the presence of pre-diabetes, diabetes, or dyslipidemia, or consider switching to a different antidepressant

- EKGs may be useful for selected patients (e.g., those with personal or family history of QTc prolongation; cardiac arrhythmia; recent myocardial infarction; uncompensated heart failure; or taking agents that prolong QTc interval such as pimozide, thioridazine, selected antiarrhythmics, moxifloxacin, sparfloxacin, etc.)
- Patients at risk for electrolyte disturbances (e.g., patients on diuretic therapy) should have baseline and periodic serum potassium and magnesium measurements

SIDE EFFECTS

How Drug Causes Side Effects

- Anticholinergic activity may explain sedative effects, dry mouth, constipation, and blurred vision
- Sedative effects and weight gain may be due to antihistamine properties
- Blockade of alpha adrenergic 1 receptors may explain dizziness, sedation, and hypotension
- Cardiac arrhythmias and seizures, especially in overdose, may be caused by blockade of ion channels

Notable Side Effects

- Blurred vision, constipation, urinary retention, increased appetite, dry mouth, nausea, diarrhea, heartburn, unusual taste in mouth, weight gain
- Fatigue, weakness, dizziness, sedation, headache, anxiety, nervousness, restlessness
- Sexual dysfunction, sweating

 Can cause extrapyramidal symptoms, akathisia, and theoretically, tardive dyskinesia

Life Threatening or Dangerous Side Effects

- Paralytic ileus, hyperthermia (TCAs/tetracyclics + anticholinergic agents)
- Lowered seizure threshold and rare seizures
- Orthostatic hypotension, sudden death, arrhythmias, tachycardia
- QTc prolongation
- Hepatic failure, extrapyramidal symptoms
- Increased intraocular pressure
- Rare induction of mania
- Rare activation of suicidal ideation and behavior (suicidality)

Weight Gain

unusual   not unusual   common   problematic

- Many experience and/or can be significant in amount
- Can increase appetite and carbohydrate craving

Sedation

unusual   not unusual   common   problematic

- Many experience and/or can be significant in amount
- Tolerance to sedative effect may develop with long-term use

What To Do About Side Effects

- Wait
- Wait
- Wait
- Lower the dose
- Switch to an SSRI or newer antidepressant

Best Augmenting Agents for Side Effects
- Many side effects cannot be improved with an augmenting agent
- May use anticholinergics for extrapyramidal symptoms, or switch to another antidepressant

DOSING AND USE

Usual Dosage Range
- 200–300 mg/day

Dosage Forms
- Tablets 25 mg, 50 mg, 100 mg, 150 mg

How to Dose
- Initial 25 mg 2–3 times/day; increase gradually to 100 mg 2–3 times/day or a single dose at bedtime; maximum 400 mg/day (may dose up to 600 mg/day in inpatients)

 Dosing Tips
- If given in a single dose, should generally be administered at bedtime because of its sedative properties
- If given in split doses, largest dose should generally be given at bedtime because of its sedative properties
- If patients experience nightmares, split dose and do not give large dose at bedtime
- If intolerable anxiety, insomnia, agitation, akathisia, or activation occur either upon dosing initiation or discontinuation, consider the possibility of activated bipolar disorder, and switch to a mood stabilizer or an atypical antipsychotic

Overdose
- Death may occur; convulsions, cardiac dysrhythmias, severe hypotension, CNS depression, coma, changes in ECG

Long-Term Use
- Generally safe
- Some patients may develop withdrawal dyskinesias when discontinuing amoxapine after long-term use

Habit Forming
- Some patients may develop tolerance

How to Stop
- Taper to avoid withdrawal effects
- Even with gradual dose reduction some withdrawal symptoms may appear within the first 2 weeks
- Many patients tolerate 50% dose reduction for 3 days, then another 50% reduction for 3 days, then discontinuation
- If withdrawal symptoms emerge during discontinuation, raise dose to stop symptoms and then restart withdrawal much more slowly

Pharmacokinetics
- Substrate for CYP450 2D6
- Half-life of parent drug approximately 8 hours
- 7- and 8-hydroxymetabolites are active and possess serotonin 2A and dopamine 2 antagonist properties, similar to atypical antipsychotics
- Amoxapine is the N-desmethyl metabolite of the conventional antipsychotic loxapine
- Half-life of the active metabolites approximately 24 hours

 Drug Interactions
- Tramadol increases the risk of seizures in patients taking TCAs
- Use of TCAs/tetracyclics with anticholinergic drugs may result in paralytic ileus or hyperthermia
- Fluoxetine, paroxetine, bupropion, duloxetine, and other CYP450 2D6 inhibitors may increase TCA/tetracyclic concentrations
- Cimetidine may increase plasma concentrations of TCAs/tetracyclics and cause anticholinergic symptoms
- Phenothiazines or haloperidol may raise TCA/tetracyclic blood concentrations
- May alter effects of antihypertensive drugs; may inhibit hypotensive effects of clonidine
- Use of TCAs/tetracyclics with sympathomimetic agents may increase sympathetic activity
- Methylphenidate may inhibit metabolism of TCAs/tetracyclics
- Activation and agitation, especially following switching or adding antidepressants, may represent the induction of a bipolar state, especially a mixed dysphoric bipolar II condition

sometimes associated with suicidal ideation, and require the addition of lithium, a mood stabilizer or an atypical antipsychotic, and/or discontinuation of amoxapine

 Other Warnings/ Precautions

- Add or initiate other antidepressants with caution for up to 2 weeks after discontinuing amoxapine
- Generally, do not use with MAO inhibitors, including 14 days after MAOIs are stopped; do not start an MAOI until 2 weeks after discontinuing amoxapine, but see Pearls
- Use with caution in patients with history of seizure, urinary retention, narrow angle-closure glaucoma, hyperthyroidism
- TCAs/tetracyclics can increase QTc interval, especially at toxic doses, which can be attained not only by overdose but also by combining with drugs that inhibit its metabolism via CYP450 2D6, potentially causing torsade de pointes-type arrhythmia or sudden death
- Because TCAs/tetracyclics can prolong QTc interval, use with caution in patients who have bradycardia or who are taking drugs that can induce bradycardia (e.g., beta blockers, calcium channel blockers, clonidine, digitalis)
- Because TCAs/tetracyclics can prolong QTc interval, use with caution in patients who have hypokalemia and/or hypomagnesemia, or who are taking drugs that can induce hypokalemia and/or magnesemia (e.g., diuretics, stimulant laxatives, intravenous amphotericin B, glucocorticoids, tetracosactide)
- When treating children, carefully weigh the risks and benefits of pharmacological treatment against the risks and benefits of nontreatment with antidepressants and make sure to document this in the patient's chart
- Distribute the brochures provided by the FDA and the drug companies
- Warn patients and their caregivers about the possibility of activating side effects and advise them to report such symptoms immediately
- Monitor patients for activation of suicidal ideation, especially children and adolescents

Do Not Use

- If patient is recovering from myocardial infarction
- If patient is taking agents capable of significantly prolonging QTc interval (e.g., pimozide, thioridazine, selected antiarrhythmics, moxifloxacin, sparfloxacin)
- If there is a history of QTc prolongation or cardiac arrhythmia, recent acute myocardial infarction, uncompensated heart failure
- If patient is taking drugs that inhibit TCA/tetracyclic metabolism, including CYP450 2D6 inhibitors, except by an expert
- If there is reduced CYP450 2D6 function, such as patients who are poor 2D6 metabolizers, except by an expert and at low doses
- If there is a proven allergy to amoxapine or loxapine

Renal Impairment
- Use with caution – may require lower than usual adult dose

Hepatic Impairment
- Use with caution – may require lower than usual adult dose

Cardiac Impairment
- TCAs/tetracyclics have been reported to cause arrhythmias, prolongation of conduction time, orthostatic hypotension, sinus tachycardia, and heart failure, especially in the diseased heart
- Myocardial infarction and stroke have been reported with TCAs/tetracyclics
- TCAs/tetracyclics produce QTc prolongation, which may be enhanced by the existence of bradycardia, hypokalemia, congenital or acquired long QTc interval, which should be evaluated prior to administering amoxapine
- Use with caution if treating concomitantly with a medication likely to produce prolonged bradycardia, hypokalemia, slowing of intracardiac conduction, or prolongation of the QTc interval
- Avoid TCAs/tetracyclics in patients with a known history of QTc prolongation, recent

acute myocardial infarction, and uncompensated heart failure
- TCAs/tetracyclics may cause a sustained increase in heart rate in patients with ischemic heart disease and may worsen (decrease) heart rate variability, an independent risk of mortality in cardiac populations
- Since SSRIs may improve (increase) heart rate variability in patients following a myocardial infarct and may improve survival as well as mood in patients with acute angina or following a myocardial infarction, these are more appropriate agents for cardiac population than tricyclic/tetracyclic antidepressants
- ✳ Risk/benefit ratio may not justify use of TCAs/tetracyclics in cardiac impairment

Elderly
- May be more sensitive to anticholinergic, cardiovascular, hypotensive, and sedative effects
- Initial dose 25 mg/day at bedtime; increase by 25 mg/day each week; maximum dose 300 mg/day

Children and Adolescents
- Carefully weigh the risks and benefits of pharmacological treatment against the risks and benefits of nontreatment with antidepressants and make sure to document this in the patient's chart
- Use with caution, observing for activation of known or unknown bipolar disorder and/or suicidal ideation, and inform parents or guardian of this risk so they can help observe child or adolescent patients
- Monitor patients face-to-face regularly, particularly during the first several weeks of treatment
- Not generally recommended for use under age 16
- Several studies show lack of efficacy of TCAs/tetracyclics for depression
- May be used to treat enuresis or hyperactive/impulsive behaviors
- Some cases of sudden death have occurred in children taking TCAs/tetracyclics
- Adolescents: initial 25–50 mg/day; increase gradually to 100 mg/day in divided doses or single dose at bedtime

Pregnancy
- Risk Category C [some animal studies show adverse effects, no controlled studies in humans]
- Amoxapine crosses the placenta
- Adverse effects have been reported in infants whose mothers took a TCA (lethargy, withdrawal symptoms, fetal malformations)
- Evaluate for treatment with an antidepressant with a better risk/benefit ratio

Breast Feeding
- Some drug is found in mother's breast milk
- ✳ Recommended either to discontinue drug or bottle feed
- Immediate postpartum period is a high-risk time for depression, especially in women who have had prior depressive episodes, so drug may need to be reinstituted late in the third trimester or shortly after childbirth to prevent a recurrence during the postpartum period
- Evaluate for treatment with an antidepressant with a better risk/benefit ratio

---

THE ART OF PSYCHOPHARMACOLOGY

Potential Advantages
- Severe or treatment-resistant depression
- Treatment-resistant psychotic depression

Potential Disadvantages
- Pediatric and geriatric patients
- Patients concerned with weight gain
- Cardiac patients
- Patients with Parkinson's disease or tardive dyskinesia

Primary Target Symptoms
- Depressed mood

Pearls
- Tricyclic/tetracyclic antidepressants are no longer generally considered a first-line treatment option for depression because of their side effect profile

- Tricyclic/tetracyclic antidepressants continue to be useful for severe or treatment-resistant depression
* Because of potential extrapyramidal symptoms, akathisia, and theoretical risk of tardive dyskinesia, first consider other TCAs/tetracyclics for long-term use in general and for treatment of chronic patients
- TCAs may aggravate psychotic symptoms
- Alcohol should be avoided because of additive CNS effects
- Underweight patients may be more susceptible to adverse cardiovascular effects
- Children, patients with inadequate hydration, and patients with cardiac disease may be more susceptible to TCA-induced cardiotoxicity than healthy adults
- For the expert only: although generally prohibited, a heroic but potentially dangerous treatment for severely treatment-resistant patients is to give a tricyclic/tetracyclic antidepressant other than clomipramine simultaneously with an MAO inhibitor for patients who fail to respond to numerous other antidepressants
- Use of MAOIs with clomipramine is always prohibited because of the risk of serotonin syndrome and death
- Amoxapine may be the preferred trycyclic/tetracyclic antidepressant to combine with an MAOI in heroic cases due to its theoretically protective 5HT2A antagonist properties
- If this option is elected, start the MAOI with the tricyclic/tetracyclic antidepressant simultaneously at low doses after appropriate drug washout, then alternately increase doses of these agents every few days to a week as tolerated
- Although very strict dietary and concomitant drug restrictions must be observed to prevent hypertensive crises

and serotonin syndrome, the most common side effects of MAOI/tricyclic or tetracyclic combinations may be weight gain and orthostatic hypotention
- Patients on TCAs/tetracyclics should be aware that they may experience symptoms such as photosensitivity or blue-green urine
- SSRIs may be more effective than TCAs/tetracyclics in women, and TCAs/tetracyclics may be more effective than SSRIs in men
* May cause some motor effects, possibly due to effects on dopamine receptors
* Amoxapine may have a faster onset of action than some other antidepressants
* May be pharmacologically similar to an atypical antipsychotic in some patients
* At high doses, patients who form high concentrations of active metabolites may have akathisia, extrapyramidal symptoms, and possibly develop tardive dyskinesia
* Structurally and pharmacologically related to the antipsychotic loxapine
- Since tricyclic/tetracyclic antidepressants are substrates for CYP450 2D6, and 7% of the population (especially Caucasians) may have a genetic variant leading to reduced activity of 2D6, such patients may not safely tolerate normal doses of tricyclic/tetracyclic antidepressants and may require dose reduction
- Phenotypic testing may be necessary to detect this genetic variant prior to dosing with a tricyclic/tetracyclic antidepressant, especially in vulnerable populations such as children, elderly, cardiac populations, and those on concomitant medications
- Patients who seem to have extraordinarily severe side effects at normal or low doses may have this phenotypic CYP450 2D6 variant and require low doses or switching to another antidepressant not metabolized by 2D6

Suggested Reading

Anderson IM. Meta-analytical studies on new antidepressants. Br Med Bull 2001; 57:161–178.

Anderson IM. Selective serotonin reuptake inhibitors versus tricyclic antidepressants: a meta-analysis of efficacy and tolerability. J Aff Disorders 2000;58:19–36.

Hayes PE, Kristoff CA. Adverse reactions to five new antidepressants. Clin Pharm 1986; 5:471–80.

Jue SG, Dawson GW, Brogden RN. Amoxapine: a review of its pharmacology and efficacy in depressed states. Drugs 1982; 24:1–23.

ATOMOXETINE

THERAPEUTICS

Brands • Strattera
see index for additional brand names

Generic? No

 Class
• Selective norepinephrine reuptake inhibitor (NRI)

Commonly Prescribed For
(bold for FDA approved)
• **Attention deficit hyperactivity disorder (ADHD) in adults and children over 6**
• Treatment-resistant depression

 How The Drug Works
• Boosts neurotransmitter norepinephrine/noradrenaline and may also increase dopamine in profrontal cortex
• Blocks norepinephrine reuptake pumps, also known as norepinephrine transporters
• Presumably this increases noradrenergic neurotransmission
• Since dopamine is inactivated by norepinephrine reuptake in frontal cortex, which largely lacks dopamine transporters, atomoxetine can also increase dopamine neurotransmission in this part of the brain

How Long Until It Works
❋ Onset of therapeutic actions in ADHD can be seen as early as the first day of dosing
• Therapeutic actions may continue to improve for 8 to 12 weeks
• If it is not working within 6 to 8 weeks, it may not work at all

If It Works
• The goal of treatment of ADHD is reduction of symptoms of inattentiveness, motor hyperactivity, and/or impulsiveness that disrupt social, school, and/or occupational functioning
• Continue treatment until all symptoms are under control or improvement is stable and then continue treatment indefinitely as long as improvement persists
• Reevaluate the need for treatment periodically
• Treatment for ADHD begun in childhood may need to be continued into adolescence and adulthood if continued benefit is documented

If It Doesn't Work
• Consider adjusting dose or switching to another agent
• Consider behavioral therapy
• Consider the presence of noncompliance and counsel patient and parents
• Consider evaluation for another diagnosis or for a comorbid condition (e.g., bipolar disorder, substance abuse, medical illness, etc.)
• Some patients may experience apparent lack of consistent efficacy due to activation of latent or underlying bipolar disorder, and require atomoxetine discontinuation and a switch to a mood stabilizer

 Best Augmenting Combos for Partial Response or Treatment-Resistance
❋ Best to attempt other monotherapies prior to augmenting
• SSRIs, SNRIs, or mirtazapine for treatment-resistant depression (use combinations of antidepressants with atomoxetine with caution as this may theoretically activate bipolar disorder and suicidal ideation)
• Mood stabilizers or atypical antipsychotics for comorbid bipolar disorder
• For the expert, can combine with modafinil, methylphenidate, or amphetamine for ADHD

Tests
• None recommended for healthy patients
• May be prudent to monitor blood pressure and pulse when initiating treatment and until dosage increments have stabilized

SIDE EFFECTS

How Drug Causes Side Effects
• Norepinephrine increases in parts of the brain and body and at receptors other than those that cause therapeutic actions (e.g., unwanted actions of norepinephrine on acetylcholine release causing decreased appetite, increased heart rate and blood pressure, dry mouth, urinary retention, etc.)

- Most side effects are immediate but often go away with time
- Lack of enhancing dopamine activity in limbic areas theoretically explains atomoxetine's lack of abuse potential

Notable Side Effects

❊ Sedation, fatigue (particularly in children)
❊ Decreased appetite
- Increased heart rate (6–9 beats/min)
- Increased blood pressure (2–4 mm Hg)
- Insomnia, dizziness, anxiety, agitation, aggression, irritability
- Dry mouth, constipation, nausea, vomiting, abdominal pain, dyspepsia
- Urinary hesitancy, urinary retention (older men)
- Dysmenorrhea, sweating
- Sexual dysfunction (men: decreased libido, erectile disturbance, impotence, ejaculatory dysfunction, abnormal orgasm; women: decreased libido, abnormal orgasm)

 Life Threatening or Dangerous Side Effects

- Increased heart rate and hypertension
- Orthostatic hypotension
- Severe liver damage (rare)
- Hypomania and, theoretically, rare induction of mania
- Rare activation of suicidal ideation and behavior (suicidality)

Weight Gain

unusual   not unusual   common   problematic

- Reported but not expected
- Patients may experience weight loss

Sedation

unusual   not unusual   common   problematic

- Occurs in significant minority, particularly in children

What To Do About Side Effects

- Wait
- Wait
- Wait
- Lower the dose
- If giving once daily, can change to split dose twice daily

- If atomoxetine is sedating, take at night to reduce daytime drowsiness
- In a few weeks, switch or add other drugs

Best Augmenting Agents for Side Effects

- For urinary hesitancy, give an alpha 1 blocker such as tamsulosin
- Often best to try another monotherapy prior to resorting to augmentation strategies to treat side effects
- Many side effects are dose-dependent (i.e., they increase as dose increases, or they reemerge until tolerance re-develops)
- Many side effects are time-dependent (i.e., they start immediately upon dosing and upon each dose increase, but go away with time)
- Activation and agitation may represent the induction of a bipolar state, especially a mixed dysphoric bipolar II condition sometimes associated with suicidal ideation, and require the addition of lithium, a mood stabilizer or an atypical antipsychotic, and/or discontinuation of atomoxetine

DOSING AND USE

Usual Dosage Range

- 0.5–1.2 mg/kg/day in children up to 70 kg; 40–100 mg/day in adults

Dosage Forms

- Capsule 10 mg, 18 mg, 25 mg, 40 mg, 60 mg, 80 mg, 100 mg

How to Dose

- For children 70 kg or less: initial dose 0.5 mg/kg/day; after 7 days can increase to 1.2 mg/kg/day either once in the morning or divided; maximum dose 1.4 mg/kg/day or 100 mg/day, whichever is less
- For adults and children over 70 kg: initial dose 40 mg/day; after 7 days can increase to 80 mg/day once in the morning or divided; after 2–4 weeks can increase to 100 mg/day if necessary; maximum daily dose 100 mg

 Dosing Tips

- Can be given once a day in the morning

* Efficacy with once-daily dosing despite a half-life of 5 hours suggests therapeutic effects persist beyond direct pharmacologic effects, unlike stimulants whose effects are generally closely correlated with plasma drug levels
* Once-daily dosing may increase gastrointestinal side effects
* Lower starting dose allows detection of those patients who may be especially sensitive to side effects such as tachycardia and increased blood pressure
* Patients especially sensitive to the side effects of atomoxetine may include those individuals deficient in the enzyme that metabolizes atomoxetine, CYP450 2D6 (i.e., 7% of Caucasians and 2% of African Americans)
* In such individuals, drug should be titrated slowly to tolerability and effectiveness
* Other individuals may require up to 1.8 mg/kg total daily dose

Overdose
* No fatalities have been reported as monotherapy; sedation, agitation, hyperactivity, abnormal behavior, gastrointestinal symptoms

Long-Term Use
* Safe

Habit Forming
* No

How to Stop
* Taper not necessary

Pharmacokinetics
* Metabolized by CYP450 2D6
* Half-life approximately 5 hours

 Drug Interactions
* Tramadol increases the risk of seizures in patients taking an antidepressant
* Plasma concentrations of atomoxetine may be increased by drugs that inhibit CYP450 2D6 (e.g., paroxetine, fluoxetine), so atomoxetine dose may need to be reduced if co-administered
* Co-administration of atomoxetine and oral or I.V. albuterol may lead to increases in heart rate and blood pressure

* Co-administration with methylphenidate does not increase cardiovascular side effects beyond those seen with methylphenidate alone
* Do not use with MAO inhibitors, including 14 days after MAOIs are stopped

 Other Warnings/ Precautions
* Growth (height and weight) should be monitored during treatment with atomoxetine; for patients who are not growing or gaining weight satisfactorily, interruption of treatment should be considered
* Use with caution in patients with hypertension, tachycardia, cardiovascular disease, or cerebrovascular disease
* Use with caution in patients with bipolar disorder
* Use with caution in patients with urinary retention, benign prostatic hypertrophy
* Use with caution with antihypertensive drugs
* When treating children, carefully weigh the risks and benefits of pharmacological treatment against the risks and benefits of nontreatment and make sure to document this in the patient's chart
* Distribute the brochures provided by the FDA and the drug companies
* Warn patients and their caregivers about the possibility of activating side effects and advise them to report such symptoms immediately
* Monitor patients for activation of suicidal ideation, especially children and adolescents

Do Not Use
* If patient is taking an MAO inhibitor
* If patient has narrow angle-closure glaucoma
* If there is a proven allergy to atomoxetine

Renal Impairment
* Dose adjustment not generally necessary

Hepatic Impairment

- For patients with moderate liver impairment, dose should be reduced to 50% of normal dose
- For patients with severe liver impairment, dose should be reduced to 25% of normal dose

Cardiac Impairment
- Use with caution because atomoxetine can increase heart rate and blood pressure

Elderly
- Some patients may tolerate lower doses better

Children and Adolescents
- Approved to treat ADHD in children over age 6
- Recommended target dose is 1.2 mg/kg/day
- Carefully weigh the risks and benefits of pharmacological treatment against the risks and benefits of nontreatment and make sure to document this in the patient's chart
- Monitor patients face-to-face regularly, particularly during the first several weeks of treatment

Pregnancy
- Risk Category C [some animal studies show adverse effects, no controlled studies in humans]
- Use in women of childbearing potential requires weighing potential benefits to the mother against potential risks to the fetus
- * For women of childbearing potential, atomoxetine should generally be discontinued before anticipated pregnancies

Breast Feeding
- Unknown if atomoxetine is secreted in human breast milk, but all psychotropics assumed to be secreted in breast milk
- * Recommend either to discontinue drug or bottle feed

THE ART OF PSYCHOPHARMACOLOGY

Potential Advantages
- No known abuse potential

Potential Disadvantages
- May not act as rapidly as stimulants when initiating treatment in some patients

Primary Target Symptoms
- Concentration, attention span
- Motor hyperactivity
- Depressed mood

Pearls
- * Unlike other agents approved for ADHD, atomoxetine does not have abuse potential and is not a scheduled substance
- * Despite its name as a selective norepinephrine reuptake inhibitor, atomoxetine enhances both dopamine and norepinephrine in frontal cortex, presumably accounting for its therapeutic actions on attention and concentration
- Since dopamine is inactivated by norepinephrine reuptake in frontal cortex, which largely lacks dopamine transporters, atomoxetine can increase dopamine as well as norepinephrine in this part of the brain, presumably causing therapeutic actions in ADHD
- Since dopamine is inactivated by dopamine reuptake in nucleus accumbens, which largely lacks norepinephrine transporters, atomoxetine does not increase dopamine in this part of the brain, presumably explaining why atomoxetine lacks abuse potential
- Atomoxetine's known mechanism of action as a selective norepinephrine reuptake inhibitor suggests its efficacy as an antidepressant
- Pro-noradrenergic actions may be theoretically useful for the treatment of chronic pain
- Atomoxetine's mechanism of action and its potential antidepressant actions suggest it has the potential to de-stabilize latent or undiagnosed bipolar disorder, similar to the known actions of proven antidepressants
- Thus, administer with caution to ADHD patients who may also have bipolar disorder

- Unlike stimulants, atomoxetine may not exacerbate tics in Tourette's Syndrome patients with comorbid ADHD
- Urinary retention in men over 50 with borderline urine flow has been observed with other agents with potent norepinephrine reuptake blocking properties (e.g., reboxetine, milnacipran),

so administer atomoxetine with caution to these patients
- Atomoxetine was originally called tomoxetine but the name was changed to avoid potential confusion with tamoxifen, which might lead to errors in drug dispensing

 Suggested Reading

Kelsey D, Sumner C, Casat C, Coury D, Quintana H, Saylor K et al. Once daily atomoxetine treatment for children with attention deficit hyperactivity behavior including an assessment of evening and morning behavior: a double-blind, placebo-controlled trial. Pediatrics 2004; 114: el-8.

Kratochvil CJ, Vaughan BS, Harrington MJ, Burke WJ. Atomoxetine: a selective noradrenaline reuptake inhibitor for the treatment of attention-deficit/hyperactivity disorder. Expert Opin Pharmacother 2003;4(7):1165–74.

Michelson D, Adler L, Spencer T, Reimherr FW, West SA, Allen AJ, Kelsey D, Wernicke J, Dietrich A, Milton D. Atomoxetine in adults with ADHD: two randomized, placebo-controlled studies. Biol Psychiatry 2003;53(2):112–20.

Michelson D, Buitelaar JK, Danckaerts M, Gillberg C, Spencer TJ, Zuddas A et al. Relapse prevention in pediatric patients with ADHD treated with atomoxetine: a randomized, double-blind, placebo-controlled study. J Am Acad Child Adolesc Psychiatry 2004;43(7): 896–904.

Simpson D, Perry CM. Atomoxetine. Paediatr Drugs 2003;5(6):407–15.

Wernicke JF, Kratochvil CJ. Safety profile of atomoxetine in the treatment of children and adolescents with ADHD. J Clin Psychiatry 2002;63 Suppl 12:50–5.

BUPROPION

THERAPEUTICS

Brands • Wellbutrin, Wellbutrin SR, Wellbutrin XL
• Zyban

Generic? Yes (bupropion and bupropion SR)

Class
• NDRI (norepinephrine dopamine reuptake inhibitor); antidepressant; smoking cessation treatment

Commonly Prescribed For
(bold for FDA approved)
• **Major depressive disorder (bupropion, bupropion SR, and bupropion XL)**
• **Nicotine addiction (bupropion SR)**
• Bipolar depression
• Attention deficit / hyperactivity disorder
• Sexual dysfunction

How The Drug Works
• Boosts neurotransmitters norepinephrine/noradrenaline and dopamine
• Blocks norepinephrine reuptake pump (norepinephrine transporter), presumably increasing norepinephrine neurotransmission
• Since dopamine is inactivated by norepinephrine reuptake in frontal cortex, which largely lacks dopamine transporters, bupropion can increase dopamine neurotransmission in this part of the brain
• Blocks dopamine reuptake pump (dopamine transporter), presumably increasing dopaminergic neurotransmission

How Long Until It Works
• Onset of therapeutic actions usually not immediate, but often delayed 2 to 4 weeks
• If it is not working within 6 to 8 weeks for depression, it may require a dosage increase or it may not work at all
• May continue to work for many years to prevent relapse of symptoms

If It Works
• The goal of treatment of depression is complete remission of current symptoms as well as prevention of future relapses
• Treatment of depression most often reduces or even eliminates symptoms, but is not a cure since symptoms can recur after medicine stopped
• Continue treatment of depression until all symptoms are gone (remission)
• Once symptoms of depression are gone, continue treating for 1 year for the first episode of depression
• For second and subsequent episodes of depression, treatment may need to be indefinite
• Treatment for nicotine addiction should consist of a single treatment for 6 weeks

If It Doesn't Work
• Many patients only have a partial response where some symptoms are improved but others persist (especially insomnia, fatigue, and problems concentrating)
• Other patients may be nonresponders, sometimes called treatment-resistant or treatment-refractory
• Some patients who have an initial response may relapse even though they continue treatment, sometimes called "poop-out"
• Consider increasing dose, switching to another agent or adding an appropriate augmenting agent
• Consider psychotherapy
• Consider evaluation for another diagnosis or for a comorbid condition (e.g., medical illness, substance abuse, etc.)
• Some patients may experience apparent lack of consistent efficacy due to activation of latent or underlying bipolar disorder, and require antidepressant discontinuation and a switch to a mood stabilizer, although this may be a less frequent problem with bupropion than with other antidepressants

Best Augmenting Combos for Partial Response or Treatment-Resistance
• Trazodone for residual insomnia
• Benzodiazepines for residual anxiety
✳ Can be added to SSRIs to reverse SSRI-induced sexual dysfunction, SSRI-induced apathy (use combinations of antidepressants with caution as this may activate bipolar disorder and suicidal ideation)

✳ Can be added to SSRIs to treat partial responders

✳ Often used as an augmenting agent to mood stabilizers and/or atypical antipsychotics in bipolar depression

• Mood stabilizers or atypical antipsychotics can also be added to bupropion for psychotic depression or treatment-resistant depression

• Hypnotics for insomnia

• Mirtazapine, modafinil, atomoxetine (add with caution and at lower doses since bupropion could theoretically raise atomoxetine levels) both for residual symptoms of depression and attention deficit disorder

Tests

• None for healthy individuals

SIDE EFFECTS

How Drug Causes Side Effects

• Side effects are probably caused in part by actions of norepinephrine and dopamine in brain areas with undesired effects (e.g., insomnia, tremor, agitation, headache, dizziness)

• Side effects are probably also caused in part by actions of norepinephrine in the periphery with undesired effects (e.g., sympathetic and parasympathetic effects such as dry mouth, constipation, nausea, anorexia, sweating)

• Most side effects are immediate but often go away with time

Notable Side Effects

• Dry mouth, constipation, nausea, weight loss, anorexia, myalgia

• Insomnia, dizziness, headache, agitation, anxiety, tremor, abdominal pain, tinnitus

• Sweating, rash

• Hypertension

Life Threatening or Dangerous Side Effects

• Rare seizures (higher incidence for immediate release than for sustained release; risk increases with doses above the recommended maximums; risk increases for patients with predisposing factors)

• Hypomania (more likely in bipolar patients but perhaps less common than with some other antidepressants)

• Rare induction of mania

• Rare activation of suicidal ideation and behavior (suicidality)

Weight Gain

unusual not unusual common problematic

• Reported but not expected

✳ Patients may experience weight loss

Sedation

unusual not unusual common problematic

• Reported but not expected

What To Do About Side Effects

• Wait

• Wait

• Wait

• Keep dose as low as possible

• Take no later than mid-afternoon to avoid insomnia

• Switch to another drug

Best Augmenting Agents for Side Effects

• Often best to try another antidepressant monotherapy prior to resorting to augmentation strategies to treat side effects

• Trazodone or a hypnotic for drug-induced insomnia

• Mirtazapine for insomnia, agitation, and gastrointestinal side effects

• Benzodiazepines or buspirone for drug-induced anxiety, agitation

• Many side effects are dose-dependent (i.e., they increase as dose increases, or they reemerge until tolerance re-develops)

• Many side effects are time-dependent (i.e., they start immediately upon dosing and upon each dose increase, but go away with time)

• Activation and agitation may represent the induction of a bipolar state, especially a mixed dysphoric bipolar II condition sometimes associated with suicidal ideation, and require the addition of lithium, a mood stabilizer or an atypical antipsychotic, and/or discontinuation of bupropion

DOSING AND USE

Usual Dosage Range
- Bupropion: 225–450 mg in 3 divided doses (maximum single dose 150 mg)
- Bupropion SR: 200–450 mg in 2 divided doses (maximum single dose 200 mg)
- Bupropion XL: 150–450 mg once daily (maximum single dose 450 mg)

Dosage Forms
- Bupropion: tablet 75 mg, 100 mg
- Bupropion SR (sustained release): tablet 100 mg, 150 mg, 200 mg
- Bupropion XL (extended release): tablet 150 mg, 300 mg

How to Dose
- Depression: for bupropion immediate release, dosing should be in divided doses, starting at 75 mg twice daily, increasing to 100 mg twice daily, then to 100 mg 3 times daily; maximum dose 450 mg per day
- Depression: for bupropion SR, initial dose 100 mg twice a day, increase to 150 mg twice a day after at least 3 days; wait 4 weeks or longer to ensure drug effects before increasing dose; maximum dose 400 mg total per day
- Depression: for bupropion XL, initial dose 150 mg once daily in the morning; can increase to 300 mg once daily after 4 days; maximum single dose 450 mg once daily
- Nicotine addiction [for bupropion SR]: Initial dose 150 mg/day once a day, increase to 150 mg twice a day after at least 3 days; maximum dose 300 mg/day; bupropion treatment should begin 1–2 weeks before smoking is discontinued

 Dosing Tips
- XL formulation has replaced immediate release and SR formulations as the preferred option
- XL is best dosed once a day, whereas SR is best dosed twice daily, and immediate release is best dosed 3 times daily
- Dosing higher than 450 mg/day (400 mg/day SR) increases seizure risk
- Patients who do not respond to 450 mg/day should discontinue use or get blood levels of bupropion and its major active metabolite 6-hydroxy-bupropion

- If levels of parent drug and active metabolite are low despite dosing at 450 mg/day, experts can prudently increase dosing beyond the therapeutic range while monitoring closely, informing the patient of the potential risk of seizures and weighing risk benefit ratios in difficult-to-treat patients
- When used for bipolar depression, it is usually as an augmenting agent to mood stabilizers, lithium, and/or atypical antipsychotics
- For smoking cessation, may be used in conjunction with nicotine replacement therapy
- Do not break or chew SR or XL tablets as this will alter controlled release properties
- The more anxious and agitated the patient, the lower the starting dose, the slower the titration, and the more likely the need for a concomitant agent such as trazodone or a benzodiazepine
- If intolerable anxiety, insomnia, agitation, akathisia, or activation occur either upon dosing initiation or discontinuation, consider the possibility of activated bipolar disorder and switch to a mood stabilizer or an atypical antipsychotic

Overdose
- Rarely lethal; seizures, cardiac disturbances, hallucinations, loss of consciousness

Long-Term Use
- For smoking cessation, treatment for up to 6 months has been found effective
- For depression, treatment up to one year has been found to decrease rate of relapse

Habit Forming
- No

How to Stop
- Tapering is prudent to avoid withdrawal effects, but no well-documented tolerance, dependence, or withdrawal reactions

Pharmacokinetics
- Inhibits CYP450 2D6
- Parent half-life 10–14 hours
- Metabolite half-life 20–27 hours

Drug Interactions

- Tramadol increases the risk of seizures in patients taking an antidepressant
- Can increase tricyclic antidepressant levels; use with caution with tricyclic antidepressants or when switching from a TCA to bupropion
- Can be fatal when combined with MAO inhibitors, so do not use with MAO inhibitors or for at least 14 days after MAOIs are stopped
- Do not start an MAO inhibitor for at least two weeks after discontinuing bupropion
- Via CYP450 2D6 inhibition, bupropion could theoretically interfere with the analgesic actions of codeine, and increase the plasma levels of some beta blockers and of atomoxetine
- Via CYP450 2D6 inhibition, bupropion could theoretically increase concentrations of thioridazine and cause dangerous cardiac arrhythmias

 Other Warnings/ Precautions

- Use cautiously with other drugs that increase seizure risk (TCAs, lithium, phenothiazines, thioxanthenes, some antipsychotics)
- Bupropion should be used with caution in patients taking levodopa or amantadine, as these agents can potentially enhance dopamine neurotransmission and be activating
- Do not use if patient has severe insomnia
- Use with caution in patients with bipolar disorder unless treated with concomitant mood stabilizing agent
- When treating children, carefully weigh the risks and benefits of pharmacological treatment against the risks and benefits of nontreatment and make sure to document this in the patient's chart
- Distribute the brochures provided by the FDA and the drug companies
- Warn patients and their caregivers about the possibility of activating side effects and advise them to report such symptoms immediately
- Monitor patients for activation of suicidal ideation, especially children and adolescents

Do Not Use

- Zyban in combination with any formulation of Wellbutrin
- If patient has history of seizures
- If patient is anorexic or bulimic, either currently or in the past, but see Pearls
- If patient is abruptly discontinuing alcohol or sedative use
- If patient has had recent head injury
- If patient has a nervous system tumor
- If patient is taking an MAO inhibitor
- If patient is taking thioridazine
- If there is a proven allergy to bupropion

SPECIAL POPULATIONS

Renal Impairment

- Lower initial dose, perhaps give less frequently
- Drug concentration may be increased
- Patient should be monitored closely

Hepatic Impairment

- Lower initial dose, perhaps give less frequently
- Patient should be monitored closely
- In severe hepatic cirrhosis, bupropion XL should be administered at no more than 150 mg every other day

Cardiac Impairment

- Limited available data
- Evidence of rise in supine blood pressure
- Use with caution

Elderly

- Some patients may tolerate lower doses better

 Children and Adolescents

- Carefully weigh the risks and benefits of pharmacological treatment against the risks and benefits of nontreatment with antidepressants and make sure to document this in the patient's chart
- Monitor patients face-to-face regularly, particularly during the first several weeks of treatment
- Use with caution, observing for activation of known or unknown bipolar disorder and/or suicidal ideation, and inform parents

or guardian of this risk so they can help observe child or adolescent patients
- Safety and efficacy have not been established
- May be used for ADHD in children or adolescents
- May be used for smoking cessation in adolescents
- Preliminary research suggests efficacy in comorbid depression and ADHD
- Dosage may follow adult pattern for adolescents
- Children may require lower doses initially, with a maximum dose of 300 mg/day

 Pregnancy

- Risk Category B [animal studies do not show adverse effects; no controlled studies in humans]
- Pregnant women wishing to stop smoking may consider behavioral therapy before pharmacotherapy
- Not generally recommended for use during pregnancy, especially during first trimester
- Must weigh the risk of treatment (first trimester fetal development, third trimester newborn delivery) to the child against the risk of no treatment (recurrence of depression, maternal health, infant bonding) to the mother and child
- For many patients this may mean continuing treatment during pregnancy

Breast Feeding
- Some drug is found in mother's breast milk
- If child becomes irritable or sedated, breast feeding or drug may need to be discontinued
- Immediate postpartum period is a high-risk time for depression, especially in women who have had prior depressive episodes, so drug may need to be reinstituted late in the third trimester or shortly after childbirth to prevent a recurrence during the postpartum period
- Must weigh benefits of breast feeding with risks and benefits of antidepressant treatment versus non-treatment to both the infant and the mother
- For many patients, this may mean continuing treatment during breast feeding

THE ART OF PSYCHOPHARMACOLOGY

Potential Advantages
- Retarded depression
- Atypical depression
- Bipolar depression
- Patients concerned about sexual dysfunction
- Patients concerned about weight gain

Potential Disadvantages
- Patients experiencing weight loss associated with their depression
- Patients who are excessively activated

Primary Target Symptoms
- Depressed mood
- Sleep disturbance, especially hypersomnia
- Cravings associated with nicotine withdrawal
- Cognitive functioning

 Pearls

* May be effective if SSRIs have failed or for SSRI "poop-out"
- Less likely to produce hypomania than some other antidepressants
* May improve cognitive slowing/pseudodementia
* Reduces hypersomnia and fatigue
- Approved to help reduce craving during smoking cessation
- Anecdotal use in attention deficit disorder
- May cause sexual dysfunction only infrequently
- May exacerbate tics
- Bupropion may not be as effective in anxiety disorders as many other antidepressants
- Prohibition for use in eating disorders due to increased risk of seizures is related to past observations when bupropion immediate release was dosed at especially high levels to low body weight patients with active anorexia nervosa
- Current practice suggests that patients of normal BMI without additional risk factors for seizures can benefit from bupropion, especially if given prudent doses of the XL formulation; such treatment should be administered by experts, and patients should be monitored closely and informed of the potential risks

- The active enantiomer of the principle active metabolite (+6-hydroxy-bupropion) is in clinical development as a novel antidepressant

Suggested Reading

Ferry L, Johnston JA. Efficacy and safety of bupropion SR for smoking cessation: data from clinical trials and five years of postmarketing experience. Int J Clin Pract 2003;57(3):224–30.

Hirschfeld RM. Efficacy of SSRIs and newer antidepressants in severe depression: comparison with TCAs. Journal of Clinical Psychiatry 1999;60:326–335.

Horst WD, Preskorn SH. Mechanisms of action and clinical characteristics of three atypical antidepressants: venlafaxine, nefazodone, bupropion. Journal of Affective Disorders 1998;51:237–254.

Masand PS, Gupta S. Long-term side effects of newer-generation antidepressants: SSRIs, venlafaxine, nefazodone, bupropion, and mirtazapine. Ann Clin Psychiatry 2002;14(3):175–82.

Nieuwstraten CE, Dolovich LR. Bupropion versus selective serotonin-reuptake inhibitors for treatment of depression. Ann Pharmacother 2001;35(12):1608–13.

CITALOPRAM

THERAPEUTICS

Brands • Celexa
see index for additional brand names

`Generic?` Yes

Class
• SSRI (selective serotonin reuptake inhibitor); often classified as an antidepressant, but it is not just an antidepressant

Commonly Prescribed For
(bold for FDA approved)
• **Depression**
• Premenstrual dysphoric disorder (PMDD)
• Obsessive-compulsive disorder (OCD)
• Panic disorder
• Generalized anxiety disorder
• Posttraumatic stress disorder (PTSD)
• Social anxiety disorder (social phobia)

How The Drug Works
• Boosts neurotransmitter serotonin
• Blocks serotonin reuptake pump (serotonin transporter)
• Desensitizes serotonin receptors, especially serotonin 1A autoreceptors
• Presumably increases serotonergic neurotransmission
✷ Citalopram also has mild antagonist actions at H1 histamine receptors
✷ Citalopram's inactive R enantiomer may interfere with the therapeutic actions of the active S enantiomer at serotonin reuptake pumps

How Long Until It Works
• Onset of therapeutic actions usually not immediate, but often delayed 2 to 4 weeks
• If it is not working within 6 to 8 weeks, it may require a dosage increase or it may not work at all
• May continue to work for many years to prevent relapse of symptoms

If It Works
• The goal of treatment is complete remission of current symptoms as well as prevention of future relapses
• Treatment most often reduces or even eliminates symptoms, but not a cure since symptoms can recur after medicine stopped
• Continue treatment until all symptoms are gone (remission) or significantly reduced (e.g., OCD, PTSD)
• Once symptoms are gone, continue treating for 1 year for the first episode of depression
• For second and subsequent episodes of depression, treatment may need to be indefinite
• Use in anxiety disorders may also need to be indefinite

If It Doesn't Work
• Many patients only have a partial response where some symptoms are improved but others persist (especially insomnia, fatigue, and problems concentrating in depression)
• Other patients may be nonresponders, sometimes called treatment-resistant or treatment-refractory
• Some patients who have an initial response may relapse even though they continue treatment, sometimes called "poop-out"
• Consider increasing dose, switching to another agent or adding an appropriate augmenting agent
• Consider psychotherapy
• Consider evaluation for another diagnosis or for a comorbid condition (e.g., medical illness, substance abuse, etc.)
• Some patients may experience apparent lack of consistent efficacy due to activation of latent or underlying bipolar disorder, and require antidepressant discontinuation and a switch to a mood stabilizer

Best Augmenting Combos for Partial Response or Treatment-Resistance

• Trazodone, especially for insomnia
• Bupropion, mirtazapine, reboxetine, or atomoxetine (add with caution and at lower doses since citalopram could theoretically raise atomoxetine levels); use combinations of antidepressants with caution as this may activate bipolar disorder and suicidal ideation
• Modafinil, especially for fatigue, sleepiness, and lack of concentration
• Mood stabilizers or atypical antipsychotics for bipolar depression, psychotic depression, treatment-resistant depression, or treatment-resistant anxiety disorders

- Benzodiazepines
- If all else fails for anxiety disorders, consider gabapentin or tiagabine
- Hypnotics for insomnia
- Classically, lithium, buspirone, or thyroid hormone

Tests

- None for healthy individuals

SIDE EFFECTS

How Drug Causes Side Effects

- Theoretically due to increases in serotonin concentrations at serotonin receptors in parts of the brain and body other than those that cause therapeutic actions (e.g., unwanted actions of serotonin in sleep centers causing insomnia, unwanted actions of serotonin in the gut causing diarrhea, etc.)
- Increasing serotonin can cause diminished dopamine release and might contribute to emotional flattening, cognitive slowing, and apathy in some patients
- Most side effects are immediate but often go away with time, in contrast to most therapeutic effects which are delayed and are enhanced over time
- * Citalopram's unique mild antihistamine properties may contribute to sedation and fatigue in some patients

Notable Side Effects

- Sexual dysfunction (men: delayed ejaculation, erectile dysfunction; men and women: decreased sexual desire, anorgasmia)
- Gastrointestinal (decreased appetite, nausea, diarrhea, constipation, dry mouth)
- Mostly central nervous system (insomnia but also sedation, agitation, tremors, headache, dizziness)
- Note: patients with diagnosed or undiagnosed bipolar or psychotic disorders may be more vulnerable to CNS-activating actions of SSRIs
- Autonomic (sweating)
- Bruising and rare bleeding
- Rare hyponatremia (mostly in elderly patients and generally reversible on discontinuation of citalopram)
- SIADH (syndrome of inappropriate antidiuretic hormone secretion)

 Life Threatening or Dangerous Side Effects

- Rare seizures
- Rare induction of mania
- Rare activation of suicidal ideation and behavior (suicidality)

Weight Gain

unusual   not unusual   common   problematic

- Reported but not expected
- Citalopram has been associated with both weight gain and weight loss in various studies, but is relatively weight neutral overall

Sedation

unusual   not unusual   common   problematic

- Occurs in significant minority

What To Do About Side Effects

- Wait
- Wait
- Wait
- Take in the morning if nighttime insomnia
- Take at night if daytime sedation
- In a few weeks, switch to another agent or add other drugs

Best Augmenting Agents for Side Effects

- Often best to try another SSRI or another antidepressant monotherapy prior to resorting to augmentation strategies to treat side effects
- Trazodone or a hypnotic for insomnia
- Bupropion, sildenafil, vardenafil, or tadalafil for sexual dysfunction
- Bupropion for emotional flattening, cognitive slowing, or apathy
- Mirtazapine for insomnia, agitation, and gastrointestinal side effects
- Benzodiazepines for jitteriness and anxiety, especially at initiation of treatment and especially for anxious patients
- Many side effects are dose-dependent (i.e., they increase as dose increases, or they reemerge until tolerance re-develops)
- Many side effects are time-dependent (i.e., they start immediately upon dosing and upon each dose increase, but go away with time)

- Activation and agitation may represent the induction of a bipolar state, especially a mixed dysphoric bipolar II condition sometimes associated with suicidal ideation, and require the addition of lithium, a mood stabilizer or an atypical antipsychotic, and/or discontinuation of citalopram

DOSING AND USE

Usual Dosage Range
- 20–60 mg/day

Dosage Forms
- Tablets 10 mg, 20 mg scored, 40 mg scored

How to Dose
- Initial 20 mg/day; increase by 20 mg/day after 1 or more weeks until desired efficacy is reached; maximum usually 60 mg/day; single dose administration, morning or evening

 Dosing Tips
- Tablets are scored, so to save costs, give 10 mg as half of 20 mg tablet or 20 mg as half of 40 mg tablet, since the tablets cost about the same in many markets
- Many patients respond better to 40 mg than to 20 mg
- Given once daily, any time of day when best tolerated by the individual
- If intolerable anxiety, insomnia, agitation, akathisia, or activation occur either upon dosing initiation or discontinuation, consider the possibility of activated bipolar disorder and switch to a mood stabilizer or an atypical antipsychotic

Overdose
- Rare fatalities have been reported with citalopram overdose, both alone and in combination with other drugs
- Vomiting, sedation, heart rhythm disturbances, dizziness, sweating, nausea, tremor
- Rarely amnesia, confusion, coma, convulsions

Long-Term Use
- Safe

Habit Forming
- No

How to Stop
- Taper not usually necessary
- However, tapering to avoid potential withdrawal reactions generally prudent
- Many patients tolerate 50% dose reduction for 3 days, then another 50% reduction for 3 days, then discontinuation
- If withdrawal symptoms emerge during discontinuation, raise dose to stop symptoms and then restart withdrawal much more slowly

Pharmacokinetics
- Parent drug has 23–45 hour half-life
- Weak inhibitor of CYP450 2D6

 Drug Interactions
- Tramadol increases the risk of seizures in patients taking an antidepressant
- Can increase tricyclic antidepressant levels; use with caution with tricyclic antidepressants
- Can cause a fatal "serotonin syndrome" when combined with MAO inhibitors, so do not use with MAO inhibitors or at least for 14 days after MAOIs are stopped
- Do not start an MAO inhibitor for at least 2 weeks after discontinuing citalopram
- May displace highly protein bound drugs (e.g., warfarin)
- Can rarely cause weakness, hyperreflexia, and incoordination when combined with sumatriptan or possibly other triptans, requiring careful monitoring of patient
- Via CYP450 2D6 inhibition, citalopram could theoretically interfere with the analgesic actions of codeine, and increase the plasma levels of some beta blockers and of atomoxetine
- Via CYP450 2D6 inhibition, citalopram could theoretically increase concentrations of thioridazine and cause dangerous cardiac arrhythmias

Other Warnings/ Precautions

- Use with caution in patients with history of seizures
- Use with caution in patients with bipolar disorder unless treated with concomitant mood stabilizing agent
- When treating children, carefully weigh the risks and benefits of pharmacological treatment against the risks and benefits of nontreatment with antidepressants and make sure to document this in the patient's chart
- Distribute the brochures provided by the FDA and the drug companies
- Warn patients and their caregivers about the possibility of activating side effects and advise them to report such symptoms immediately
- Monitor patients for activation of suicidal ideation, especially children and adolescents

Do Not Use

- If patient is taking an MAO inhibitor
- If patient is taking thioridazine
- If there is a proven allergy to citalopram or escitalopram

SPECIAL POPULATIONS

Renal Impairment

- No dose adjustment for mild to moderate impairment
- Use cautiously in patients with severe impairment

Hepatic Impairment

- Recommended dose 20 mg/day; can be raised to 40 mg/day for nonresponders
- May need to dose cautiously at the lower end of the dose range in some patients for maximal tolerability

Cardiac Impairment

- Clinical experience suggests that citalopram is safe in these patients
- Treating depression with SSRIs in patients with acute angina or following myocardial infarction may reduce cardiac events and improve survival as well as mood

Elderly

- 20 mg/day; 40 mg/day for nonresponders
- May need to dose at the lower end of the dose range in some patients for maximal tolerability
- Citalopram may be an especially well-tolerated SSRI in the elderly

 Children and Adolescents

- Carefully weigh the risks and benefits of pharmacological treatment against the risks and benefits of nontreatment with antidepressants and make sure to document this in the patient's chart
- Monitor patients face-to-face regularly, particularly during the first several weeks of treatment
- Use with caution, observing for activation of known or unknown bipolar disorder and/or suicidal ideation, and inform parents or guardian of this risk so they can help observe child or adolescent patients
- Not specifically approved, but preliminary data suggest citalopram is safe and effective in children and adolescents with OCD and with depression

 Pregnancy

- Risk Category C [some animal studies show adverse effects, no controlled studies in humans]
- Not generally recommended for use during pregnancy, especially during first trimester
- Nonetheless, continuous treatment during pregnancy may be necessary and has not been proven to be harmful to the fetus
- At delivery there may be more bleeding in the mother and transient irritability or sedation in the newborn
- Must weigh the risk of treatment (first trimester fetal development, third trimester newborn delivery) to the child against the risk of no treatment (recurrence of depression, maternal health, infant bonding) to the mother and child
- For many patients, this may mean continuing treatment during pregnancy
- Neonates exposed to SSRIs or SNRIs late in the third trimester have developed complications requiring prolonged hospitalization, respiratory support, and tube feeding; reported symptoms are

consistent with either a direct toxic effect of SSRIs and SNRIs or, possibly, a drug discontinuation syndrome, and include respiratory distress, cyanosis, apnea, seizures, temperature instability, feeding difficulty, vomiting, hypoglycemia, hypotonia, hypertonia, hyperreflexia, tremor, jitteriness, irritability, and constant crying

Breast Feeding
- Some drug is found in mother's breast milk
- Trace amounts may be present in nursing children whose mothers are on citalopram
- If child becomes irritable or sedated, breast feeding or drug may need to be discontinued
- Immediate postpartum period is a high-risk time for depression, especially in women who have had prior depressive episodes, so drug may need to be reinstituted late in the third trimester or shortly after childbirth to prevent a recurrence during the postpartum period
- Must weigh benefits of breast feeding with risks and benefits of antidepressant treatment versus non-treatment to both the infant and the mother
- For many patients, this may mean continuing treatment during breast feeding

THE ART OF PSYCHOPHARMACOLOGY

Potential Advantages
- Elderly patients
- Patients excessively activated or sedated by other SSRIs

Potential Disadvantages
- May require dosage titration to attain optimal efficacy

- Can be sedating in some patients

Primary Target Symptoms
- Depressed mood
- Anxiety
- Panic attacks, avoidant behavior, re-experiencing, hyperarousal
- Sleep disturbance, both insomnia and hypersomnia

 Pearls

* May be more tolerable than some other antidepressants
- May have less sexual dysfunction than some other SSRIs
- May be especially well tolerated in the elderly

* May be less well tolerated than escitalopram
- Documentation of efficacy in anxiety disorders is less comprehensive than for escitalopram and other SSRIs
- Can cause cognitive and affective "flattening"
- Some evidence suggests that citalopram treatment during only the luteal phase may be more effective than continuous treatment for patients with PMDD
- SSRIs may be less effective in women over 50, especially if they are not taking estrogen
- SSRIs may be useful for hot flushes in perimenopausal women
- Nonresponse to citalopram in elderly may require consideration of mild cognitive impairment or Alzheimer disease

Suggested Reading

Bezchlibnyk-Butler K, Aleksic I, Kennedy SH. Citalopram – a review of pharmacological and clinical effects. Journal of Psychiatry and Neuroscience 2000;25:241–254.

Edwards JG, Anderson I. Systematic review and guide to selection of selective serotonin reuptake inhibitors. Drugs 1999;57:507–533.

Keller MB. Citalopram therapy for depression: a review of 10 years of European experience and data from U.S. clinical trials. Journal of Clinical Psychiatry 2000;61:896–908.

Pollock BG. Citalopram: a comprehensive review. Expert Opin Pharmacother 2001;2:681–98.

Stahl SM. Placebo-controlled comparison of the selective serotonin reuptake inhibitors citalopram and sertraline. Biol Psychiatry 2000;48:894–901.

CLOMIPRAMINE

THERAPEUTICS

Brands • Anafranil

see index for additional brand names

Generic? Yes

Class

- Tricyclic antidepressant (TCA)
- Parent drug is a potent serotonin reuptake inhibitor
- Active metabolite is a potent norepinephrine/noradrenaline reuptake inhibitor

Commonly Prescribed For

(bold for FDA approved)

- ✻ **Obsessive-compulsive disorder**
- Depression
- ✻ Severe and treatment-resistant depression
- ✻ Cataplexy syndrome
- Anxiety
- Insomnia
- Neuropathic pain/chronic pain

How The Drug Works

- Boosts neurotransmitters serotonin and norepinephrine/noradrenaline
- Blocks serotonin reuptake pump (serotonin transporter), presumably increasing serotonergic neurotransmission
- Blocks norepinephrine reuptake pump (norepinephrine transporter), presumably increasing noradrenergic neurotransmission
- Presumably desensitizes both serotonin 1A receptors and beta adrenergic receptors
- Since dopamine is inactivated by norepinephrine reuptake in frontal cortex, which largely lacks dopamine transporters, clomipramine can increase dopamine neurotransmission in this part of the brain

How Long Until It Works

- May have immediate effects in treating insomnia or anxiety
- Onset of therapeutic actions in depression usually not immediate, but often delayed 2 to 4 weeks
- Onset of therapeutic action in OCD can be delayed 6 to 12 weeks
- If it is not working within 6 to 8 weeks for depression, it may require a dosage increase or it may not work at all
- If it is not working within 12 weeks for OCD, it may not work at all
- May continue to work for many years to prevent relapse of symptoms

If It Works

- The goal of treatment of depression is complete remission of current symptoms as well as prevention of future relapses
- Treatment most often reduces or even eliminates symptoms, but not a cure since symptoms can recur after medicine stopped
- Although the goal of treatment of OCD is also complete remission of symptoms, this may be less likely than in depression
- The goal of treatment of chronic neuropathic pain is to reduce symptoms as much as possible, especially in combination with other treatments
- Continue treatment of depression until all symptoms are gone (remission)
- Once symptoms of depression are gone, continue treating for 1 year for the first episode of depression
- For second and subsequent episodes of depression, treatment may need to be indefinite
- Use in OCD may also need to be indefinite, starting from the time of initial treatment
- Use in other anxiety disorders and chronic pain may also need to be indefinite, but long-term treatment is not well studied in these conditions

If It Doesn't Work

- Many patients only have a partial response where some symptoms are improved but others persist (especially insomnia, fatigue, and problems concentrating)
- Other patients may be nonresponders, sometimes called treatment-resistant or treatment-refractory
- Consider increasing dose, switching to another agent or adding an appropriate augmenting agent
- Consider psychotherapy, especially behavioral therapy in OCD
- Consider evaluation for another diagnosis or for a comorbid condition (e.g., medical illness, substance abuse, etc.)
- Some patients may experience apparent lack of consistent efficacy due to activation

of latent or underlying bipolar disorder, and require antidepressant discontinuation and a switch to a mood stabilizer

Best Augmenting Combos for Partial Response or Treatment-Resistance

- Lithium, buspirone, hormone (for depression and OCD)
- For the expert: consider cautious addition of fluvoxamine for treatment-resistant OCD
- Thyroid hormone (for depression)
- Atypical antipsychotics (for OCD)

Tests

✳ None for healthy individuals, although monitoring of plasma drug levels is potentially available at specialty laboratories for the expert

✳ Since tricyclic and tetracyclic antidepressants are frequently associated with weight gain, before starting treatment, weigh all patients and determine if the patient is already overweight (BMI 25.0–29.9) or obese (BMI ≥30)

- Before giving a drug that can cause weight gain to an overweight or obese patient, consider determining whether the patient already has pre-diabetes (fasting plasma glucose 100–125 mg/dl), diabetes (fasting plasma glucose >126 mg/dl), or dyslipidemia (increased total cholesterol, LDL cholesterol and triglycerides; decreased HDL cholesterol), and treat or refer such patients for treatment, including nutrition and weight management, physical activity counseling, smoking cessation, and medical management

✳ Monitor weight and BMI during treatment

✳ While giving a drug to a patient who has gained >5% of initial weight, consider evaluating for the presence of pre-diabetes, diabetes, or dyslipidemia, or consider switching to a different antidepressant

- EKGs may be useful for selected patients (e.g., those with personal or family history of QTc prolongation; cardiac arrhythmia; recent myocardial infarction; uncompensated heart failure; or taking agents that prolong QTc interval such as pimozide, thioridazine, selected antiarrhythmics, moxifloxacin, sparfloxacin, etc.)
- Patients at risk for electrolyte disturbances (e.g., patients on diuretic therapy) should have baseline and periodic serum potassium and magnesium measurements

SIDE EFFECTS

How Drug Causes Side Effects

- Anticholinergic activity may explain sedative effects, dry mouth, constipation, and blurred vision
- Sedative effects and weight gain may be due to antihistamine properties
- Blockade of alpha adrenergic 1 receptors may explain dizziness, sedation, and hypotension
- Cardiac arrhythmias and seizures, especially in overdose, may be caused by blockade of ion channels

Notable Side Effects

- Blurred vision, constipation, urinary retention, increased appetite, dry mouth, nausea, diarrhea, heartburn, unusual taste in mouth, weight gain
- Fatigue, weakness, dizziness, sedation, headache, anxiety, nervousness, restlessness
- Sexual dysfunction, sweating

Life Threatening or Dangerous Side Effects

- Paralytic ileus, hyperthermia (TCAs + anticholinergic agents)
- Lowered seizure threshold and rare seizures
- Orthostatic hypotension, sudden death, arrhythmias, tachycardia
- QTc prolongation
- Hepatic failure, extrapyramidal symptoms
- Increased intraocular pressure
- Rare induction of mania
- Rare activation of suicidal ideation and behavior (suicidality)

Weight Gain

unusual   not unusual   common   problematic

- Many experience and/or can be significant in amount
- Can increase appetite and carbohydrate craving

Sedation

unusual   not unusual   common   problematic

- Many experience and/or can be significant in amount

- Tolerance to sedative effect may develop with long-term use

What To Do About Side Effects
- Wait
- Wait
- Wait
- Lower the dose
- Switch to an SSRI or newer antidepressant

Best Augmenting Agents for Side Effects
- Many side effects cannot be improved with an augmenting agent

DOSING AND USE

Usual Dosage Range
- 100 mg/day – 200 mg/day

Dosage Forms
- Capsule 25 mg, 50 mg, 75 mg

How to Dose
- Initial 25 mg/day; increase over 2 weeks to 100 mg/day; maximum dose generally 250 mg/day

 Dosing Tips
- If given in a single dose, should generally be administered at bedtime because of its sedative properties
- If given in split doses, largest dose should generally be given at bedtime because of its sedative properties
- If patients experience nightmares, split dose and do not give large dose at bedtime
- Patients treated for chronic pain may only require lower doses
- ✳ Patients treated for OCD may often require doses at the high end of the range (e.g., 200–250 mg/day)
- Risk of seizure increases with dose, especially with clomipramine at doses above 250 mg/day
- ✳ Dose of 300 mg may be associated with up to 7/1000 incidence of seizures, a generally unacceptable risk
- If intolerable anxiety, insomnia, agitation, akathisia, or activation occur either upon dosing initiation or discontinuation, consider the possibility of activated bipolar disorder, and switch to a mood stabilizer or an atypical antipsychotic

Overdose
- Death may occur; convulsions, cardiac dysrhythmias, severe hypotension, CNS depression, coma, changes in ECG

Long-Term Use
- Limited data but appears to be efficacious and safe long-term

Habit Forming
- No

How to Stop
- Taper to avoid withdrawal effects
- Even with gradual dose reduction some withdrawal symptoms may appear within the first 2 weeks
- Many patients tolerate 50% dose reduction for 3 days, then another 50% reduction for 3 days, then discontinuation
- If withdrawal symptoms emerge during discontinuation, raise dose to stop symptoms and then restart withdrawal much more slowly

Pharmacokinetics
- Substrate for CYP450 2D6 and 1A2
- Metabolized to an active metabolite, desmethyl-clomipramine, a predominantly norepinephrine reuptake inhibitor, by demethylation via CYP450 1A2
- Half-life approximately 17–28 hours

 Drug Interactions
- Tramadol increases the risk of seizures in patients taking TCAs
- Use of TCAs with anticholinergic drugs may result in paralytic ileus or hyperthermia
- Fluoxetine, paroxetine, bupropion, duloxetine, and other CYP450 2D6 inhibitors may increase TCA concentrations
- Fluvoxamine, a CYP450 1A2 inhibitor, can decrease the conversion of clomipramine to desmethyl-clomipramine, and increase clomipramine plasma concentrations
- Cimetidine may increase plasma concentrations of TCAs and cause anticholinergic symptoms
- Phenothiazines or haloperidol may raise TCA blood concentrations

- May alter effects of antihypertensive drugs
- Use of TCAs with sympathomimetic agents may increase sympathetic activity
- TCAs may inhibit hypotensive effects of clonidine
- Methylphenidate may inhibit metabolism of TCAs
- Activation and agitation, especially following switching or adding antidepressants, may represent the induction of a bipolar state, especially a mixed dysphoric bipolar II condition sometimes associated with suicidal ideation, and require the addition of lithium, a mood stabilizer or an atypical antipsychotic, and/or discontinuation of clomipramine

Other Warnings/ Precautions

- Add or initiate other antidepressants with caution for up to 2 weeks after discontinuing clomipramine
- Generally, do not use with MAO inhibitors, including 14 days after MAOIs are stopped; do not start an MAOI until 2 weeks after discontinuing clomipramine, but see Pearls
- Use with caution in patients with history of seizures, urinary retention, narrow angle-closure glaucoma, hyperthyroidism
- TCAs can increase QTc interval, especially at toxic doses, which can be attained not only by overdose but also by combining with drugs that inhibit TCA metabolism via CYP450 2D6, potentially causing torsade de pointes-type arrhythmia or sudden death
- Because TCAs can prolong QTc interval, use with caution in patients who have bradycardia or who are taking drugs that can induce bradycardia (e.g., beta blockers, calcium channel blockers, clonidine, digitalis)
- Because TCAs can prolong QTc interval, use with caution in patients who have hypokalemia and/or hypomagnesemia or who are taking drugs that can induce hypokalemia and/or magnesemia (e.g., diuretics, stimulant laxatives, intravenous amphotericin B, glucocorticoids, tetracosactide)
- When treating children, carefully weigh the risks and benefits of pharmacological treatment against the risks and benefits of nontreatment with antidepressants and make sure to document this in the patient's chart
- Distribute the brochures provided by the FDA and the drug companies
- Warn patients and their caregivers about the possibility of activating side effects and advise them to report such symptoms immediately
- Monitor patients for activation of suicidal ideation, especially children and adolescents

Do Not Use

- If patient is recovering from myocardial infarction
- If patient is taking agents capable of significantly prolonging QTc interval (e.g., pimozide, thioridazine, selected antiarrhythmics, moxifloxacin, sparfloxacin)
- If there is a history of QTc prolongation or cardiac arrhythmia, recent acute myocardial infarction, uncompensated heart failure
- If patient is taking drugs that inhibit TCA metabolism, including CYP450 2D6 inhibitors, except by an expert
- If there is reduced CYP450 2D6 function, such as patients who are poor 2D6 metabolizers, except by an expert and at low doses
- If there is a proven allergy to clomipramine

SPECIAL POPULATIONS

Renal Impairment
- Use with caution

Hepatic Impairment
- Use with caution

Cardiac Impairment
- TCAs have been reported to cause arrhythmias, prolongation of conduction time, orthostatic hypotension, sinus tachycardia, and heart failure, especially in the diseased heart
- Myocardial infarction and stroke have been reported with TCAs
- TCAs produce QTc prolongation, which may be enhanced by the existence of bradycardia, hypokalemia, congenital or acquired long QTc interval, which should

be evaluated prior to administering clomipramine

- Use with caution if treating concomitantly with a medication likely to produce prolonged bradycardia, hypokalemia, slowing of intracardiac conduction, or prolongation of the QTc interval
- Avoid TCAs in patients with a known history of QTc prolongation, recent acute myocardial infarction, and uncompensated heart failure
- TCAs may cause a sustained increase in heart rate in patients with ischemic heart disease and may worsen (decrease) heart rate variability, an independent risk of mortality in cardiac populations
- Since SSRIs may improve (increase) heart rate variability in patients following a myocardial infarct and may improve survival as well as mood in patients with acute angina or following a myocardial infarction, these are more appropriate agents for cardiac population than tricyclic/tetracyclic antidepressants
- ❋ Risk/benefit ratio may not justify use of TCAs in cardiac impairment

Elderly

- May be more sensitive to anticholinergic, cardiovascular, hypotensive, and sedative effects
- Dose may need to be lower than usual adult dose, at least initially

 Children and Adolescents

- Carefully weigh the risks and benefits of pharmacological treatment against the risks and benefits of nontreatment with antidepressants and make sure to document this in the patient's chart
- Monitor patients face-to-face regularly, particularly during the first several weeks of treatment
- Use with caution, observing for activation of known or unknown bipolar disorder and/or suicidal ideation, and inform parents or guardian of this risk so they can help observe child or adolescent patients
- Not recommended for use under age 10
- Several studies show lack of efficacy of TCAs for depression
- May be used to treat enuresis or hyperactive/impulsive behaviors

- Effective for OCD in children
- Some cases of sudden death have occurred in children taking TCAs
- Dose in children/adolescents should be titrated to a maximum of 100 mg/day or 3 mg/kg/day after 2 weeks, after which dose can then be titrated up to a maximum of 200 mg/day or 3 mg/kg/day

 Pregnancy

- Risk Category C [some animal studies show adverse effects, no controlled studies in humans]
- Clomipramine crosses the placenta
- Adverse effects have been reported in infants whose mothers took a TCA (lethargy, withdrawal symptoms, fetal malformations)
- Must weigh the risk of treatment (first trimester fetal development, third trimester newborn delivery) to the child against the risk of no treatment (recurrence of depression, worsening of OCD, maternal health, infant bonding) to the mother and child
- For many patients this may mean continuing treatment during pregnancy

Breast Feeding

- Some drug is found in mother's breast milk
- ❋ Recommended either to discontinue drug or bottle feed
- Immediate postpartum period is a high-risk time for depression and worsening of OCD, especially in women who have had prior depressive episodes or OCD symptoms, so drug may need to be reinstituted late in the third trimester or shortly after childbirth to prevent a recurrence or exacerbation during the postpartum period
- Must weigh benefits of breast feeding with risks and benefits of antidepressant treatment versus non-treatment to both the infant and the mother
- For many patients this may mean continuing treatment during breast feeding

THE ART OF PSYCHOPHARMACOLOGY

Potential Advantages

- Patients with insomnia
- Severe or treatment-resistant depression

- Patients with comorbid OCD and depression
- Patients with cataplexy

Potential Disadvantages

- Pediatric and geriatric patients
- Patients concerned with weight gain
- Cardiac patients
- Patients with seizure disorders

Primary Target Symptoms

- Depressed mood
- Obsessive thoughts
- Compulsive behaviors

Pearls

* The only TCA with proven efficacy in OCD

- Normally, clomipramine (CMI), a potent serotonin reuptake blocker, at steady state is metabolized extensively to its active metabolite desmethyl-clomipramine (de-CMI), a potent nonadrenaline reuptake blocker, by the enzyme CYP450 1A2
- Thus, at steady state, plasma drug activity is generally more noradrenergic (with higher de-CMI levels) than serotonergic (with lower parent CMI levels)
- Addition of the SSRI and CYP450 1A2 inhibitor fluvoxamine blocks this conversion and results in higher CMI levels than de-CMI levels
- For the expert only: addition of the SSRI fluvoxamine to CMI in treatment-resistant OCD can powerfully enhance serotonergic activity, not only due to the inherent additive pharmacodynamic serotonergic activity of fluvoxamine added to CMI, but also due to a favorable pharmacokinetic interaction inhibiting CYP450 1A2 and thus converting CMI's metabolism to a more powerful serotonergic portfolio of parent drug

* One of the most favored TCAs for treating severe depression

- Tricyclic antidepressants are no longer generally considered a first-line treatment option for depression because of their side effect profile
- Tricyclic antidepressants continue to be useful for severe or treatment-resistant depression
- Tricyclic antidepressants are often a first-line treatment option for chronic pain

* Unique among TCAs, clomipramine has a potentially fatal interaction with MAOIs in addition to the danger of hypertension characteristic of all MAOI-TCA combinations

* A potentially fatal serotonin syndrome with high fever, seizures, and coma, analogous to that caused by SSRIs and MAOIs, can occur with clomipramine and SSRIs, presumably due to clomipramine's potent serotonin reuptake blocking properties

- TCAs may aggravate psychotic symptoms
- Alcohol should be avoided because of additive CNS effects
- Underweight patients may be more susceptible to adverse cardiovascular effects
- Children, patients with inadequate hydration, and patients with cardiac disease may be more susceptible to TCA-induced cardiotoxicity than healthy adults
- Patients on TCAs should be aware that they may experience symptoms such as photosensitivity or blue-green urine
- SSRIs may be more effective than TCAs in women, and TCAs may be more effective than SSRIs in men
- Since tricyclic/tetracyclic antidepressants are substrates for CYP450 2D6, and 7% of the population (especially Caucasians) may have a genetic variant leading to reduced activity of 2D6, such patients may not safely tolerate normal doses of tricyclic/tetracyclic antidepressants and may require dose reduction
- Phenotypic testing may be necessary to detect this genetic variant prior to dosing with a tricyclic/tetracyclic antidepressant, especially in vulnerable populations such as children, elderly, cardiac populations, and those on concomitant medications
- Patients who seem to have extraordinarily severe side effects at normal or low doses may have this phenotypic CYP450 2D6 variant and require low doses or switching to another antidepressant not metabolized by 2D6

Suggested Reading

Anderson IM. Meta-analytical studies on new antidepressants. Br Med Bull 2001; 57:161–178.

Anderson IM. Selective serotonin reuptake inhibitors versus tricyclic antidepressants: a meta-analysis of efficacy and tolerability. J Aff Disorders 2000;58:19–36.

Cox BJ, Swinson RP, Morrison B, Lee PS. Clomipramine, fluoxetine, and behavior therapy in the treatment of obsessive-compulsive disorder: a meta-analysis. J Behav Ther Exp Psychiatry 1993;24:149–53.

Feinberg M. Clomipramine for obsessive-compulsive disorder. Am Fam Physician 1991; 43:1735–8.

DESIPRAMINE

Brands • Norpramin
see index for additional brand names

Generic? Yes

Class

- Tricyclic antidepressant (TCA)
- Predominantly a norepinephrine/ noradrenaline reuptake inhibitor

Commonly Prescribed For
(bold for FDA approved)
- **Depression**
- Anxiety
- Insomnia
- Neuropathic pain/chronic pain
- Treatment-resistant depression

How The Drug Works
- Boosts neurotransmitter norepinephrine/noradrenaline
- Blocks norepinephrine reuptake pump (norepinephrine transporter), presumably increasing noradrenergic neurotransmission
- Since dopamine is inactivated by norepinephrine reuptake in frontal cortex, which largely lacks dopamine transporters, desipramine can thus increase dopamine neurotransmission in this part of the brain
- A more potent inhibitor of norepinephrine reuptake pump than serotonin reuptake pump (serotonin transporter)
- At high doses may also boost neurotransmitter serotonin and presumably increase serotonergic neurotransmission

How Long Until It Works
- May have immediate effects in treating insomnia or anxiety
- Onset of therapeutic actions usually not immediate, but often delayed 2 to 4 weeks
- If it is not working within 6 to 8 weeks for depression, it may require a dosage increase or it may not work at all
- May continue to work for many years to prevent relapse of symptoms

If It Works
- The goal of treatment of depression is complete remission of current symptoms as well as prevention of future relapses
- The goal of treatment of chronic neuropathic pain is to reduce symptoms as much as possible, especially in combination with other treatments
- Treatment of depression most often reduces or even eliminates symptoms, but not a cure since symptoms can recur after medicine stopped
- Treatment of chronic neuropathic pain may reduce symptoms, but rarely eliminates them completely, and is not a cure since symptoms can recur after medicine is stopped
- Continue treatment of depression until all symptoms are gone (remission)
- Once symptoms of depression are gone, continue treating for 1 year for the first episode of depression
- For second and subsequent episodes of depression, treatment may need to be indefinite
- Use in anxiety disorders and chronic pain may also need to be indefinite, but long-term treatment is not well studied in these conditions

If It Doesn't Work
- Many depressed patients only have a partial response where some symptoms are improved but others persist (especially insomnia, fatigue, and problems concentrating)
- Other depressed patients may be nonresponders, sometimes called treatment-resistant or treatment-refractory
- Consider increasing dose, switching to another agent or adding an appropriate augmenting agent
- Consider psychotherapy
- Consider evaluation for another diagnosis or for a comorbid condition (e.g., medical illness, substance abuse, etc.)
- Some patients may experience apparent lack of consistent efficacy due to activation of latent or underlying bipolar disorder, and require antidepressant discontinuation and a switch to a mood stabilizer

Best Augmenting Combos for Partial Response or Treatment-Resistance

- Lithium, buspirone, thyroid hormone (for depression)
- Gabapentin, tiagabine, other anticonvulsants, even opiates if done by experts while monitoring carefully in difficult cases (for chronic pain)

Tests

* None for healthy individuals, although monitoring of plasma drug levels is available
* Since tricyclic and tetracyclic antidepressants are frequently associated with weight gain, before starting treatment, weigh all patients and determine if the patient is already overweight (BMI 25.0–29.9) or obese (BMI ≥30)
- Before giving a drug that can cause weight gain to an overweight or obese patient, consider determining whether the patient already has pre-diabetes (fasting plasma glucose 100–125 mg/dl), diabetes (fasting plasma glucose >126 mg/dl), or dyslipidemia (increased total cholesterol, LDL cholesterol and triglycerides; decreased HDL cholesterol), and treat or refer such patients for treatment, including nutrition and weight management, physical activity counseling, smoking cessation, and medical management
* Monitor weight and BMI during treatment
* While giving a drug to a patient who has gained >5% of initial weight, consider evaluating for the presence of pre-diabetes, diabetes, or dyslipidemia, or consider switching to a different antidepressant
- EKGs may be useful for selected patients (e.g., those with personal or family history of QTc prolongation; cardiac arrhythmia; recent myocardial infarction; uncompensated heart failure; or taking agents that prolong QTc interval such as pimozide, thioridazine, selected antiarrhythmics, moxifloxacin, sparfloxacin, etc.)
- Patients at risk for electrolyte disturbances (e.g., patients on diuretic therapy) should have baseline and periodic serum potassium and magnesium measurements

SIDE EFFECTS

How Drug Causes Side Effects

* Anticholinergic activity for desipramine may be somewhat less than for some other TCAs, yet can still explain the presence, if lower incidence, of sedative effects, dry mouth, constipation, and blurred vision
- Sedative effects and weight gain may be due to antihistamine properties
- Blockade of alpha adrenergic 1 receptors may explain dizziness, sedation, and hypotension
- Cardiac arrhythmias and seizures, especially in overdose, may be caused by blockade of ion channels

Notable Side Effects

- Blurred vision, constipation, urinary retention, increased appetite, dry mouth, nausea, diarrhea, heartburn, unusual taste in mouth, weight gain
- Fatigue, weakness, dizziness, sedation, headache, anxiety, nervousness, restlessness
- Sexual dysfunction, sweating

Life Threatening or Dangerous Side Effects

- Paralytic ileus, hyperthermia (TCAs + anticholinergic agents)
- Lowered seizure threshold and rare seizures
- Orthostatic hypotension, sudden death, arrhythmias, tachycardia
- QTc prolongation
- Hepatic failure, extrapyramidal symptoms
- Increased intraocular pressure
- Blood dyscrasias
- Rare induction of mania
- Rare activation of suicidal ideation and behavior (suicidality)

Weight Gain

unusual not unusual common problematic

- Many experience and/or can be significant in amount
- Can increase appetite and carbohydrate craving

Sedation

unusual not unusual common problematic

- Many experience and/or can be significant in amount
- Tolerance to sedative effects may develop with long-term use

What To Do About Side Effects
- Wait
- Wait
- Wait
- Lower the dose
- Switch to an SSRI or newer antidepressant

Best Augmenting Agents for Side Effects
- Many side effects cannot be improved with an augmenting agent

DOSING AND USE

Usual Dosage Range
- 100–200 mg/day (for depression)
- 50–150 mg/day (for chronic pain)

Dosage Forms
- Tablets 10 mg, 25 mg, 50 mg, 75 mg, 100 mg, 150 mg

How to Dose
- Initial 25 mg/day at bedtime; increase by 25 mg every 3–7 days
- 75 mg/day once daily or in divided doses; gradually increase dose to achieve desired therapeutic effect; maximum dose 300 mg/day

 Dosing Tips
- If given in a single dose, should generally be administered at bedtime because of its sedative properties
- If given in split doses, largest dose should generally be given at bedtime because of its sedative properties
- If patients experience nightmares, split dose and do not give large dose at bedtime
- Patients treated for chronic pain may only require lower doses (e.g., 50–75 mg/day)
- Risk of seizure increases with dose
- ✳ Monitoring plasma levels of desipramine is recommended in patients who do not respond to the usual dose or whose treatment is regarded as urgent

- If intolerable anxiety, insomnia, agitation, akathisia, or activation occur either upon dosing initiation or discontinuation, consider the possibility of activated bipolar disorder, and switch to a mood stabilizer or an atypical antipsychotic

Overdose
- Death may occur; convulsions, cardiac dysrhythmias, severe hypotension, CNS depression, coma, changes in ECG

Long-Term Use
- Safe

Habit Forming
- No

How to Stop
- Taper to avoid withdrawal effects
- Even with gradual dose reduction some withdrawal symptoms may appear within the first 2 weeks
- Many patients tolerate 50% dose reduction for 3 days, then another 50% reduction for 3 days, then discontinuation
- If withdrawal symptoms emerge during discontinuation, raise dose to stop symptoms and then restart withdrawal much more slowly

Pharmacokinetics
- Substrate for CYP450 2D6 and 1A2
- Is the active metabolite of imipramine, formed by demethylation via CYP450 1A2
- Half-life approximately 24 hours

 Drug Interactions
- Tramadol increases the risk of seizures in patients taking TCAs
- Use of TCAs with anticholinergic drugs may result in paralytic ileus or hyperthermia
- Fluoxetine, paroxetine, bupropion, duloxetine, and other CYP450 2D6 inhibitors may increase TCA concentrations
- Cimetidine may increase plasma concentrations of TCAs and cause anticholinergic symptoms
- Phenothiazines or haloperidol may raise TCA blood concentrations
- May alter effects of antihypertensive drugs; may inhibit hypotensive effects of clonidine

- Use of TCAs with sympathomimetic agents may increase sympathetic activity
- Methylphenidate may inhibit metabolism of TCAs
- Activation and agitation, especially following switching or adding antidepressants, may represent the induction of a bipolar state, especially a mixed dysphoric bipolar II condition sometimes associated with suicidal ideation, and require the addition of lithium, a mood stabilizer or an atypical antipsychotic, and/or discontinuation of desipramine

 Other Warnings/ Precautions

- Add or initiate other antidepressants with caution for up to 2 weeks after discontinuing desipramine
- Generally, do not use with MAO inhibitors, including 14 days after MAOIs are stopped; do not start an MAOI until 2 weeks after discontinuing desipramine, but see Pearls
- Use with caution in patients with history of seizures, urinary retention, narrow angle-closure glaucoma, hyperthyroidism
- TCAs can increase QTc interval, especially at toxic doses, which can be attained not only by overdose but also by combining with drugs that inhibit TCA metabolism via CYP450 2D6, potentially causing torsade de pointes-type arrhythmia or sudden death
- Because TCAs can prolong QTc interval, use with caution in patients who have bradycardia or who are taking drugs that can induce bradycardia (e.g., beta blockers, calcium channel blockers, clonidine, digitalis)
- Because TCAs can prolong QTc interval, use with caution in patients who have hypokalemia and/or hypomagnesemia or who are taking drugs that can induce hypokalemia and/or magnesemia (e.g., diuretics, stimulant laxatives, intravenous amphotericin B, glucocorticoids, tetracosactide)
- When treating children, carefully weigh the risks and benefits of pharmacological treatment against the risks and benefits of nontreatment with antidepressants and make sure to document this in the patient's chart

- Distribute the brochures provided by the FDA and the drug companies
- Warn patients and their caregivers about the possibility of activating side effects and advise them to report such symptoms immediately
- Monitor patients for activation of suicidal ideation, especially children and adolescents

Do Not Use

- If patient is recovering from myocardial infarction
- If patient is taking agents capable of significantly prolonging QTc interval (e.g., pimozide, thioridazine, selected antiarrhythmics, moxifloxacin, sparfloxacin)
- If there is a history of QTc prolongation or cardiac arrhythmia, recent acute myocardial infarction, uncompensated heart failure
- If patient is taking drugs that inhibit TCA metabolism, including CYP450 2D6 inhibitors, except by an expert
- If there is reduced CYP450 2D6 function, such as patients who are poor 2D6 metabolizers, except by an expert and at low doses
- If there is a proven allergy to desipramine, imipramine, or lofepramine

SPECIAL POPULATIONS

Renal Impairment
- Use with caution; may need to lower dose
- May need to monitor plasma levels

Hepatic Impairment
- Use with caution; may need to lower dose
- May need to monitor plasma levels

Cardiac Impairment
- TCAs have been reported to cause arrhythmias, prolongation of conduction time, orthostatic hypotension, sinus tachycardia, and heart failure, especially in the diseased heart
- Myocardial infarction and stroke have been reported with TCAs
- TCAs produce QTc prolongation, which may be enhanced by the existence of bradycardia, hypokalemia, congenital or acquired long QTc interval, which should

be evaluated prior to administering desipramine
- Use with caution if treating concomitantly with a medication likely to produce prolonged bradycardia, hypokalemia, slowing of intracardiac conduction, or prolongation of the QTc interval
- Avoid TCAs in patients with a known history of QTc prolongation, recent acute myocardial infarction, and uncompensated heart failure
- TCAs may cause a sustained increase in heart rate in patients with ischemic heart disease and may worsen (decrease) heart rate variability, an independent risk of mortality in cardiac populations
- Since SSRIs may improve (increase) heart rate variability in patients following a myocardial infarct and may improve survival as well as mood in patients with acute angina or following a myocardial infarction, these are more appropriate agents for cardiac population than tricyclic/tetracyclic antidepressants
- ✳ Risk/benefit ratio may not justify use of TCAs in cardiac impairment

Elderly
- May be more sensitive to anticholinergic, cardiovascular, hypotensive, and sedative effects
- Initial dose 25–50 mg/day, raise to 100 mg/day; maximum 150 mg/day
- May be useful to monitor plasma levels in elderly patients

Children and Adolescents
- Carefully weigh the risks and benefits of pharmacological treatment against the risks and benefits of nontreatment with antidepressants and make sure to document this in the patient's chart
- Monitor patients face-to-face regularly, particularly during the first several weeks of treatment
- Use with caution, observing for activation of known or unknown bipolar disorder and/or suicidal ideation, and inform parents or guardian of this risk so they can help observe child or adolescent patients
- Not recommended for use under age 12
- Several studies show lack of efficacy of TCAs for depression

- May be used to treat enuresis or hyperactive/impulsive behaviors
- May reduce tic symptoms
- Some cases of sudden death have occurred in children taking TCAs
- Adolescents: initial dose 25–50 mg/day, increase to 100 mg/day; maximum dose 150 mg/day
- May be useful to monitor plasma levels in children and adolescents

Pregnancy
- Risk Category C [some animal studies show adverse effects, no controlled studies in humans]
- Crosses the placenta
- Adverse effects have been reported in infants whose mothers took a TCA (lethargy, withdrawal symptoms, fetal malformations)
- Must weigh the risk of treatment (first trimester fetal development, third trimester newborn delivery) to the child against the risk of no treatment (recurrence of depression, maternal health, infant bonding) to the mother and child
- For many patients this may mean continuing treatment during pregnancy

Breast Feeding
- Some drug is found in mother's breast milk
- ✳ Recommended either to discontinue drug or bottle feed
- Immediate postpartum period is a high-risk time for depression, especially in women who have had prior depressive episodes, so drug may need to be reinstituted late in the third trimester or shortly after childbirth to prevent a recurrence during the postpartum period
- Must weigh benefits of breast feeding with risks and benefits of antidepressant treatment versus non-treatment to both the infant and the mother
- For many patients this may mean continuing treatment during breast feeding

THE ART OF PSYCHOPHARMACOLOGY

Potential Advantages
- Patients with insomnia
- Severe or treatment-resistant depression

DESIPRAMINE (continued)

- Patients for whom therapeutic drug monitoring is desirable

Potential Disadvantages
- Pediatric and geriatric patients
- Patients concerned with weight gain
- Cardiac patients

Primary Target Symptoms
- Depressed mood
- Chronic pain

Pearls

- Tricyclic antidepressants are often a first-line treatment option for chronic pain
- Tricyclic antidepressants are no longer generally considered a first-line option for depression because of their side effect profile
- Tricyclic antidepressants continue to be useful for severe or treatment-resistant depression
- Noradrenergic reuptake inhibitors such as desipramine can be used as a second-line treatment for smoking cessation, cocaine dependence, and attention deficit disorder
- TCAs may aggravate psychotic symptoms
- Alcohol should be avoided because of additive CNS effects
- Underweight patients may be more susceptible to adverse cardiovascular effects
- Children, patients with inadequate hydration, and patients with cardiac disease may be more susceptible to TCA-induced cardiotoxicity than healthy adults
- For the expert only: although generally prohibited, a heroic but potentially dangerous treatment for severely treatment-resistant patients is to give a tricyclic/tetracyclic antidepressant other than clomipramine simultaneously with an MAO inhibitor for patients who fail to respond to numerous other antidepressants
- If this option is elected, start the MAOI with the tricyclic/tetracyclic antidepressant

simultaneously at low doses after appropriate drug washout, then alternately increase doses of these agents every few days to a week as tolerated
- Although very strict dietary and concomitant drug restrictions must be observed to prevent hypertensive crises and serotonin syndrome, the most common side effects of MAOI/tricyclic or tetracyclic combinations may be weight gain and orthostatic hypotension
- Patients on TCAs should be aware that they may experience symptoms such as photosensitivity or blue-green urine
- SSRIs may be more effective than TCAs in women, and TCAs may be more effective than SSRIs in men
- Not recommended for first-line use in children with ADHD because of the availability of safer treatments with better documented efficacy and because of desipramine's potential for sudden death in children
- ✱ Desipramine is one of the few TCAs where monitoring of plasma drug levels has been well studied
- ✱ Fewer anticholinergic side effects than some other TCAs
- Since tricyclic/tetracyclic antidepressants are substrates for CYP450 2D6, and 7% of the population (especially Caucasians) may have a genetic variant leading to reduced activity of 2D6, such patients may not safely tolerate normal doses of tricyclic/tetracyclic antidepressants and may require dose reduction
- Phenotypic testing may be necessary to detect this genetic variant prior to dosing with a tricyclic/tetracyclic antidepressant, especially in vulnerable populations such as children, elderly, cardiac populations, and those on concomitant medications
- Patients who seem to have extraordinarily severe side effects at normal or low doses may have this phenotypic CYP450 2D6 variant and require low doses or switching to another antidepressant not metabolized by 2D6

Suggested Reading

Anderson IM. Meta-analytical studies on new antidepressants. Br Med Bull 2001; 57:161–178.

Anderson IM. Selective serotonin reuptake inhibitors versus tricyclic antidepressants: a meta-analysis of efficacy and tolerability. J Aff Disorders 2000;58:19–36.

Janowsky DS, Byerley B. Desipramine: an overview. J Clin Psychiatry 1984;45:3–9.

Levin FR, Lehman AF. Meta-analysis of desipramine as an adjunct in the treatment of cocaine addiction. J Clin Psychopharmacol 1991;11:374–8.

DOTHIEPIN

THERAPEUTICS

Brands • Prothiaden
see index for additional brand names

Generic? In United Kingdom

Class
• Tricyclic antidepressant (TCA)
• Serotonin and norepinephrine/
  noradrenaline reuptake inhibitor

Commonly Prescribed For
(bold for FDA approved)
• Major depressive disorder
• Anxiety
• Insomnia
• Neuropathic pain/chronic pain
• Treatment-resistant depression

How The Drug Works
• Boosts neurotransmitters serotonin and
  norepinephrine/noradrenaline
• Blocks serotonin reuptake pump (serotonin
  transporter), presumably increasing
  serotonergic neurotransmission
• Blocks norepinephrine reuptake pump
  (norepinephrine transporter), presumably
  increasing noradrenergic
  neurotransmission
• Presumably desensitizes both serotonin 1A
  receptors and beta adrenergic receptors
• Since dopamine is inactivated by
  norepinephrine reuptake in frontal cortex,
  which largely lacks dopamine transporters,
  dothiepin can increase dopamine
  neurotransmission in this part of the brain

How Long Until It Works
• May have immediate effects in treating
  insomnia or anxiety
• Onset of therapeutic actions usually not
  immediate, but often delayed 2 to 4 weeks
• If it is not working within 6 to 8 weeks for
  depression, it may require a dosage
  increase or it may not work at all
• May continue to work for many years to
  prevent relapse of symptoms

If It Works
• The goal of treatment of depression is
  complete remission of current symptoms
  as well as prevention of future relapses
• The goal of treatment of chronic
  neuropathic pain is to reduce symptoms as
  much as possible, especially in
  combination with other treatments
• Treatment of depression most often
  reduces or even eliminates symptoms, but
  not a cure since symptoms can recur after
  medicine stopped
• Treatment of chronic neuropathic pain may
  reduce symptoms, but rarely eliminates
  them completely, and is not a cure since
  symptoms can recur after medicine is
  stopped
• Continue treatment of depression until all
  symptoms are gone (remission)
• Once symptoms of depression are gone,
  continue treating for 1 year for the first
  episode of depression
• For second and subsequent episodes of
  depression, treatment may need to be
  indefinite
• Use in anxiety disorders and chronic pain
  may also need to be indefinite, but long-
  term treatment is not well studied in these
  conditions

If It Doesn't Work
• Many depressed patients only have a
  partial response where some symptoms
  are improved but others persist (especially
  insomnia, fatigue, and problems
  concentrating)
• Other depressed patients may be
  nonresponders, sometimes called
  treatment-resistant or treatment-refractory
• Consider increasing dose, switching to
  another agent or adding an appropriate
  augmenting agent
• Consider psychotherapy
• Consider evaluation for another diagnosis
  or for a comorbid condition (e.g, medical
  illness, substance abuse, etc.)
• Some patients may experience apparent
  lack of consistent efficacy due to activation
  of latent or underlying bipolar disorder, and
  require antidepressant discontinuation and
  a switch to a mood stabilizer

Best Augmenting Combos for Partial Response or Treatment-Resistance

- Lithium, buspirone, thyroid hormone (for depression)
- Gabapentin, tiagabine, other anticonvulsants, even opiates if done by experts while monitoring carefully in difficult cases (for chronic pain)

Tests

- None for healthy individuals
- ✳ Since tricyclic and tetracyclic antidepressants are frequently associated with weight gain, before starting treatment, weigh all patients and determine if the patient is already overweight (BMI 25.0–29.9) or obese (BMI ≥30)
- Before giving a drug that can cause weight gain to an overweight or obese patient, consider determining whether the patient already has pre-diabetes (fasting plasma glucose 100–125 mg/dl), diabetes (fasting plasma glucose >126 mg/dl), or dyslipidemia (increased total cholesterol, LDL cholesterol and triglycerides; decreased HDL cholesterol), and treat or refer such patients for treatment including nutrition and weight management, physical activity counseling, smoking cessation, and medical management
- ✳ Monitor weight and BMI during treatment
- ✳ While giving a drug to a patient who has gained >5% of initial weight, consider evaluating for the presence of pre-diabetes, diabetes, or dyslipidemia, or consider switching to a different antidepressant
- EKGs may be useful for selected patients (e.g., those with personal or family history of QTc prolongation; cardiac arrhythmia; recent myocardial infarction; uncompensated heart failure; or taking agents that prolong QTc interval such as pimozide, thioridazine, selected antiarrhythmics, moxifloxacin, sparfloxacin, etc.)
- Patients at risk for electrolyte disturbances (e.g., patients on diuretic therapy) should have baseline and periodic serum potassium and magnesium measurements

SIDE EFFECTS

How Drug Causes Side Effects

- Anticholinergic activity may explain sedative effects, dry mouth, constipation, and blurred vision
- Sedative effects and weight gain may be due to antihistamine properties
- Blockade of alpha adrenergic 1 receptors may explain dizziness, sedation, and hypotension
- Cardiac arrhythmias and seizures, especially in overdose, may be caused by blockade of ion channels

Notable Side Effects

- Blurred vision, constipation, urinary retention, increased appetite, dry mouth, nausea, diarrhea, heartburn, unusual taste in mouth, weight gain
- Fatigue, weakness, dizziness, sedation, headache, anxiety, nervousness, restlessness
- Sexual dysfunction, sweating

Life Threatening or Dangerous Side Effects

- Paralytic ileus, hyperthermia (TCAs + anticholinergic agents)
- Lowered seizure threshold and rare seizures
- Orthostatic hypotension, sudden death, arrhythmias, tachycardia
- QTc prolongation
- Hepatic failure, extrapyramidal symptoms
- Increased intraocular pressure
- Rare induction of mania
- Rare activation of suicidal ideation and behavior (suicidality)

Weight Gain

unusual   not unusual   common   problematic

- Many experience and/or can be significant in amount
- Can increase appetite and carbohydrate craving

Sedation

unusual   not unusual   common   problematic

- Many experience and/or can be significant in amount

- Tolerance to sedative effect may develop with long-term use

What To Do About Side Effects
- Wait
- Wait
- Wait
- Lower the dose
- Switch to an SSRI or newer antidepressant

Best Augmenting Agents for Side Effects
- Many side effects cannot be improved with an augmenting agent

DOSING AND USE

Usual Dosage Range
- 75–150 mg/day

Dosage Forms
- Capsule 25 mg
- Tablet 75 mg

How to Dose
- 75 mg/day once daily or in divided doses; gradually increase dose to achieve desired therapeutic effect; maximum dose 300 mg/day

 Dosing Tips
- If given in a single dose, should generally be administered at bedtime because of its sedative properties
- If given in split doses, largest dose should generally be given at bedtime because of its sedative properties
- If patients experience nightmares, split dose and do not give large dose at bedtime
- Patients treated for chronic pain may only require lower doses
- Risk of seizure increases with dose
- If intolerable anxiety, insomnia, agitation, akathisia, or activation occur either upon dosing initiation or discontinuation, consider the possibility of activated bipolar disorder, and switch to a mood stabilizer or an atypical antipsychotic

Overdose
- Death may occur; convulsions, cardiac dysrhythmias, severe hypotension, CNS depression, coma, changes in ECG

Long-Term Use
- Safe

Habit Forming
- No

How to Stop
- Taper to avoid withdrawal effects
- Even with gradual dose reduction some withdrawal symptoms may appear within the first 2 weeks
- Many patients tolerate 50% dose reduction for 3 days, then another 50% reduction for 3 days, then discontinuation
- If withdrawal symptoms emerge during discontinuation, raise dose to stop symptoms and then restart withdrawal much more slowly

Pharmacokinetics
- Substrate for CYP450 2D6
- Half-life approximately 14–40 hours

 Drug Interactions
- Tramadol increases the risk of seizures in patients taking TCAs
- Use of TCAs with anticholinergic drugs may result in paralytic ileus or hyperthermia
- Fluoxetine, paroxetine, bupropion, duloxetine, and other CYP450 2D6 inhibitors may increase TCA concentrations
- Cimetidine may increase plasma concentrations of TCAs and cause anticholinergic symptoms
- Phenothiazines or haloperidol may raise TCA blood concentrations
- May alter effects of antihypertensive drugs; may inhibit hypotensive effects of clonidine
- Use of TCAs with sympathomimetic agents may increase sympathetic activity
- Methylphenidate may inhibit metabolism of TCAs
- Activation and agitation, especially following switching or adding antidepressants, may represent the induction of a bipolar state, especially a mixed dysphoric bipolar II condition sometimes associated with suicidal ideation, and require the addition of lithium, a mood stabilizer or an atypical antipsychotic, and/or discontinuation of dothiepin

Other Warnings/ Precautions

- Add or initiate other antidepressants with caution for up to 2 weeks after discontinuing dothiepin
- Generally, do not use with MAO inhibitors, including 14 days after MAOIs are stopped; do not start an MAOI until 2 weeks after discontinuing dothiepin, but see Pearls
- Use with caution in patients with history of seizures, urinary retention, narrow angle-closure glaucoma, hyperthyroidism, and in patients recovering from myocardial infarction
- TCAs can increase QTc interval, especially at toxic doses, which can be attained not only by overdose but also by combining with drugs that inhibit TCA metabolism via CYP450 2D6, potentially causing torsade de pointes-type arrhythmia or sudden death
- Because TCAs can prolong QTc interval, use with caution in patients who have bradycardia or who are taking drugs that can induce bradycardia (e.g., beta blockers, calcium channel blockers, clonidine, digitalis)
- Because TCAs can prolong QTc interval, use with caution in patients who have hypokalemia and/or hypomagnesemia or who are taking drugs that can induce hypokalemia and/or magnesemia (e.g., diuretics, stimulant laxatives, intravenous amphotericin B, glucocorticoids, tetracosactide)
- When treating children, carefully weigh the risks and benefits of pharmacological treatment against the risks and benefits of nontreatment with antidepressants and make sure to document this in the patient's chart
- Distribute the brochures provided by the FDA and the drug companies
- Warn patients and their caregivers about the possibility of activating side effects and advise them to report such symptoms immediately
- Monitor patients for activation of suicidal ideation, especially children and adolescents

Do Not Use

- If patient is recovering from myocardial infarction

- If patient is taking agents capable of significantly prolonging QTc interval (e.g., pimozide, thioridazine, selected antiarrhythmics, moxifloxacin, sparfloxacin)
- If there is a history of QTc prolongation or cardiac arrhythmia, recent acute myocardial infarction, uncompensated heart failure
- If patient is taking drugs that inhibit TCA metabolism, including CYP450 2D6 inhibitors, except by an expert
- If there is reduced CYP450 2D6 function, such as patients who are poor 2D6 metabolizers, except by an expert and at low doses
- If there is a proven allergy to dothiepin

SPECIAL POPULATIONS

Renal Impairment
- Use with caution

Hepatic Impairment
- Use with caution

Cardiac Impairment

- TCAs have been reported to cause arrhythmias, prolongation of conduction time, orthostatic hypotension, sinus tachycardia, and heart failure, especially in the diseased heart
- Myocardial infarction and stroke have been reported with TCAs
- TCAs produce QTc prolongation, which may be enhanced by the existence of bradycardia, hypokalemia, congenital or acquired long QTc interval, which should be evaluated prior to administering dothiepin
- Use with caution if treating concomitantly with a medication likely to produce prolonged bradycardia, hypokalemia, slowing of intracardiac conduction, or prolongation of the QTc interval
- Avoid TCAs in patients with a known history of QTc prolongation, recent acute myocardial infarction, and uncompensated heart failure
- TCAs may cause a sustained increase in heart rate in patients with ischemic heart disease and may worsen (decrease) heart rate variability, an independent risk of mortality in cardiac populations

- Since SSRIs may improve (increase) heart rate variability in patients following a myocardial infarct and may improve survival as well as mood in patients with acute angina or following a myocardial infarction, these are more appropriate agents for cardiac population than tricyclic/tetracyclic antidepressants
- ✳ Risk/benefit ratio may not justify use of TCAs in cardiac impairment

Elderly

- May be more sensitive to anticholinergic, cardiovascular, hypotensive, and sedative effects

 Children and Adolescents

- Carefully weigh the risks and benefits of pharmacological treatment against the risks and benefits of nontreatment with antidepressants and make sure to document this in the patient's chart
- Monitor patients face-to-face regularly, particularly during the first several weeks of treatment
- Use with caution, observing for activation of known or unknown bipolar disorder and/or suicidal ideation, and inform parents or guardian of this risk so they can help observe child or adolescent patients
- Not recommended for use under age 18
- Several studies show lack of efficacy of TCAs for depression
- May be used to treat enuresis or hyperactive/impulsive behaviors
- Some cases of sudden death have occurred in children taking TCAs

 Pregnancy

- Risk Category C [some animal studies show adverse effects, no controlled studies in humans]
- Crosses the placenta
- Adverse effects have been reported in infants whose mothers took a TCA (lethargy, withdrawal symptoms, fetal malformations)
- Not generally recommended for use during pregnancy, especially during first trimester
- Must weigh the risk of treatment (first trimester fetal development, third trimester newborn delivery) to the child against the

risk of no treatment (recurrence of depression, maternal health, infant bonding) to the mother and child
- For many patients this may mean continuing treatment during pregnancy

Breast Feeding

- Some drug is found in mother's breast milk
- ✳ Recommended either to discontinue drug or bottle feed
- Immediate postpartum period is a high-risk time for depression, especially in women who have had prior depressive episodes, so drug may need to be reinstituted late in the third trimester or shortly after childbirth to prevent a recurrence during the postpartum period
- Must weigh benefits of breast feeding with risks and benefits of antidepressant treatment versus non-treatment to both the infant and the mother
- For many patients this may mean continuing treatment during breast feeding

THE ART OF PSYCHOPHARMACOLOGY

Potential Advantages
- Patients with insomnia
- Severe or treatment-resistant depression
- Anxious depression

Potential Disadvantages
- Pediatric and geriatric patients
- Patients concerned with weight gain
- Cardiac patients

Primary Target Symptoms
- Depressed mood
- Chronic pain

 Pearls

- ✳ Close structural similarity to amitriptyline
- Tricyclic antidepressants are often a first-line treatment option for chronic pain
- Tricyclic antidepressants are no longer generally considered a first-line option for depression because of their side effect profile
- Tricyclic antidepressants continue to be useful for severe or treatment-resistant depression
- TCAs may aggravate psychotic symptoms

- Alcohol should be avoided because of additive CNS effects
- Underweight patients may be more susceptible to adverse cardiovascular effects
- Children, patients with inadequate hydration, and patients with cardiac disease may be more susceptible to TCA-induced cardiotoxicity than healthy adults
- For the expert only: a heroic treatment (but potentially dangerous) for severely treatment-resistant patients is to give simultaneously with monoamine oxidase inhibitors for patients who fail to respond to numerous other antidepressants, but generally recommend a different TCA than dothiepin for this use
- If this option is elected, start the MAOI with the tricyclic/tetracyclic antidepressant simultaneously at low doses after appropriate drug washout, then alternately increase doses of these agents every few days to a week as tolerated
- Although very strict dietary and concomitant drug restrictions must be observed to prevent hypertensive crises and serotonin syndrome, the most common side effects of MAOI and tricyclic/tetracyclic antidepressant combinations may be weight gain and orthostatic hypotension
- Patients on TCAs should be aware that they may experience symptoms such as photosensitivity or blue-green urine
- SSRIs may be more effective than TCAs in women, and TCAs may be more effective than SSRIs in men
- Since tricyclic/tetracyclic antidepressants are substrates for CYP450 2D6, and 7% of the population (especially Caucasians) may have a genetic variant leading to reduced activity of 2D6, such patients may not safely tolerate normal doses of tricyclic/tetracyclic antidepressants and may require dose reduction
- Phenotypic testing may be necessary to detect this genetic variant prior to dosing with a tricyclic/tetracyclic antidepressant, especially in vulnerable populations such as children, elderly, cardiac populations, and those on concomitant medications
- Patients who seem to have extraordinarily severe side effects at normal or low doses may have this phenotypic CYP450 2D6 variant and require low doses or switching to another antidepressant not metabolized by 2D6

 Suggested Reading

Anderson IM. Meta-analytical studies on new antidepressants. Br Med Bull. 2001; 57:161–178.

Anderson IM. Selective serotonin reuptake inhibitors versus tricyclic antidepressants: a meta-analysis of efficacy and tolerability. J Aff Disorders. 2000;58:19–36.

Donovan S, Dearden L, Richardson L. The tolerability of dothiepin: a review of clinical studies between 1963 and 1990 in over 13,000 depressed patients. Prog Neuropsychopharmacol Biol Psychiatry. 1994; 18:1143–62.

Lancaster SG, Gonzalez JP. Dothiepin. A review of its pharmacodynamic and pharmacokinetic properties, and therapeutic efficacy in depressive illness. Drugs. 1989; 38:123–47.

DOXEPIN

THERAPEUTICS

Brands • Sinequan
see index for additional brand names

Generic? Yes

Class
- Tricyclic antidepressant (TCA)
- Serotonin and norepinephrine/noradrenaline reuptake inhibitor

Commonly Prescribed For
(bold for FDA approved)
- **Psychoneurotic patient with depression and/or anxiety**
- **Depression and/or anxiety associated with alcoholism**
- **Depression and/or anxiety associated with organic disease**
- **Psychotic depressive disorders with associated anxiety**
- **Involutional depression**
- **Manic-depressive disorder**
- ✳ Pruritus/itching (topical)
- Dermatitis, atopic (topical)
- Lichen simplex chronicus (topical)
- Anxiety
- Insomnia
- Neuropathic pain/chronic pain
- Treatment-resistant depression

How The Drug Works
- Boosts neurotransmitters serotonin and norepinephrine/noradrenaline
- Blocks serotonin reuptake pump (serotonin transporter), presumably increasing serotonergic neurotransmission
- Blocks norepinephrine reuptake pump (norepinephrine transporter), presumably increasing noradrenergic neurotransmission
- Presumably desensitizes both serotonin 1A receptors and beta adrenergic receptors
- Since dopamine is inactivated by norepinephrine reuptake in frontal cortex, which largely lacks dopamine transporters, doxepin can thus increase dopamine neurotransmission in this part of the brain
- May be effective in treating skin conditions because of its strong antihistamine properties

How Long Until It Works
- May have immediate effects in treating insomnia or anxiety
- Onset of therapeutic actions usually not immediate, but often delayed 2 to 4 weeks
- If it is not working within 6 to 8 weeks for depression, it may require a dosage increase or it may not work at all
- May continue to work for many years to prevent relapse of symptoms

If It Works
- The goal of treatment of depression is complete remission of current symptoms as well as prevention of future relapses
- The goal of treatment of chronic neuropathic pain is to reduce symptoms as much as possible, especially in combination with other treatments
- Treatment of depression most often reduces or even eliminates symptoms, but not a cure since symptoms can recur after medicine stopped
- Treatment of chronic neuropathic pain may reduce symptoms, but rarely eliminates them completely, and is not a cure since symptoms can recur after medicine is stopped
- Continue treatment of depression until all symptoms are gone (remission)
- Once symptoms of depression are gone, continue treating for 1 year for the first episode of depression
- For second and subsequent episodes of depression, treatment may need to be indefinite
- Use in anxiety disorders, chronic pain, and skin conditions may also need to be indefinite, but long-term treatment is not well studied in these conditions

If It Doesn't Work
- Many depressed patients only have a partial response where some symptoms are improved but others persist (especially insomnia, fatigue, and problems concentrating)
- Other depressed patients may be nonresponders, sometimes called treatment-resistant or treatment-refractory
- Consider increasing dose, switching to another agent or adding an appropriate augmenting agent
- Consider psychotherapy

- Consider evaluation for another diagnosis or for a comorbid condition (e.g., medical illness, substance abuse, etc.)
- Some patients may experience apparent lack of consistent efficacy due to activation of latent or underlying bipolar disorder, and require antidepressant discontinuation and a switch to a mood stabilizer

 ### Best Augmenting Combos for Partial Response or Treatment-Resistance

- Lithium, buspirone, thyroid hormone (for depression)
- Gabapentin, tiagabine, other anticonvulsants, even opiates if done by experts while monitoring carefully in difficult cases (for chronic pain)

Tests

- None for healthy individuals
- ✱ Since tricyclic and tetracyclic antidepressants are frequently associated with weight gain, before starting treatment, weigh all patients and determine if the patient is already overweight (BMI 25.0–29.9) or obese (BMI ≥30)
- Before giving a drug that can cause weight gain to an overweight or obese patient, consider determining whether the patient already has pre-diabetes (fasting plasma glucose 100–125 mg/dl), diabetes (fasting plasma glucose >126 mg/dl), or dyslipidemia (increased total cholesterol, LDL cholesterol and triglycerides; decreased HDL cholesterol), and treat or refer such patients for treatment including nutrition and weight management, physical activity counseling, smoking cessation, and medical management
- ✱ Monitor weight and BMI during treatment
- ✱ While giving a drug to a patient who has gained >5% of initial weight, consider evaluating for the presence of pre-diabetes, diabetes, or dyslipidemia, or consider switching to a different antidepressant
- EKGs may be useful for selected patients (e.g., those with personal or family history of QTc prolongation; cardiac arrhythmia; recent myocardial infarction; uncompensated heart failure; or taking agents that prolong QTc interval such as pimozide, thioridazine, selected antiarrhythmics, moxifloxacin, sparfloxacin, etc.)

- Patients at risk for electrolyte disturbances (e.g., patients on diuretic therapy) should have baseline and periodic serum potassium and magnesium measurements

SIDE EFFECTS

How Drug Causes Side Effects

- Anticholinergic activity may explain sedative effects, dry mouth, constipation, and blurred vision
- Sedative effects and weight gain may be due to antihistamine properties
- Blockade of alpha adrenergic 1 receptors may explain dizziness, sedation, and hypotension
- Cardiac arrhythmias and seizures, especially in overdose, may be caused by blockade of ion channels

Notable Side Effects

- Blurred vision, constipation, urinary retention, increased appetite, dry mouth, nausea, diarrhea, heartburn, unusual taste in mouth, weight gain
- Fatigue, weakness, dizziness, sedation, headache, anxiety, nervousness, restlessness
- Sexual dysfunction, sweating
- Topical: burning, stinging, itching, or swelling at application site

 ### Life Threatening or Dangerous Side Effects

- Paralytic ileus, hyperthermia (TCAs + anticholinergic agents)
- Lowered seizure threshold and rare seizures
- Orthostatic hypotension, sudden death, arrhythmias, tachycardia
- QTc prolongation
- Hepatic failure, extrapyramidal symptoms
- Increased intraocular pressure, increased psychotic symptoms
- Rare induction of mania
- Rare activation of suicidal ideation and behavior (suicidality)

Weight Gain

unusual · not unusual · common · problematic

- Many experience and/or can be significant in amount
- Can increase appetite and carbohydrate craving

Sedation

unusual | not unusual | **common** | problematic

- Many experience and/or can be significant in amount
- Tolerance to sedative effect may develop with long-term use

What To Do About Side Effects

- Wait
- Wait
- Wait
- Lower the dose
- Switch to an SSRI or newer antidepressant

Best Augmenting Agents for Side Effects

- Many side effects cannot be improved with an augmenting agent

DOSING AND USE

Usual Dosage Range

- 75–150 mg/day

Dosage Forms

- Capsule 10 mg, 25 mg, 50 mg, 75 mg, 100 mg, 150 mg
- Solution 10 mg/mL
- Topical 5%

How to Dose

- Initial 25 mg/day at bedtime; increase by 25 mg every 3–7 days
- 75 mg/day; increase gradually until desired efficacy is achieved; can be dosed once a day at bedtime or in divided doses; maximum dose 300 mg/day
- Topical: apply thin film 4 times a day (or every 3–4 hours while awake)

 Dosing Tips

- If given in a single dose, should generally be administered at bedtime because of its sedative properties
- If given in split doses, largest dose should generally be given at bedtime because of its sedative properties
- If patients experience nightmares, split dose and do not give large dose at bedtime
- Patients treated for chronic pain may only require lower doses

- Liquid formulation should be diluted with water or juice, excluding grape juice
- 150 mg capsule available only for maintenance use, not initial therapy
- ✳ Topical administration is absorbed systematically and can cause the same systematic side effects as oral administration
- If intolerable anxiety, insomnia, agitation, akathisia, or activation occur either upon dosing initiation or discontinuation, consider the possibility of activated bipolar disorder, and switch to a mood stabilizer or an atypical antipsychotic

Overdose

- Death may occur; convulsions, cardiac dysrhythmias, severe hypotension, CNS depression, coma, changes in ECG

Long-Term Use

- Safe

Habit Forming

- No

How to Stop

- Taper to avoid withdrawal effects
- Even with gradual dose reduction some withdrawal symptoms may appear within the first 2 weeks
- Many patients tolerate 50% dose reduction for 3 days, then another 50% reduction for 3 days, then discontinuation
- If withdrawal symptoms emerge during discontinuation, raise dose to stop symptoms and then restart withdrawal much more slowly

Pharmacokinetics

- Substrate for CYP450 2D6
- Half-life approximately 8–24 hours

 Drug Interactions

- Tramadol increases the risk of seizures in patients taking TCAs
- Use of TCAs with anticholinergic drugs may result in paralytic ileus or hyperthermia
- Fluoxetine, paroxetine, bupropion, duloxetine, and other CYP450 2D6 inhibitors may increase TCA concentrations

- Cimetidine may increase plasma concentrations of TCAs and cause anticholinergic symptoms
- Phenothiazines or haloperidol may raise TCA blood concentrations
- May alter effects of antihypertensive drugs; may inhibit hypotensive effects of clonidine
- Use with sympathomimetic agents may increase sympathetic activity
- Methylphenidate may inhibit metabolism of TCAs
- Activation and agitation, especially following switching or adding antidepressants, may represent the induction of a bipolar state, especially a mixed dysphoric bipolar II condition sometimes associated with suicidal ideation, and require the addition of lithium, a mood stabilizer or an atypical antipsychotic, and/or discontinuation of doxepin

 Other Warnings/ Precautions

- Add or initiate other antidepressants with caution for up to 2 weeks after discontinuing doxepin
- Generally, do not use with MAO inhibitors, including 14 days after MAOIs are stopped; do not start an MAOI until 2 weeks after discontinuing doxepin, but see Pearls
- Use with caution in patients with history of seizures, urinary retention, narrow angle-closure glaucoma, hyperthyroidism
- TCAs can increase QTc interval, especially at toxic doses, which can be attained not only by overdose but also by combining with drugs that inhibit TCA metabolism via CYP450 2D6, potentially causing torsade de pointes-type arrhythmia or sudden death
- Because TCAs can prolong QTc interval, use with caution in patients who have bradycardia or who are taking drugs that can induce bradycardia (e.g., beta blockers, calcium channel blockers, clonidine, digitalis)
- Because TCAs can prolong QTc interval, use with caution in patients who have hypokalemia and/or hypomagnesemia or who are taking drugs that can induce hypokalemia and/or magnesemia (e.g., diuretics, stimulant laxatives, intravenous amphotericin B, glucocorticoids, tetracosactide)

- When treating children, carefully weigh the risks and benefits of pharmacological treatment against the risks and benefits of nontreatment with antidepressants and make sure to document this in the patient's chart
- Distribute the brochures provided by the FDA and the drug companies
- Warn patients and their caregivers about the possibility of activating side effects and advise them to report such symptoms immediately
- Monitor patients for activation of suicidal ideation, especially children and adolescents

Do Not Use
- If patient is recovering from myocardial infarction
- If patient is taking agents capable of significantly prolonging QTc interval (e.g., pimozide, thioridazine, selected antiarrhythmics, moxifloxacin, sparfloxacin)
- If there is a history of QTc prolongation or cardiac arrhythmia, recent acute myocardial infarction, uncompensated heart failure
- If patient is taking drugs that inhibit TCA metabolism, including CYP450 2D6 inhibitors, except by an expert
- If there is reduced CYP450 2D6 function, such as patients who are poor 2D6 metabolizers, except by an expert and at low doses
- If patient has narrow angle-closure glaucoma
- If there is a proven allergy to doxepin

SPECIAL POPULATIONS

Renal Impairment
- Use with caution

Hepatic Impairment
- Use with caution – may need lower than usual adult dose

Cardiac Impairment
- TCAs have been reported to cause arrhythmias, prolongation of conduction time, orthostatic hypotension, sinus tachycardia, and heart failure, especially in the diseased heart

- Myocardial infarction and stroke have been reported with TCAs
- TCAs produce QTc prolongation, which may be enhanced by the existence of bradycardia, hypokalemia, congenital or acquired long QTc interval, which should be evaluated prior to administering doxepin
- Use with caution if treating concomitantly with a medication likely to produce prolonged bradycardia, hypokalemia, slowing of intracardiac conduction, or prolongation of the QTc interval
- Avoid TCAs in patients with a known history of QTc prolongation, recent acute myocardial infarction, and uncompensated heart failure
- TCAs may cause a sustained increase in heart rate in patients with ischemic heart disease and may worsen (decrease) heart rate variability, an independent risk of mortality in cardiac populations
- Since SSRIs may improve (increase) heart rate variability in patients following a myocardial infarct and may improve survival as well as mood in patients with acute angina or following a myocardial infarction, these are more appropriate agents for cardiac population than tricyclic/tetracyclic antidepressants
- ✳ Risk/benefit ratio may not justify use of TCAs in cardiac impairment

Elderly

- May be more sensitive to anticholinergic, cardiovascular, hypotensive, and sedative effects

 Children and Adolescents

- Carefully weigh the risks and benefits of pharmacological treatment against the risks and benefits of nontreatment with antidepressants and make sure to document this in the patient's chart
- Monitor patients face-to-face regularly, particularly during the first several weeks of treatment
- Use with caution, observing for activation of known or unknown bipolar disorder and/or suicidal ideation, and inform parents or guardian of this risk so they can help observe child or adolescent patients
- Not recommended for use under age 12

- Several studies show lack of efficacy of TCAs for depression
- May be used to treat enuresis or hyperactive/impulsive behaviors
- Some cases of sudden death have occurred in children taking TCAs
- Initial dose 25–50 mg/day; maximum 100 mg/day

 Pregnancy

- Risk Category C [some animal studies show adverse effects, no controlled studies in humans]
- Crosses the placenta
- Adverse effects have been reported in infants whose mothers took a TCA (lethargy, withdrawal symptoms, fetal malformations)
- Not generally recommended for use during pregnancy, especially during first trimester
- Must weigh the risk of treatment (first trimester fetal development, third trimester newborn delivery) to the child against the risk of no treatment (recurrence of depression, maternal health, infant bonding) to the mother and child
- For many patients this may mean continuing treatment during pregnancy

Breast Feeding

- Some drug is found in mother's breast milk
- Significant drug levels have been detected in some nursing infants
- ✳ Recommended either to discontinue drug or bottle feed
- Immediate postpartum period is a high-risk time for depression, especially in women who have had prior depressive episodes, so drug may need to be reinstituted late in the third trimester or shortly after childbirth to prevent a recurrence during the postpartum period
- Must weigh benefits of breast feeding with risks and benefits of antidepressant treatment versus non-treatment to both the infant and the mother
- For many patients this may mean continuing treatment during breast feeding

THE ART OF PSYCHOPHARMACOLOGY

Potential Advantages
- Patients with insomnia
- Severe or treatment-resistant depression
- Patients with neuro-dermatitis and itching

Potential Disadvantages
- Pediatric and geriatric patients
- Patients concerned with weight gain
- Cardiac patients

Primary Target Symptoms
- Depressed mood
- Anxiety
- Disturbed sleep, energy
- Somatic symptoms
- Itching skin

 Pearls

* Only TCA available in topical formulation
* Topical administration may reduce symptoms in patients with various neuro-dermatitis syndromes, especially itching
- Tricyclic antidepressants are often a first-line treatment option for chronic pain
- Tricyclic antidepressants are no longer generally considered a first-line option for depression because of their side effect profile
- Tricyclic antidepressants continue to be useful for severe or treatment-resistant depression
- TCAs may aggravate psychotic symptoms
- Alcohol should be avoided because of additive CNS effects
- Underweight patients may be more susceptible to adverse cardiovascular effects
- Children, patients with inadequate hydration, and patients with cardiac disease may be more susceptible to TCA-induced cardiotoxicity than healthy adults
- For the expert only: although generally prohibited, a heroic but potentially dangerous treatment for severely treatment-resistant patients is to give a tricyclic/tetracyclic antidepressant other than clomipramine simultaneously with an MAO inhibitor for patients who fail to respond to numerous other antidepressants
- If this option is elected, start the MAOI with the tricyclic/tetracyclic antidepressant simultaneously at low doses after appropriate drug washout, then alternately increase doses of these agents every few days to a week as tolerated
- Although very strict dietary and concomitant drug restrictions must be observed to prevent hypertensive crises and serotonin syndrome, the most common side effects of MAOI/tricyclic or tetracyclic combinations may be weight gain and orthostatic hypotension
- Patients on TCAs should be aware that they may experience symptoms such as photosensitivity or blue-green urine
- SSRIs may be more effective than TCAs in women, and TCAs may be more effective than SSRIs in men
- Since tricyclic/tetracyclic antidepressants are substrates for CYP450 2D6, and 7% of the population (especially Caucasians) may have a genetic variant leading to reduced activity of 2D6, such patients may not safely tolerate normal doses of tricyclic/tetracyclic antidepressants and may require dose reduction
- Phenotypic testing may be necessary to detect this genetic variant prior to dosing with a tricyclic/tetracyclic antidepressant, especially in vulnerable populations such as children, elderly, cardiac populations, and those on concomitant medications
- Patients who seem to have extraordinarily severe side effects at normal or low doses may have this phenotypic CYP450 2D6 variant and require low doses or switching to another antidepressant not metabolized by 2D6

Suggested Reading

Anderson IM. Meta-analytical studies on new antidepressants. Br Med Bull 2001; 57:161–178.

Anderson IM. Selective serotonin reuptake inhibitors versus tricyclic antidepressants: a meta-analysis of efficacy and tolerability. J Aff Disorders 2000;58:19–36.

Godfrey RG. A guide to the understanding and use of tricyclic antidepressants in the overall management of fibromyalgia and other chronic pain syndromes. Arch Intern Med 1996; 156:1047–52.

DULOXETINE

Brands • Cymbalta
see index for additional brand names

Generic? No

 Class

- SNRI (dual serotonin and norepinephrine reuptake inhibitor); may be classified as an antidepressant, but it is not just an antidepressant

Commonly Prescribed For

(bold for FDA approved)
- **Major depressive disorder**
- **Diabetic peripheral neuropathic pain (DPNP)**
- Stress urinary incontinence
- Neuropathic pain/chronic pain
- Fibromyalgia
- Generalized anxiety disorder
- Other anxiety disorders

 How The Drug Works

- Boosts neurotransmitters serotonin, norepinephrine/noradrenaline, and dopamine
- Blocks serotonin reuptake pump (serotonin transporter), presumably increasing serotonergic neurotransmission
- Blocks norepinephrine reuptake pump (norepinephrine transporter), presumably increasing noradrenergic neurotransmission
- Presumably desensitizes both serotonin 1A receptors and beta adrenergic receptors
- Since dopamine is inactivated by norepinephrine reuptake in frontal cortex, which largely lacks dopamine transporters, duloxetine can increase dopamine neurotransmission in this part of the brain
- Weakly blocks dopamine reuptake pump (dopamine transporter), and may increase dopamine neurotransmission

How Long Until It Works

- Onset of therapeutic actions usually not immediate, but often delayed 2 to 4 weeks for depression
- If it is not working within 6 to 8 weeks for depression, it may require a dosage increase or it may not work at all

- Can reduce neuropathic pain within a week, but onset can take longer
- May continue to work for many years to prevent relapse of depressive symptoms or prevent worsening of painful symptoms

If It Works

- The goal of treatment of depression and anxiety disorders is complete remission of current symptoms as well as prevention of future relapses
- The goal of treatment of diabetic peripheral neuropathic pain and fibromyalgia and chronic neuropathic pain is to reduce symptoms as much as possible, especially in combination with other treatments
- Treatment of depression most often reduces or even eliminates symptoms, but is not a cure since symptoms can recur after medicine stopped
- Treatment of diabetic peripheral neuropathic pain, fibromyalgia, and chronic neuropathic pain may reduce symptoms, but rarely eliminates them completely, and is not a cure since symptoms can recur after medicine is stopped
- Continue treatment of depression and anxiety disorders until all symptoms are gone (remission)
- Once symptoms of depression are gone, continue treating for 1 year for the first episode of depression
- For second and subsequent episodes of depression, treatment may need to be indefinite
- Use in diabetic peripheral neuropathic pain, fibromyalgia, and chronic neuropathic pain may also need to be indefinite, but long-term treatment is not well studied in these conditions

If It Doesn't Work

- Many patients only have a partial response where some symptoms are improved but others persist (especially insomnia, fatigue, and problems concentrating)
- Other patients may be nonresponders, sometimes called treatment-resistant or treatment-refractory
- Some depressed patients who have an initial response may relapse even though they continue treatment, sometimes called "poop-out"

- Consider increasing dose, switching to another agent or adding an appropriate augmenting agent
- Consider psychotherapy for depression or biofeedback or hypnosis for pain
- Consider evaluation for another diagnosis or for a comorbid condition (e.g., medical illness, substance abuse, etc.)
- Consider the presence of noncompliance and counsel the patient
- Some patients may experience apparent lack of consistent efficacy due to activation of latent or underlying bipolar disorder, and require antidepressant discontinuation and a switch to a mood stabilizer

Best Augmenting Combos for Partial Response or Treatment-Resistance

* Augmentation experience is limited compared to other antidepressants and treatments for neuropathic pain

* Adding other agents to duloxetine for treating depression could follow the same practice for augmenting SSRIs or other SNRIs if done by experts while monitoring carefully in difficult cases

- Although no controlled studies and little clinical experience, adding other agents for treating diabetic peripheral neuropathic pain and fibromyalgia and neuropathic pain could theoretically include gabapentin, pregabalin, and tiagabine, if done by experts while monitoring carefully in difficult cases
- Mirtazapine ("California rocket fuel" for depression; a potentially powerful dual serotonin and norepinephrine combination, but observe for activation of bipolar disorder and suicidal ideation)
- Bupropion, reboxetine, nortriptyline, desipramine, maprotiline, atomoxetine (all potentially powerful enhancers of noradrenergic action for depression, but observe for activation of bipolar disorder and suicidal ideation)
- Modafinil, especially for fatigue, sleepiness, and lack of concentration
- Mood stabilizers or atypical antipsychotics for bipolar depression, psychotic depression or treatment-resistant depression
- Benzodiazepines

- If all else fails for anxiety disorders, consider gabapentin, pregabalin, or tiagabine
- Hypnotics or trazodone for insomnia
- Classically, lithium, buspirone, or thyroid hormone for depression

Tests
- Check blood pressure before initiating treatment and regularly during treatment

SIDE EFFECTS

How Drug Causes Side Effects
- Theoretically due to increases in serotonin and norepinephrine concentrations at receptors in parts of the brain and body other than those that cause therapeutic actions (e.g., unwanted actions of serotonin in sleep centers causing insomnia, unwanted actions of norepinephrine on acetylcholine release causing decreased appetite, increased blood pressure, urinary retention, etc.)
- Most side effects are immediate but often go away with time

Notable Side Effects
- Nausea, diarrhea, decreased appetite
- Insomnia, sedation
- Sexual dysfunction (men: abnormal ejaculation/orgasm, impotence, decreased libido; women: abnormal orgasm)
- Sweating
- Increase in blood pressure (up to 2 mm Hg)

Life Threatening or Dangerous Side Effects
- Rare seizures
- Rare induction of hypomania
- Rare activation of suicidal ideation, suicide attempts, and completed suicide

Weight Gain

 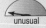

unusual | not unusual | common | problematic

- Reported but not expected

Sedation

unusual | not unusual | common | problematic

- Occurs in significant minority

• May also be activating in some patients

What To Do About Side Effects
• Wait
• Wait
• Wait
• Lower the dose
• In a few weeks, switch or add other drugs

Best Augmenting Agents for Side Effects
• For urinary hesitancy, give an alpha 1 blocker such as tamsulosin
• Often best to try another antidepressant monotherapy prior to resorting to augmentation strategies to treat side effects
• Trazodone or a hypnotic for insomnia
• Bupropion, sildenafil, vardenafil, or tadalafil for sexual dysfunction
• Benzodiazepines for jitteriness and anxiety, especially at initiation of treatment and especially for anxious patients
• Mirtazapine for insomnia, agitation, and gastrointestinal side effects
• Many side effects are dose-dependent (i.e., they increase as dose increases, or they reemerge until tolerance re-develops)
• Many side effects are time-dependent (i.e., they start immediately upon dosing and upon each dose increase, but go away with time)
• Activation and agitation may represent the induction of a bipolar state, especially a mixed dysphoric bipolar II condition sometimes associated with suicidal ideation, and require the addition of lithium, a mood stabilizer or an atypical antipsychotic, and/or discontinuation of duloxetine

DOSING AND USE

Usual Dosage Range
• 40–60 mg/day in 1–2 doses for depression
• 60 mg once daily for diabetic peripheral neuropathic pain
• 40 mg twice daily for stress urinary incontinence

Dosage Forms
• Capsule 20 mg, 30 mg, 60 mg

How to Dose
• Initial 40 mg/day in 1–2 doses; can increase to 60 mg/day if necessary; maximum dose generally 120 mg/day

 Dosing Tips
• Studies have not demonstrated increased efficacy beyond 60 mg/day
∗ Some patients may require up to or more than 120 mg/day, but clinical experience is quite limited with high dosing
• In relapse prevention studies in depression, a significant percentage of patients who relapsed on 60 mg/day responded and remitted when the dose was increased to 120 mg/day
• Dosing for neuropathic pain and fibromyalgia may be similar to that for depression but different from dosing for stress urinary incontinence, but clinical experience is still evolving
• Some studies suggest that both serotonin and norepinephrine reuptake blockade are present at 40–60 mg/day
• Do not chew or crush and do not sprinkle on food or mix with food, but rather always swallow whole to avoid affecting enteric coating
• Some patients may require dosing above 120 mg/day in 2 divided doses, but this should be done with caution and by experts

Overdose
• No fatalities have been reported as monotherapy

Long-Term Use
• Blood pressure should be monitored regularly

Habit Forming
• No

How to Stop
• Taper to avoid withdrawal effects (dizziness, nausea, vomiting, headache, paresthesias, irritability)
• Many patients tolerate 50% dose reduction for 3 days, then another 50% reduction for 3 days, then discontinuation
∗ If withdrawal symptoms emerge during discontinuation, raise dose to stop

symptoms and then restart withdrawal much more slowly

Pharmacokinetics

- Elimination half-life approximately 12 hours
- Metabolized mainly by CYP450 2D6 and CYP450 1A2
- Inhibitor of CYP450 2D6 (probably clinically significant) and CYP450 1A2 (probably not clinically significant)
- Absorption may be delayed by up to 3 hours and clearance may be increased by one-third after an evening dose as compared to a morning dose

 Drug Interactions

- Can increase tricyclic antidepressant levels; use with caution with tricyclic antidepressants or when switching from a TCA to duloxetine
- Can cause a fatal "serotonin syndrome" when combined with MAO inhibitors, so do not use with MAO inhibitors or for at least 14 days after MAOIs are stopped
- Do not start an MAO inhibitor for at least 5 days after discontinuing duloxetine
- Inhibitors of CYP450 1A2, such as fluvoxamine, increase plasma levels of duloxetine and may require a dosage reduction of duloxetine
- Cigarette smoking induces CYP450 1A2 and may reduce plasma levels of duloxetine, but dosage modifications are not recommended for smokers
- ✳ Inhibitors of CYP450 2D6, such as paroxetine, fluoxetine, and quinidine, may increase plasma levels of duloxetine and require a dosage reduction of duloxetine
- Via CYP450 1A2 inhibition, duloxetine could theoretically reduce clearance of theophylline and clozapine; however, studies of co-administration with theophylline did not demonstrate significant effects of duloxetine on theophylline pharmacokinetics
- Via CYP450 2D6 inhibition, duloxetine could theoretically interfere with the analgesic actions of codeine, and increase the plasma levels of some beta blockers and of atomoxetine
- Via CYP450 2D6 inhibition, duloxetine could theoretically increase concentrations

of thioridazine and cause dangerous cardiac arrhythmias

 Other Warnings/ Precautions

- Use with caution in patients with history of seizures
- Use with caution in patients with bipolar disorder unless treated with concomitant mood stabilizing agent
- When treating children, carefully weigh the risks and benefits of pharmacological treatment against the risks and benefits of nontreatment with antidepressants and make sure to document this in the patient's chart
- Distribute the brochures provided by the FDA and the drug companies
- Warn patients and their caregivers about the possibility of activating side effects and advise them to report such symptoms immediately
- Monitor patients for activation of suicidal ideation, especially children and adolescents
- Duloxetine may increase blood pressure, so blood pressure should be monitored during treatment

Do Not Use

- If patient has uncontrolled narrow angle-closure glaucoma
- If patient has substantial alcohol use
- If patient is taking an MAO inhibitor
- If patient is taking thioridazine
- If there is a proven allergy to duloxetine

SPECIAL POPULATIONS

Renal Impairment

- Dose adjustment generally not necessary for mild to moderate impairment
- Not recommended for use in patients with end-stage renal disease (requiring dialysis) or severe renal impairment

Hepatic Impairment

- Not to be administered to patients with any hepatic insufficiency
- Not recommended for use in patients with substantial alcohol use
- Increased risk of elevation of serum transaminase levels

Cardiac Impairment
- Drug should be used with caution
- Duloxetine may raise blood pressure

Elderly
- Some patients may tolerate lower doses better

 Children and Adolescents
- Carefully weigh the risks and benefits of pharmacological treatment against the risks and benefits of nontreatment with antidepressants and make sure to document this in the patient's chart
- Monitor patients face-to-face regularly, particularly during the first several weeks of treatment
- Use with caution, observing for activation of known or unknown bipolar disorder and/or suicidal ideation, and inform parents or guardian of this risk so they can help observe child or adolescent patients
- Not studied, but can be used by experts

 Pregnancy
- Risk Category C [some animal studies show adverse effects, no controlled studies in humans]
- Not generally recommended for use during pregnancy, especially during first trimester
- Nonetheless, continuous treatment during pregnancy may be necessary and has not been proven to be harmful to the fetus
- Must weigh the risk of treatment (first trimester fetal development, third trimester newborn delivery) to the child against the risk of no treatment (recurrence of depression, maternal health, infant bonding) to the mother and child
- For many patients this may mean continuing treatment during pregnancy
- Neonates exposed to SSRIs or SNRIs late in the third trimester have developed complications requiring prolonged hospitalization, respiratory support, and tube feeding; reported symptoms are consistent with either a direct toxic effect of SSRIs and SNRIs or, possibly, a drug discontinuation syndrome, and include respiratory distress, cyanosis, apnea, seizures, temperature instability, feeding difficulty, vomiting, hypoglycemia, hypotonia, hypertonia, hyperreflexia, tremor, jitteriness, irritability, and constant crying

Breast Feeding
- Unknown if duloxetine is secreted in human breast milk, but all psychotropics assumed to be secreted in breast milk
- If child becomes irritable or sedated, breast feeding or drug may need to be discontinued
- Immediate postpartum period is a high-risk time for depression, especially in women who have had prior depressive episodes, so drug may need to be reinstituted late in the third trimester or shortly after childbirth to prevent a recurrence during the postpartum period
- Must weigh benefits of breast feeding with risks and benefits of antidepressant treatment versus non-treatment to both the infant and the mother
- For many patients, this may mean continuing treatment during breast feeding

THE ART OF PSYCHOPHARMACOLOGY

Potential Advantages
- Patients with physical symptoms of depression
- Patients with retarded depression
- Patients with atypical depression
- Patients with depression may have higher remission rates on SNRIs than on SSRIs
- Depressed patients with somatic symptoms, fatigue, and pain
- Patients who do not respond or do not remit on treatment with SSRIs

Potential Disadvantages
- Patients with urologic disorders, prostate disorders (e.g., older men)
- Patients sensitive to nausea

Primary Target Symptoms
- Depressed mood
- Energy, motivation, and interest
- Sleep disturbance
- Physical symptoms
- Pain

Pearls

* Duloxetine has well-documented efficacy for the painful physical symptoms of depression
* Duloxetine has only somewhat greater potency for serotonin reuptake blockade than for norepinephrine reuptake blockade, but this is of unclear clinical significance as a differentiator from other SNRIs
* No head-to-head studies, but may have less hypertension than venlafaxine XR
* Powerful pro-noradrenergic actions may occur at doses greater than 60 mg/day
* Not well-studied in ADHD or anxiety disorders, but may be effective
* Approved in many countries for stress urinary incontinence
* Patients may have higher remission rate for depression on SNRIs than on SSRIs
* Add or switch to or from pro-noradrenergic agents (e.g., atomoxetine, reboxetine, other SNRIs, mirtazapine, maprotiline, nortriptyline, desipramine, bupropion) with caution
* Add or switch to or from CYP450 2D6 substrates with caution (e.g., atomoxetine, maprotiline, nortriptyline, desipramine)
* Mechanism of action as SNRI suggests it may be effective in some patients who fail to respond to SSRIs

Suggested Reading

Bymaster FP, Dreshfield-Ahmad LJ, Threlkeld PG, Shaw JL, Thompson L, Nelson DL, Hemrick-Luecke SK, Wong DT. Comparative affinity of duloxetine and venlafaxine for serotonin and norepinephrine transporters in vitro and in vivo, human serotonin receptor subtypes, and other neuronal receptors. Neuropsychopharmacology 2001; 25(6):871–80.

Detke MJ, Lu Y, Goldstein DJ, Hayes JR, Demitrack MA. Duloxetine, 60 mg once daily, for major depressive disorder: a randomized double-blind placebo-controlled trial. J Clin Psychiatry 2002;63(4):308–15.

Goldstein DJ, Mallinckrodt C, Lu Y, Demitrack MA. Duloxetine in the treatment of major depressive disorder: a double-blind clinical trial. J Clin Psychiatry 2002;63(3):225–31.

Karpa KD, Cavanaugh JE, Lakoski JM. Duloxetine pharmacology: profile of a dual monoamine modulator. CNS Drug Rev 2002;8(4):361–76.

Zinner NR. Duloxetine: a serotonin-noradrenaline re-uptake inhibitor for the treatment of stress urinary incontinence. Expert Opin Investig Drugs 2003; 12(9):1559–66.

ESCITALOPRAM

THERAPEUTICS

Brands • Lexapro
see index for additional brand names

Generic? Not in the U.S. or Europe

Class
- SSRI (selective serotonin reuptake inhibitor); often classified as an antidepressant, but it is not just an antidepressant

Commonly Prescribed For
(bold for FDA approved)
- **Major depressive disorder**
- **Generalized anxiety disorder**
- Panic disorder
- Obsessive-compulsive disorder (OCD)
- Posttraumatic stress disorder (PTSD)
- Social anxiety disorder (social phobia)
- Premenstrual dysphoric disorder (PMDD)

How The Drug Works
- Boosts neurotransmitter serotonin
- Blocks serotonin reuptake pump (serotonin transporter)
- Desensitizes serotonin receptors, especially serotonin 1A autoreceptors
- Presumably increases serotonergic neurotransmission

How Long Until It Works
- Onset of therapeutic actions usually not immediate, but often delayed 2 to 4 weeks
- If it is not working within 6 to 8 weeks, it may require a dosage increase or it may not work at all
- May continue to work for many years to prevent relapse of symptoms

If It Works
- The goal of treatment is complete remission of current symptoms as well as prevention of future relapses
- Treatment most often reduces or even eliminates symptoms, but not a cure since symptoms can recur after medicine stopped
- Continue treatment until all symptoms are gone (remission) or significantly reduced (e.g., OCD, PTSD)

- Once symptoms gone, continue treating for 1 year for the first episode of depression
- For second and subsequent episodes of depression, treatment may need to be indefinite
- Use in anxiety disorders may also need to be indefinite

If It Doesn't Work
- Many patients only have a partial response where some symptoms are improved but others persist (especially insomnia, fatigue, and problems concentrating in depression)
- Other patients may be nonresponders, sometimes called treatment-resistant or treatment-refractory
- Some patients who have an initial response may relapse even though they continue treatment, sometimes called "poop-out"
- Consider increasing dose, switching to another agent or adding an appropriate augmenting agent
- Consider psychotherapy
- Consider evaluation for another diagnosis or for a comorbid condition (e.g., medical illness, substance abuse, etc.)
- Some patients may experience apparent lack of consistent efficacy due to activation of latent or underlying bipolar disorder, and require antidepressant discontinuation and a switch to a mood stabilizer

Best Augmenting Combos for Partial Response or Treatment-Resistance

- Trazodone, especially for insomnia
- Bupropion, mirtazapine, reboxetine, or atomoxetine (use combinations of antidepressants with caution as this may activate bipolar disorder and suicidal ideation)
- Modafinil, especially for fatigue, sleepiness, and lack of concentration
- Mood stabilizers or atypical antipsychotics for bipolar depression, psychotic depression, treatment-resistant depression, or treatment-resistant anxiety disorders
- Benzodiazepines
- If all else fails for anxiety disorders, consider gabapentin or tiagabine
- Hypnotics for insomnia
- Classically, lithium, buspirone, or thyroid hormone

Tests
• None for healthy individuals

SIDE EFFECTS

How Drug Causes Side Effects
• Theoretically due to increases in serotonin concentrations at serotonin receptors in parts of the brain and body other than those that cause therapeutic actions (e.g., unwanted actions of serotonin in sleep centers causing insomnia, unwanted actions of serotonin in the gut causing diarrhea, etc.)
• Increasing serotonin can cause diminished dopamine release and might contribute to emotional flattening, cognitive slowing, and apathy in some patients
• Most side effects are immediate but often go away with time, in contrast to most therapeutic effects which are delayed and are enhanced over time
✳ As escitalopram has no known important secondary pharmacologic properties, its side effects are presumably all mediated by its serotonin reuptake blockade

Notable Side Effects
• Sexual dysfunction (men: delayed ejaculation, erectile dysfunction; men and women: decreased sexual desire, anorgasmia)
• Gastrointestinal (decreased appetite, nausea, diarrhea, constipation, dry mouth)
• Mostly central nervous system (insomnia but also sedation, agitation, tremors, headache, dizziness)
• Note: patients with diagnosed or undiagnosed bipolar or psychotic disorders may be more vulnerable to CNS-activating actions of SSRIs
• Autonomic (sweating)
• Bruising and rare bleeding
• Rare hyponatremia (mostly in elderly patients and generally reversible on discontinuation of escitalopram

Life Threatening or Dangerous Side Effects
• Rare seizures
• Rare induction of mania
• Rare activation of suicidal ideation and behavior (suicidality)

Weight Gain

unusual   not unusual   common   problematic

• Reported but not expected

Sedation

unusual   not unusual   common   problematic

• Reported but not expected

What To Do About Side Effects
• Wait
• Wait
• Wait
• In a few weeks, switch to another agent or add other drugs

Best Augmenting Agents for Side Effects
• Often best to try another SSRI or another antidepressant monotherapy prior to resorting to augmentation strategies to treat side effects
• Trazodone or a hypnotic for insomnia
• Bupropion, sildenafil, vardenafil, or tadalafil for sexual dysfunction
• Bupropion for emotional flattening, cognitive slowing, or apathy
• Mirtazapine for insomnia, agitation, and gastrointestinal side effects
• Benzodiazepines for jitteriness and anxiety, especially at initiation of treatment and especially for anxious patients
• Many side effects are dose-dependent (i.e., they increase as dose increases, or they reemerge until tolerance re-develops)
• Many side effects are time-dependent (i.e., they start immediately upon dosing and upon each dose increase, but go away with time)
• Activation and agitation may represent the induction of a bipolar state, especially a mixed dysphoric bipolar II condition sometimes associated with suicidal ideation, and require the addition of lithium, a mood stabilizer or an atypical antipsychotic, and/or discontinuation of escitalopram

DOSING AND USE

Usual Dosage Range
- 10–20 mg/day
- Oral solution 5 mg/5 mL

Dosage Forms
- Tablets 10 mg, 20 mg

How to Dose
- Initial 10 mg/day; increase to 20 mg/day if necessary; single dose administration, morning or evening

 Dosing Tips
- Given once daily, any time of day tolerated
* 10 mg of escitalopram may be comparable in efficacy to 40 mg of citalopram with fewer side effects
- Thus, give an adequate trial of 10 mg prior to giving 20 mg
- Some patients require dosing with 30 or 40 mg
- If intolerable anxiety, insomnia, agitation, akathisia, or activation occur either upon dosing initiation or discontinuation, consider the possibility of activated bipolar disorder and switch to a mood stabilizer or an atypical antipsychotic

Overdose
- Few reports of escitalopram overdose, but probably similar to citalopram overdose
- Rare fatalities have been reported in citalopram overdose, both in combination with other drugs and alone
- Symptoms associated with citalopram overdose include vomiting, sedation, heart rhythm disturbances, dizziness, sweating, nausea, tremor, and rarely amnesia, confusion, coma, convulsions

Long-Term Use
- Safe

Habit Forming
- No

How to Stop
- Taper not usually necessary
- However, tapering to avoid potential withdrawal reactions generally prudent

- Many patients tolerate 50% dose reduction for 3 days, then another 50% reduction for 3 days, then discontinuation
- If withdrawal symptoms emerge during discontinuation, raise dose to stop symptoms and then restart withdrawal much more slowly

Pharmacokinetics
- Mean terminal half-life 27–32 hours
- Steady-state plasma concentrations achieved within 1 week
- No significant actions on CYP450 enzymes

 Drug Interactions
- Tramadol increases the risk of seizures in patients taking an antidepressant
- Can cause a fatal "serotonin syndrome" when combined with MAO inhibitors, so do not use with MAO inhibitors or for at least 14 days after MAOIs are stopped
- Do not start an MAO inhibitor for at least 2 weeks after discontinuing escitalopram
- Could theoretically cause weakness, hyperreflexia, and incoordination when combined with sumatriptan or possibly other triptans, requiring careful monitoring of patient
- Few known adverse drug interactions

 Other Warnings/ Precautions
- Use with caution in patients with history of seizures
- Use with caution in patients with bipolar disorder unless treated with concomitant mood stabilizing agent
- When treating children, carefully weigh the risks and benefits of pharmacological treatment against the risks and benefits of nontreatment with antidepressants and make sure to document this in the patient's chart
- Distribute the brochures provided by the FDA and the drug companies
- Warn patients and their caregivers about the possibility of activating side effects and advise them to report such symptoms immediately
- Monitor patients for activation of suicidal ideation, especially children and adolescents

Do Not Use

- If patient is taking an MAO inhibitor
- If there is a proven allergy to escitalopram or citalopram

Renal Impairment

- Few data available for use in patients with renal impairment, but start with 10 mg/day

Hepatic Impairment

- Recommended dose 10 mg/day

Cardiac Impairment

- Not systematically evaluated in patients with cardiac impairment
- Preliminary data suggest that citalopram is safe in patients with cardiac impairment, suggesting that escitalopram is also safe
- Treating depression with SSRIs in patients with acute angina or following myocardial infarction may reduce cardiac events and improve survival as well as mood

Elderly

- Recommended dose 10 mg/day

 Children and Adolescents

- Safety and efficacy have not been established
- Carefully weigh the risks and benefits of pharmacological treatment against the risks and benefits of nontreatment with antidepressants and make sure to document this in the patient's chart
- Monitor patients face-to-face regularly, particularly during the first several weeks of treatment
- Use with caution, observing for activation of known or unknown bipolar disorder and/or suicidal ideation, and inform parents or guardian of this risk so they can help observe child or adolescent patients

 Pregnancy

- Risk Category C [some animal studies show adverse effects, no controlled studies in humans]
- Not generally recommended for use during pregnancy, especially during first trimester
- Nonetheless, continuous treatment during pregnancy may be necessary and has not been proven to be harmful to the fetus
- At delivery there may be more bleeding in the mother and transient irritability or sedation in the newborn
- Must weigh the risk of treatment (first trimester fetal development, third trimester newborn delivery) to the child against the risk of no treatment (recurrence of depression, maternal health, infant bonding) to the mother and child
- For many patients, this may mean continuing treatment during pregnancy
- Neonates exposed to SSRIs or SNRIs late in the third trimester have developed complications requiring prolonged hospitalization, respiratory support, and tube feeding; reported symptoms are consistent with either a direct toxic effect of SSRIs and SNRIs or, possibly, a drug discontinuation syndrome, and include respiratory distress, cyanosis, apnea, seizures, temperature instability, feeding difficulty, vomiting, hypoglycemia, hypotonia, hypertonia, hyperreflexia, tremor, jitteriness, irritability, and constant crying

Breast Feeding

- Some drug is found in mother's breast milk
- Trace amounts may be present in nursing children whose mothers are on escitalopram
- If child becomes irritable or sedated, breast feeding or drug may need to be discontinued
- Immediate postpartum period is a high-risk time for depression, especially in women who have had prior depressive episodes, so drug may need to be reinstituted late in the third trimester or shortly after childbirth to prevent a recurrence during the postpartum period
- Must weigh benefits of breast feeding with risks and benefits of antidepressant treatment versus non-treatment to both the infant and the mother
- For many patients, this may mean continuing treatment during breast feeding

THE ART OF PSYCHOPHARMACOLOGY

Potential Advantages
- Patients taking concomitant medications (few drug interactions and fewer even than with citalopram)
- Patients requiring faster onset of action

Potential Disadvantages
- More expensive than citalopram in markets where citalopram is generic

Primary Target Symptoms
- Depressed mood
- Anxiety
- Panic attacks, avoidant behavior, re-experiencing, hyperarousal
- Sleep disturbance, both insomnia and hypersomnia

 Pearls

✳ May be among the best-tolerated antidepressants
- May have less sexual dysfunction than some other SSRIs
- May be better tolerated than citalopram
- Can cause cognitive and affective "flattening"
✳ R-citalopram may interfere with the binding of S-citalopram at the serotonin transporter

✳ For this reason, S-citalopram may be more than twice as potent as R,S-citalopram (i.e., citalopram)
- Thus, 10 mg starting dose of S-citalopram may have the therapeutic efficacy of 40 mg of R,S-citalopram
- Thus, escitalopram may have faster onset and better efficacy with reduced side effects compared to R,S-citalopram
- Some data may actually suggest remission rates comparable to dual serotonin and norepinephrine reuptake inhibitors, but this is not proven
✳ Escitalopram is commonly used with augmenting agents, as it is the SSRI with the least interaction at either CYP450 2D6 or 3A4, therefore causing fewer pharmacokinetically-mediated drug interactions with augmenting agents than other SSRIs
- SSRIs may be less effective in women over 50, especially if they are not taking estrogen
- SSRIs may be useful for hot flushes in perimenopausal women
- Some postmenopausal women's depression will respond better to escitalopram plus estrogen augmentation than to escitalopram alone
- Nonresponse to escitalopram in elderly may require consideration of mild cognitive impairment or Alzheimer disease

 Suggested Reading

Baldwin DS. Escitalopram: efficacy and tolerability in the treatment of depression. Hosp Med. 2002;63:668–71.

Burke WJ. Escitalopram. Expert Opin Investig Drugs. 2002;11(10):1477–86.

Edwards JG, Anderson I. Systematic review and guide to selection of selective serotonin reuptake inhibitors. Drugs. 1999;57:507–533.

Waugh J, Goa KL. Escitalopram : a review of its use in the management of major depressive and anxiety disorders. CNS Drugs. 2003;17:343–62.

FLUOXETINE

THERAPEUTICS

Brands • Prozac   • Prozac weekly
        • Sarafem
see index for additional brand names

Generic? Yes

Class
- SSRI (selective serotonin reuptake inhibitor); often classified as an antidepressant, but it is not just an antidepressant

Commonly Prescribed For
(bold for FDA approved)
- **Major depressive disorder**
- **Obsessive-compulsive disorder (OCD)**
- **Premenstrual dysphoric disorder (PMDD)**
- **Bulimia nervosa**
- **Panic disorder**
- **Bipolar depression [in combination with olanzapine (Symbyax)]**
- Social anxiety disorder (social phobia)
- Posttraumatic stress disorder (PTSD)

How The Drug Works
- Boosts neurotransmitter serotonin
- Blocks serotonin reuptake pump (serotonin transporter)
- Desensitizes serotonin receptors, especially serotonin 1A receptors
- Presumably increases serotonergic neurotransmission
- ✷ Fluoxetine also has antagonist properties at 5HT2C receptors, which could increase norepinephrine and dopamine neurotransmission

How Long Until It Works
- ✷ Some patients may experience increased energy or activation early after initiation of treatment
- Onset of therapeutic actions usually not immediate, but often delayed 2 to 4 weeks
- If it is not working within 6 to 8 weeks, it may require a dosage increase or it may not work at all
- May continue to work for many years to prevent relapse of symptoms

If It Works
- The goal of treatment is complete remission of current symptoms as well as prevention of future relapses
- Treatment most often reduces or even eliminates symptoms, but not a cure since symptoms can recur after medicine stopped
- Continue treatment until all symptoms are gone (remission) or significantly reduced (e.g., OCD, PTSD)
- Once symptoms gone, continue treating for 1 year for the first episode of depression
- For second and subsequent episodes of depression, treatment may need to be indefinite
- For anxiety disorders and bulimia, treatment may also need to be indefinite

If It Doesn't Work
- Many patients only have a partial response where some symptoms are improved but others persist (especially insomnia, fatigue, and problems concentrating in depression)
- Other patients may be nonresponders, sometimes called treatment-resistant or treatment-refractory
- Some patients who have an initial response may relapse even though they continue treatment, sometimes called "poop-out"
- Consider increasing dose, switching to another agent or adding an appropriate augmenting agent
- Consider psychotherapy
- Consider evaluation for another diagnosis or for a comorbid condition (e.g., medical illness, substance abuse, etc.)
- Some patients may experience apparent lack of consistent efficacy due to activation of latent or underlying bipolar disorder, and require antidepressant discontinuation and a switch to a mood stabilizer

Best Augmenting Combos for Partial Response or Treatment-Resistance
- Trazodone, especially for insomnia
- Bupropion, mirtazapine, reboxetine, or atomoxetine (add with caution and at lower doses since fluoxetine could theoretically raise atomoxetine levels); use combinations of antidepressants with caution as this may activate bipolar disorder and suicidal ideation

- Modafinil, especially for fatigue, sleepiness, and lack of concentration
- Mood stabilizers or atypical antipsychotics for bipolar depression, psychotic depression, treatment-resistant depression, or treatment-resistant anxiety disorders
- * Fluoxetine has been specifically studied in combination with olanzapine (olanzapine-fluoxetine combination) with excellent results for bipolar depression, treatment-resistant unipolar depression, and psychotic depression
- Benzodiazepines
- If all else fails for anxiety disorders, consider gabapentin or tiagabine
- Hypnotics for insomnia
- Classically, lithium, buspirone, or thyroid hormone

Tests
- None for healthy individuals

SIDE EFFECTS

How Drug Causes Side Effects
- Theoretically due to increases in serotonin concentrations at serotonin receptors in parts of the brain and body other than those that cause therapeutic actions (e.g., unwanted actions of serotonin in sleep centers causing insomnia, unwanted actions of serotonin in the gut causing diarrhea, etc.)
- Increasing serotonin can cause diminished dopamine release and might contribute to emotional flattening, cognitive slowing, and apathy in some patients
- Most side effects are immediate but often go away with time, in contrast to most therapeutic effects which are delayed and are enhanced over time
- * Fluoxetine's unique 5HT2C antagonist properties could contribute to agitation, anxiety, and undesirable activation, especially early in dosing

Notable Side Effects
- Sexual dysfunction (men: delayed ejaculation, erectile dysfunction; men and women: decreased sexual desire, anorgasmia)
- Gastrointestinal (decreased appetite, nausea, diarrhea, constipation, dry mouth)

RLS sx ?

- Mostly central nervous system (insomnia but also sedation, agitation, tremors, headache, dizziness)
- Note: patients with diagnosed or undiagnosed bipolar or psychotic disorders may be more vulnerable to CNS-activating actions of SSRIs
- Autonomic (sweating)
- Bruising and rare bleeding

 ### Life Threatening or Dangerous Side Effects
- Rare seizures
- Rare induction of mania
- Rare activation of suicidal ideation and behavior (suicidality)

Weight Gain

unusual   not unusual   common   problematic

- Reported but not expected
- Possible weight loss, especially short-term

Sedation

unusual   not unusual   common   problematic

- Reported but not expected

What To Do About Side Effects
- Wait
- Wait
- Wait
- If fluoxetine is activating, take in the morning to help reduce insomnia
- Reduce dose to 10 mg, and either stay at this dose if tolerated and effective, or consider increasing again to 20 mg or more if tolerated but not effective at 10 mg
- In a few weeks, switch or add other drugs

Best Augmenting Agents for Side Effects
- Often best to try another SSRI or another antidepressant monotherapy prior to resorting to augmentation strategies to treat side effects
- Trazodone or a hypnotic for insomnia
- Bupropion, sildenafil, vardenafil, or tadalafil for sexual dysfunction
- Bupropion for emotional flattening, cognitive slowing, or apathy
- Mirtazapine for insomnia, agitation, and gastrointestinal side effects

- Benzodiazepines for jitteriness and anxiety, especially at initiation of treatment and especially for anxious patients
- Many side effects are dose-dependent (i.e., they increase as dose increases, or they reemerge until tolerance re-develops)
- Many side effects are time-dependent (i.e., they start immediately upon dosing and upon each dose increase, but go away with time)
- Activation and agitation may represent the induction of a bipolar state, especially a mixed dysphoric bipolar II condition sometimes associated with suicidal ideation, and require the addition of lithium, a mood stabilizer or an atypical antipsychotic, and/or discontinuation of fluoxetine

DOSING AND USE

Usual Dosage Range
- 20–80 mg for depression and anxiety disorders
- 60–80 mg for bulimia

Dosage Forms
- Capsules 10 mg, 20 mg, 40 mg
- Tablet 10 mg
- Liquid 20 mg / 5 ml – 120 ml bottles
- Weekly capsule 90 mg

How to Dose
- Depression and OCD: Initial dose 20 mg/day in morning, usually wait a few weeks to assess drug effects before increasing dose; maximum dose generally 80 mg/day
- Bulimia: Initial dose 60 mg/day in morning; some patients may need to begin at lower dose and titrate over several days

 Dosing Tips
- The long half-lives of fluoxetine and its active metabolites mean that dose changes will not be fully reflected in plasma for several weeks, lengthening titration to final dose and extending withdrawal from treatment
- Give once daily, often in the mornings, but at any time of day tolerated

- Often available in capsules, not tablets, so unable to break capsules in half
- Occasional patients are dosed above 80 mg
- Liquid formulation easiest for doses below 10 mg when used for cases that are very intolerant to fluoxetine or for very slow up and down titration needs
* For some patients, weekly dosing with the weekly formulation may enhance compliance
- The more anxious and agitated the patient, the lower the starting dose, the slower the titration, and the more likely the need for a concomitant agent such as trazodone or a benzodiazepine
- If intolerable anxiety, insomnia, agitation, akathisia, or activation occur either upon dosing initiation or discontinuation, consider the possibility of activated bipolar disorder and switch to a mood stabilizer or an atypical antipsychotic

Overdose
- Rarely lethal in monotherapy overdose; respiratory depression especially with alcohol, ataxia, sedation, possible seizures

Long-Term Use
- Safe

Habit Forming
- No

How to Stop
- Taper rarely necessary since fluoxetine tapers itself after immediate discontinuation, due to the long half-life of fluoxetine and its active metabolites

Pharmacokinetics
- Active metabolite (norfluoxetine) has 2 week half-life
- Parent drug has 2–3 day half-life
- Inhibits CYP450 2D6
- Inhibits CYP450 3A4

 Drug Interactions
- Tramadol increases the risk of seizures in patients taking an antidepressant
- Can increase tricyclic antidepressant levels; use with caution with tricyclic antidepressants or when switching from a TCA to fluoxetine

- Can cause a fatal "serotonin syndrome" when combined with MAO inhibitors, so do not use with MAO inhibitors or for at least 14 days after MAOIs are stopped
- Do not start an MAO inhibitor for at least 5 weeks after discontinuing fluoxetine
- May displace highly protein bound drugs (e.g., warfarin)
- Can rarely cause weakness, hyperreflexia, and incoordination when combined with sumatriptan, or possibly with other triptans, requiring careful monitoring of patient
- Via CYP450 2D6 inhibition, could theoretically interfere with the analgesic actions of codeine, and increase the plasma levels of some beta blockers and of atomoxetine
- Via CYP450 2D6 inhibition, fluoxetine could theoretically increase concentrations of thioridazine and cause dangerous cardiac arrhythmias
- May reduce the clearance of diazepam or trazodone, thus increasing their levels
- Via CYP450 3A4 inhibition, may increase the levels of alprazolam, buspirone, and triazolam
- Via CYP450 3A4 inhibition, fluoxetine could theoretically increase concentrations of certain cholesterol lowering HMG CoA reductase inhibitors, especially simvastatin, atorvastatin, and lovastatin, but not pravastatin or fluvastatin, which would increase the risk of rhabdomyolysis; thus, coadministration of fluoxetine with certain HMG CoA reductase inhibitors should proceed with caution
- Via CYP450 3A4 inhibition, fluoxetine could theoretically increase the concentrations of pimozide, and cause QTc prolongation and dangerous cardiac arrhythmias

 Other Warnings/ Precautions

✳ Add or initiate other antidepressants with caution for up to 5 weeks after discontinuing fluoxetine
- Use with caution in patients with history of seizure
- Use with caution in patients with bipolar disorder unless treated with concomitant mood stabilizing agent
- When treating children, carefully weigh the risks and benefits of pharmacological

treatment against the risks and benefits of nontreatment with antidepressants and make sure to document this in the patient's chart
- Distribute the brochures provided by the FDA and the drug companies
- Warn patients and their caregivers about the possibility of activating side effects and advise them to report such symptoms immediately
- Monitor patients for activation of suicidal ideation, especially children and adolescents

Do Not Use
- If patient is taking an MAO inhibitor
- If patient is taking thioridazine
- If patient is taking pimozide
- If there is a proven allergy to fluoxetine

SPECIAL POPULATIONS

Renal Impairment
- No dose adjustment
- Not removed by hemodialysis

Hepatic Impairment
- Lower dose or give less frequently, perhaps by half

Cardiac Impairment
- Preliminary research suggests that fluoxetine is safe in these patients
- Treating depression with SSRIs in patients with acute angina or following myocardial infarction may reduce cardiac events and improve survival as well as mood

Elderly
- Some patients may tolerate lower doses better

 Children and Adolescents
- Carefully weigh the risks and benefits of pharmacological treatment against the risks and benefits of nontreatment with antidepressants and make sure to document this in the patient's chart
- Monitor patients face-to-face regularly, particularly during the first several weeks of treatment

- Use with caution, observing for activation of known or unknown bipolar disorder and/or suicidal ideation, and inform parents or guardian of this risk so they can help observe child or adolescent patients
- Approved for OCD and depression
- Adolescents often receive adult dose, but doses slightly lower for children
- Children taking fluoxetine may have slower growth; long-term effects are unknown

 Pregnancy

- Risk Category C [some animal studies show adverse effects, no controlled studies in humans]
- Not generally recommended for use during pregnancy, especially during first trimester
- Nonetheless, continuous treatment during pregnancy may be necessary and has not been proven to be harmful to the fetus
- Current patient registries of children whose mothers took fluoxetine during pregnancy do not show adverse consequences
- At delivery there may be more bleeding in the mother and transient irritability or sedation in the newborn
- Must weigh the risk of treatment (first trimester fetal development, third trimester newborn delivery) to the child against the risk of no treatment (recurrence of depression, maternal health, infant bonding) to the mother and child
- For many patients this may mean continuing treatment during pregnancy
- Neonates exposed to SSRIs or SNRIs late in the third trimester have developed complications requiring prolonged hospitalization, respiratory support, and tube feeding; reported symptoms are consistent with either a direct toxic effect of SSRIs and SNRIs or, possibly, a drug discontinuation syndrome, and include respiratory distress, cyanosis, apnea, seizures, temperature instability, feeding difficulty, vomiting, hypoglycemia, hypotonia, hypertonia, hyperreflexia, tremor, jitteriness, irritability, and constant crying

Breast Feeding

- Some drug is found in mother's breast milk
- Trace amounts may be present in nursing children whose mothers are on fluoxetine

- If child becomes irritable or sedated, breast feeding or drug may need to be discontinued
- Immediate postpartum period is a high-risk time for depression, especially in women who have had prior depressive episodes, so drug may need to be reinstituted late in the third trimester or shortly after childbirth to prevent a recurrence during the postpartum period
- Must weigh benefits of breast feeding with risks and benefits of antidepressant treatment versus non-treatment to both the infant and the mother
- For many patients this may mean continuing treatment during breast feeding

THE ART OF PSYCHOPHARMACOLOGY

Potential Advantages
- Patients with atypical depression (hypersomnia, increased appetite)
- Patients with fatigue and low energy
- Patients with comorbid eating and affective disorders
- Generic is less expensive than brand name where available
- Patients for whom weekly administration is desired
- Children with OCD or depression

Potential Disadvantages
- Patients with anorexia
- Initiating treatment in anxious, agitated patients
- Initiating treatment in severe insomnia

Primary Target Symptoms
- Depressed mood
- Energy, motivation, and interest
- Anxiety (eventually, but can actually increase anxiety, especially short-term)
- Sleep disturbance, both insomnia and hypersomnia (eventually, but may actually cause insomnia, especially short-term)

 Pearls

* May be a first-line choice for atypical depression (e.g., hypersomnia, hyperphagia, low energy, mood reactivity)
- Consider avoiding in agitated insomniacs

- Can cause cognitive and affective "flattening"
- Not as well tolerated as some other SSRIs for panic disorder and other anxiety disorders, especially when dosing is initiated, unless given with co-therapies such as benzodiazepines or trazodone
- Long half-life; even longer lasting active metabolite
- ✳ Actions at 5HT2C receptors may explain its activating properties
- ✳ Actions at 5HT2C receptors may explain in part fluoxetine's efficacy in combination with olanzapine for bipolar depression and treatment-resistant depression, since both agents have this property
- For sexual dysfunction, can augment with bupropion, sildenafil, vardenafil, or tadalafil, or switch to a non-SSRI such as bupropion or mirtazapine
- Mood disorders can be associated with eating disorders (especially in adolescent females) and be treated successfully with fluoxetine

- SSRIs may be less effective in women over 50, especially if they are not taking estrogen
- SSRIs may be useful for hot flushes in perimenopausal women
- Some postmenopausal women's depression will respond better to fluoxetine plus estrogen augmentation than to fluoxetine alone
- Nonresponse to fluoxetine in elderly may require consideration of mild cognitive impairment or Alzheimer disease
- SSRIs may not cause as many patients to attain remission of depression as some other classes of antidepressants (e.g., SNRIs)
- A single pill containing both fluoxetine and olanzapine is available for combination treatment of bipolar depression, psychotic depression, and treatment-resistant unipolar depression

Suggested Reading

Anderson IM. Selective serotonin reuptake inhibitors versus tricyclic antidepressants: a meta-analysis of efficacy and tolerability. Journal of Affective Disorders. 2000;58:19–36.

Beasley CM Jr, Koke SC, Nilsson ME, Gonzales JS. Adverse events and treatment discontinuations in clinical trials of fluoxetine in major depressive disorder: an updated meta-analysis. Clinical Therapeutics. 2000;22:1319–1330.

Calil HM. Fluoxetine: a suitable long-term treatment. J Clin Psychiatry. 2001;62 (suppl 22):24–9.

Edwards JG, Anderson I. Systematic review and guide to selection of selective serotonin reuptake inhibitors. Drugs. 1999;57:507–533.

Wagstaff AJ, Goa KL. Once-weekly fluoxetine. Drugs. 2001;61:2221–8.

FLUVOXAMINE

THERAPEUTICS

Brands • Luvox
see index for additional brand names

Generic? Yes

Class
• SSRI (selective serotonin reuptake inhibitor); often classified as an antidepressant, but it is not just an antidepressant

Commonly Prescribed For
(bold for FDA approved)
• **Obsessive-compulsive disorder (OCD)**
• Depression
• Panic disorder
• Generalized anxiety disorder (GAD)
• Social anxiety disorder (social phobia)
• Posttraumatic stress disorder (PTSD)

How The Drug Works
• Boosts neurotransmitter serotonin
• Blocks serotonin reuptake pump (serotonin transporter)
• Desensitizes serotonin receptors, especially serotonin 1A receptors
• Presumably increases serotonergic neurotransmission
✳ Fluvoxamine also has antagonist properties at sigma 1 receptors

How Long Until It Works
✳ Some patients may experience relief of insomnia or anxiety early after initiation of treatment
• Onset of therapeutic actions usually not immediate, but often delayed 2 to 4 weeks
• If it is not working within 6 to 8 weeks, it may require a dosage increase or it may not work at all
• May continue to work for many years to prevent relapse of symptoms

If It Works
• The goal of treatment is complete remission of current symptoms as well as prevention of future relapses
• Treatment most often reduces or even eliminates symptoms, but not a cure since symptoms can recur after medicine stopped

• Continue treatment until all symptoms are gone (remission) or significantly reduced (e.g., OCD)
• Once symptoms gone, continue treating for 1 year for the first episode of depression
• For second and subsequent episodes of depression, treatment may need to be indefinite
• Use in anxiety disorders may also need to be indefinite

If It Doesn't Work
• Many patients only have a partial response where some symptoms are improved but others persist (especially insomnia, fatigue, and problems concentrating in depression)
• Other patients may be nonresponders, sometimes called treatment-resistant or treatment-refractory
• Some patients who have an initial response may relapse even though they continue treatment, sometimes called "poop-out"
• Consider increasing dose, switching to another agent or adding an appropriate augmenting agent
• Consider psychotherapy
• Consider evaluation for another diagnosis or for a comorbid condition (e.g., medical illness, substance abuse, etc.)
• Some patients may experience apparent lack of consistent efficacy due to activation of latent or underlying bipolar disorder, and require antidepressant discontinuation and a switch to a mood stabilizer

Best Augmenting Combos for Partial Response or Treatment-Resistance
• For the expert, consider cautious addition of clomipramine for treatment-resistant OCD
• Trazodone, especially for insomnia
• Bupropion, mirtazapine, reboxetine, or atomoxetine (use combinations of antidepressants with caution as this may activate bipolar disorder and suicidal ideation)
• Modafinil, especially for fatigue, sleepiness, and lack of concentration
• Mood stabilizers or atypical antipsychotics for bipolar depression, psychotic depression, treatment-resistant depression, or treatment-resistant anxiety disorders
• Benzodiazepines

- If all else fails for anxiety disorders, consider gabapentin or tiagabine
- Hypnotics for insomnia
- Classically, lithium, buspirone, or thyroid hormone
- In Europe and Japan, augmentation is more commonly administered for the treatment of depression and anxiety disorders, especially with benzodiazepines and lithium
- In the US, augmentation is more commonly administered for the treatment of OCD, especially with atypical antipsychotics, buspirone, or even clomipramine; clomipramine should be added with caution and at low doses as fluvoxamine can alter clomipramine metabolism and raise its levels

Tests

- None for healthy individuals

SIDE EFFECTS

How Drug Causes Side Effects

- Theoretically due to increases in serotonin concentrations at serotonin receptors in parts of the brain and body other than those that cause therapeutic actions (e.g., unwanted actions of serotonin in sleep centers causing insomnia, unwanted actions of serotonin in the gut causing diarrhea, etc.)
- Increasing serotonin can cause diminished dopamine release and might contribute to emotional flattening, cognitive slowing, and apathy in some patients
- Most side effects are immediate but often go away with time, in contrast to most therapeutic effects which are delayed and are enhanced over time
- ✳ Fluvoxamine's sigma 1 antagonist properties may contribute to sedation and fatigue in some patients

Notable Side Effects

- Sexual dysfunction (men: delayed ejaculation, erectile dysfunction; men and women: decreased sexual desire, anorgasmia)
- Gastrointestinal (decreased appetite, nausea, diarrhea, constipation, dry mouth)

- Mostly central nervous system (insomnia but also sedation, agitation, tremors, headache, dizziness)
- Note: patients with diagnosed or undiagnosed bipolar or psychotic disorders may be more vulnerable to CNS-activating actions of SSRIs
- Autonomic (sweating)
- Bruising and rare bleeding
- Rare hyponatremia

 Life Threatening or Dangerous Side Effects

- Rare seizures
- Rare induction of mania
- Rare activation of suicidal ideation and behavior (suicidality)

Weight Gain

unusual   not unusual   common   problematic

- Reported but not expected
- Patients may actually experience weight loss

Sedation

unusual   not unusual   common   problematic

- Many experience and/or can be significant in amount

What To Do About Side Effects

- Wait
- Wait
- Wait
- If fluvoxamine is sedating, take at night to reduce drowsiness
- Reduce dose
- In a few weeks, switch or add other drugs

Best Augmenting Agents for Side Effects

- Often best to try another SSRI or another antidepressant monotherapy prior to resorting to augmentation strategies to treat side effects
- Trazodone or a hypnotic for insomnia
- Bupropion, sildenafil, vardenafil, or tadalafil for sexual dysfunction
- Bupropion for emotional flattening, cognitive slowing, or apathy
- Mirtazapine for insomnia, agitation, and gastrointestinal side effects

- Benzodiazepines for jitteriness and anxiety, especially at initiation of treatment and especially for anxious patients
- Many side effects are dose-dependent (i.e., they increase as dose increases, or they reemerge until tolerance re-develops)
- Many side effects are time-dependent (i.e., they start immediately upon dosing and upon each dose increase, but go away with time)
- Activation and agitation may represent the induction of a bipolar state, especially a mixed dysphoric bipolar II condition sometimes associated with suicidal ideation, and require the addition of lithium, a mood stabilizer or an atypical antipsychotic, and/or discontinuation of fluvoxamine

DOSING AND USE

Usual Dosage Range
- 100–300 mg/day for OCD
- 100–200 mg/day for depression

Dosage Forms
- Tablets 25 mg, 50 mg scored, 100 mg scored

How to Dose
- Initial 50 mg/day; increase by 50 mg/day in 4–7 days; usually wait a few weeks to assess drug effects before increasing dose further, but can increase by 50 mg/day every 4–7 days until desired efficacy is reached; maximum 300 mg/day
- Doses below 100 mg/day usually given as a single dose at bedtime; doses above 100 mg/day can be divided into two doses to enhance tolerability, with the larger dose administered at night, but can also be given as a single dose at bedtime

 Dosing Tips
- 50 mg and 100 mg tablets are scored, so to save costs, give 25 mg as half of 50 mg tablet, and give 50 mg as half of 100 mg tablet
- To improve tolerability, dosing can either be given once a day, usually all at night, or split either symmetrically or

asymmetrically, usually with more of the dose given at night
- Some patients take more than 300 mg/day
- If intolerable anxiety, insomnia, agitation, akathisia, or activation occur either upon dosing initiation or discontinuation, consider the possibility of activated bipolar disorder and switch to a mood stabilizer or an atypical antipsychotic

Overdose
- Rare fatalities have been reported, both in combination with other drugs and alone; sedation, dizziness, vomiting, diarrhea, irregular heartbeat, seizures, coma, breathing difficulty

Long-Term Use
- Safe

Habit Forming
- No

How to Stop
- Taper to avoid withdrawal effects (dizziness, nausea, stomach cramps, sweating, tingling, dysesthesias)
- Many patients tolerate 50% dose reduction for 3 days, then another 50% reduction for 3 days, then discontinuation
- If withdrawal symptoms emerge during discontinuation, raise dose to stop symptoms and then restart withdrawal much more slowly

Pharmacokinetics
- Parent drug has 9–28 hour half-life
- Inhibits CYP450 3A4
- Inhibits CYP450 1A2
- Inhibits CYP450 2C9/2C19

 Drug Interactions
- Tramadol increases the risk of seizures in patients taking an antidepressant
- Can increase tricyclic antidepressant levels; use with caution with tricyclic antidepressants
- Can cause a fatal "serotonin syndrome" when combined with MAO inhibitors, so do not use with MAO inhibitors or for at least 14 days after MAOIs are stopped
- Do not start an MAO inhibitor for at least 2 weeks after discontinuing fluvoxamine

- May displace highly protein bound drugs (e.g., warfarin)
- Can rarely cause weakness, hyperreflexia, and incoordination when combined with sumatriptan or possibly with other triptans, requiring careful monitoring of patient
- Via CYP450 1A2 inhibition, fluvoxamine may reduce clearance of theophylline and clozapine, thus raising their levels and requiring their dosing to be lowered
- Fluvoxamine administered with either caffeine or theophylline can thus cause jitteriness, excessive stimulation, or rarely seizures, so concomitant use should proceed cautiously
- Metabolism of fluvoxamine may be enhanced in smokers and thus its levels lowered, requiring higher dosing
- Via CYP450 3A4 inhibition, fluvoxamine may reduce clearance of carbamazepine and benzodiazepines such as alprazolam and triazolam, and thus require dosage reduction
- Via CYP450 3A4 inhibition, fluvoxamine could theoretically increase concentrations of certain cholesterol lowering HMG CoA reductase inhibitors, especially simvastatin, atorvastatin, and lovastatin, but not pravastatin or fluvastatin, which would increase the risk of rhabdomyolysis; thus, coadministration of fluvoxamine with certain HMG CoA reductase inhibitors should proceed with caution
- Via CYP450 3A4 inhibition, fluvoxamine could theoretically increase the concentrations of pimozide, and cause QTc prolongation and dangerous cardiac arrhythmias

 Other Warnings/ Precautions

- Add or initiate other antidepressants with caution for up to two weeks after discontinuing fluvoxamine
- Use with caution in patients with history of seizure
- Use with caution in patients with bipolar disorder unless treated with concomitant mood stabilizing agent
- May cause photosensitivity
- When treating children, carefully weigh the risks and benefits of pharmacological treatment against the risks and benefits of nontreatment with antidepressants and

make sure to document this in the patient's chart
- Distribute the brochures provided by the FDA and the drug companies
- Warn patients and their caregivers about the possibility of activating side effects and advise them to report such symptoms immediately
- Monitor patients for activation of suicidal ideation, especially children and adolescents

Do Not Use
- If patient is taking an MAO inhibitor
- If patient is taking thioridazine or pimozide
- If there is a proven allergy to fluvoxamine

SPECIAL POPULATIONS

Renal Impairment
- No dose adjustment

Hepatic Impairment
- Lower dose or give less frequently, perhaps by half; use slower titration

Cardiac Impairment
- Preliminary research suggests that fluvoxamine is safe in these patients
- Treating depression with SSRIs in patients with acute angina or following myocardial infarction may reduce cardiac events and improve survival as well as mood

Elderly
- May require lower initial dose and slower titration

 Children and Adolescents
- Approved for ages 8–17 for OCD
- 8–17: initial 25 mg/day at bedtime; increase by 25 mg/day every 4–7 days; maximum 200 mg/day; doses above 50 mg/day should be divided into 2 doses with the larger dose administered at bedtime
- Preliminary evidence suggests efficacy for other anxiety disorders and depression in children and adolescents
- Carefully weigh the risks and benefits of pharmacological treatment against the risks and benefits of nontreatment with

antidepressants and make sure to document this in the patient's chart
- Monitor patients face-to-face regularly, particularly during the first several weeks of treatment
- Use with caution, observing for activation of known or unknown bipolar disorder and/or suicidal ideation, and inform parents or guardian of this risk so they can help observe child or adolescent patients

 Pregnancy

- Risk Category C [some animal studies show adverse effects, no controlled studies in humans]
- Not generally recommended for use during pregnancy, especially during first trimester
- Nonetheless, continuous treatment during pregnancy may be necessary and has not been proven to be harmful to the fetus
- At delivery there may be more bleeding in the mother and transient irritability or sedation in the newborn
- Must weigh the risk of treatment (first trimester fetal development, third trimester newborn delivery) to the child against the risk of no treatment (recurrence of depression, maternal health, infant bonding) to the mother and child
- For many patients this may mean continuing treatment during pregnancy
- Neonates exposed to SSRIs or SNRIs late in the third trimester have developed complications requiring prolonged hospitalization, respiratory support, and tube feeding; reported symptoms are consistent with either a direct toxic effect of SSRIs and SNRIs or, possibly, a drug discontinuation syndrome, and include respiratory distress, cyanosis, apnea, seizures, temperature instability, feeding difficulty, vomiting, hypoglycemia, hypotonia, hypertonia, hyperreflexia, tremor, jitteriness, irritability, and constant crying

Breast Feeding
- Some drug is found in mother's breast milk
- Trace amounts may be present in nursing children whose mothers are on fluvoxamine
- If child becomes irritable or sedated, breast feeding or drug may need to be discontinued

- Immediate postpartum period is a high-risk time for depression, especially in women who have had prior depressive episodes, so drug may need to be reinstituted late in the third trimester or shortly after childbirth to prevent a recurrence during the postpartum period
- Must weigh benefits of breast feeding with risks and benefits of antidepressant treatment versus non-treatment to both the infant and the mother
- For many patients this may mean continuing treatment during breast feeding

THE ART OF PSYCHOPHARMACOLOGY

Potential Advantages
- Patients with mixed anxiety/depression
- Generic is less expensive than brand name where available

Potential Disadvantages
- Patients with irritable bowel or multiple gastrointestinal complaints
- Can require dose titration and twice daily dosing

Primary Target Symptoms
- Depressed mood
- Anxiety

 Pearls

- ✳ Often a preferred treatment of anxious depression as well as major depressive disorder comorbid with anxiety disorders
- Some withdrawal effects, especially gastrointestinal effects
- May have lower incidence of sexual dysfunction than other SSRIs
- Preliminary research suggests that fluvoxamine is efficacious in obsessive-compulsive symptoms in schizophrenia when combined with antipsychotics
- Not FDA approved for depression, but used widely for depression in many countries
- SSRIs may be less effective in women over 50, especially if they are not taking estrogen
- SSRIs may be useful for hot flushes in perimenopausal women
- ✳ Actions at sigma 1 receptors may explain in part fluvoxamine's sometimes rapid

onset effects in anxiety disorders and insomnia

✳ Actions at sigma 1 receptors may explain potential advantages of fluvoxamine for psychotic depression and delusional depression

✳ For treatment-resistant OCD, consider cautious combination of fluvoxamine and clomipramine by an expert

• Normally, clomipramine (CMI), a potent serotonin reuptake blocker, at steady state is metabolized extensively to its active metabolite desmethyl-clomipramine (de-CMI), a potent noradrenergic reuptake blocker

• Thus, at steady state, plasma drug activity is generally more noradrenergic (with higher de-CMI levels) than serotonergic (with lower parent CMI levels)

• Addition of a CYP450 1A2 inhibitor, fluvoxamine, blocks this conversion and results in higher CMI levels than de-CMI levels

• Thus, addition of the SSRI fluvoxamine to CMI in treatment-resistant OCD can powerfully enhance serotonergic activity, not only due to the inherent serotonergic activity of fluvoxamine, but also due to a favorable pharmacokinetic interaction inhibiting CYP450 1A2 and thus converting CMI's metabolism to a more powerful serotonergic portfolio of parent drug

 Suggested Reading

Cheer SM, Figgitt DP. Spotlight on fluvoxamine in anxiety disorders in children and adolescents. CNS Drugs. 2002;16:139–44.

Edwards JG, Anderson I. Systematic review and guide to selection of selective serotonin reuptake inhibitors. Drugs. 1999;57:507–533.

Figgitt DP, McClellan KJ. Fluvoxamine. An updated review of its use in the management of adults with anxiety disorders. Drugs. 2000;60:925–954.

Pigott TA, Seay SM. A review of the efficacy of selective serotonin reuptake inhibitors in obsessive-compulsive disorder. Journal of Clinical Psychiatry. 1999;60:101–106.

Wares MR. Fluvoxamine: a review of the controlled trials in depression. Journal of Clinical Psychiatry. 1997;58(suppl 5):15–23.

IMIPRAMINE

Brands • Tofranil
see index for additional brand names

Generic? Yes

Class
• Tricyclic antidepressant (TCA)
• Serotonin and norepinephrine/
noradrenaline reuptake inhibitor

Commonly Prescribed For
(bold for FDA approved)
• **Depression**
✳ Enuresis
• Anxiety
• Insomnia
• Neuropathic pain/chronic pain
• Treatment-resistant depression
• Cataplexy syndrome

How The Drug Works
• Boosts neurotransmitters serotonin and
norepinephrine/noradrenaline
• Blocks serotonin reuptake pump (serotonin
transporter), presumably increasing
serotonergic neurotransmission
• Blocks norepinephrine reuptake pump
(norepinephrine transporter), presumably
increasing noradrenergic
neurotransmission
• Presumably desensitizes both serotonin 1A
receptors and beta adrenergic receptors
• Since dopamine is inactivated by
norepinephrine reuptake in frontal cortex,
which largely lacks dopamine transporters,
imipramine can increase dopamine
neurotransmission in this part of the brain
• May be effective in treating enuresis
because of its anticholinergic properties

How Long Until It Works
• May have immediate effects in treating
insomnia or anxiety
• Onset of therapeutic actions usually not
immediate, but often delayed 2 to 4 weeks
• If it is not working within 6 to 8 weeks for
depression, it may require a dosage
increase or it may not work at all
• May continue to work for many years to
prevent relapse of symptoms

If It Works
• The goal of treatment of depression is
complete remission of current symptoms
as well as prevention of future relapses
• The goal of treatment of chronic
neuropathic pain is to reduce symptoms as
much as possible, especially in
combination with other treatments
• Treatment of depression most often
reduces or even eliminates symptoms, but
not a cure since symptoms can recur after
medicine stopped
• Treatment of chronic neuropathic pain may
reduce symptoms, but rarely eliminates
them completely, and is not a cure since
symptoms can recur after medicine is
stopped
• Continue treatment of depression until all
symptoms are gone (remission)
• Once symptoms of depression are gone,
continue treating for 1 year for the first
episode of depression
• For second and subsequent episodes of
depression, treatment may need to be
indefinite
• Use in anxiety disorders and chronic pain
may also need to be indefinite, but long-
term treatment is not well studied in these
conditions

If It Doesn't Work
• Many depressed patients only have a
partial response where some symptoms
are improved but others persist (especially
insomnia, fatigue, and problems
concentrating)
• Other depressed patients may be
nonresponders, sometimes called
treatment-resistant or treatment-refractory
• Consider increasing dose, switching to
another agent or adding an appropriate
augmenting agent
• Consider psychotherapy
• Consider evaluation for another diagnosis
or for a comorbid condition (e.g., medical
illness, substance abuse, etc.)
• Some patients may experience apparent
lack of consistent efficacy due to activation
of latent or underlying bipolar disorder, and
require antidepressant discontinuation and
a switch to a mood stabilizer

Best Augmenting Combos for Partial Response or Treatment-Resistance

- Lithium, buspirone, thyroid hormone (for depression)
- Gabapentin, tiagabine, other anticonvulsants, even opiates if done by experts while monitoring carefully in difficult cases (for chronic pain)

Tests

- None for healthy individuals
- * Since tricyclic and tetracyclic antidepressants are frequently associated with weight gain, before starting treatment, weigh all patients and determine if the patient is already overweight (BMI 25.0–29.9) or obese (BMI ≥30)
- Before giving a drug that can cause weight gain to an overweight or obese patient, consider determining whether the patient already has pre-diabetes (fasting plasma glucose 100–125 mg/dl), diabetes (fasting plasma glucose >126 mg/dl), or dyslipidemia (increased total cholesterol, LDL cholesterol and triglycerides; decreased HDL cholesterol), and treat or refer such patients for treatment, including nutrition and weight management, physical activity counseling, smoking cessation, and medical management
- * Monitor weight and BMI during treatment
- * While giving a drug to a patient who has gained >5% of initial weight, consider evaluating for the presence of pre-diabetes, diabetes, or dyslipidemia, or consider switching to a different antidepressant
- EKGs may be useful for selected patients (e.g., those with personal or family history of QTc prolongation; cardiac arrhythmia; recent myocardial infarction; uncompensated heart failure; or taking agents that prolong QTc interval such as pimozide, thioridazine, selected antiarrhythmics, moxifloxacin, sparfloxacin, etc.)
- Patients at risk for electrolyte disturbances (e.g., patients on diuretic therapy) should have baseline and periodic serum potassium and magnesium measurements

SIDE EFFECTS

How Drug Causes Side Effects

- Anticholinergic activity may explain sedative effects, dry mouth, constipation, and blurred vision
- Sedative effects and weight gain may be due to antihistamine properties
- Blockade of alpha adrenergic 1 receptors may explain dizziness, sedation, and hypotension
- Cardiac arrhythmias and seizures, especially in overdose, may be caused by blockade of ion channels

Notable Side Effects

- Blurred vision, constipation, urinary retention, increased appetite, dry mouth, nausea, diarrhea, heartburn, unusual taste in mouth, weight gain
- Fatigue, weakness, dizziness, sedation, headache, anxiety, nervousness, restlessness
- Sexual dysfunction, sweating

Life Threatening or Dangerous Side Effects

- Paralytic ileus, hyperthermia (TCAs + anticholinergic agents)
- Lowered seizure threshold and rare seizures
- Orthostatic hypotension, sudden death, arrhythmias, tachycardia
- QTc prolongation
- Hepatic failure, extrapyramidal symptoms
- Increased intraocular pressure, increased psychotic symptoms
- Rare induction of mania
- Rare activation of suicidal ideation and behavior (suicidality)

Weight Gain

unusual   not unusual   common   problematic

- Many experience and/or can be significant in amount
- Can increase appetite and carbohydrate craving

Sedation

unusual   not unusual   common   problematic

- Many experience and/or can be significant in amount

- Tolerance to sedative effects may develop with long-term use

What To Do About Side Effects
- Wait
- Wait
- Wait
- Lower the dose
- Switch to an SSRI or newer antidepressant

Best Augmenting Agents for Side Effects
- Many side effects cannot be improved with an augmenting agent

DOSING AND USE

Usual Dosage Range
- 50–150 mg/day

Dosage Forms
- Capsule 75 mg, 100 mg, 125 mg, 150 mg
- Tablet 10 mg, 25 mg, 50 mg

How to Dose
- Initial 25 mg/day at bedtime; increase by 25 mg every 3–7 days
- 75–100 mg/day once daily or in divided doses; gradually increase daily dose to achieve desired therapeutic effects; dose at bedtime for daytime sedation and in morning for insomnia; maximum dose 300 mg/day

 Dosing Tips
- If given in a single dose, should generally be administered at bedtime because of its sedative properties
- If given in split doses, largest dose should generally be given at bedtime because of its sedative properties
- If patients experience nightmares, split dose and do not give large dose at bedtime
- Patients treated for chronic pain may only require lower doses
- Tofranil-PM(r) (imipramine pamoate) 100- and 125-mg capsules contain the dye tartrazine (FD&C yellow No. 5), which may cause allergic reactions in some patients; this reaction is more likely in patients with sensitivity to aspirin

- If intolerable anxiety, insomnia, agitation, akathisia, or activation occur either upon dosing initiation or discontinuation, consider the possibility of activated bipolar disorder, and switch to a mood stabilizer or an atypical antipsychotic

Overdose
- Death may occur; convulsions, cardiac dysrhythmias, severe hypotension, CNS depression, coma, changes in ECG

Long-Term Use
- Safe

Habit Forming
- No

How to Stop
- Taper to avoid withdrawal effects
- Even with gradual dose reduction some withdrawal symptoms may appear within the first 2 weeks
- Many patients tolerate 50% dose reduction for 3 days, then another 50% reduction for 3 days, then discontinuation
- If withdrawal symptoms emerge during discontinuation, raise dose to stop symptoms and then restart withdrawal much more slowly

Pharmacokinetics
- Substrate for CYP450 2D6 and 1A2
- Metabolized to an active metabolite, desipramine, a predominantly norepinephrine reuptake inhibitor, by demethylation via CYP450 1A2

 Drug Interactions
- Tramadol increases the risk of seizures in patients taking TCAs
- Use of TCAs with anticholinergic drugs may result in paralytic ileus or hyperthermia
- Fluoxetine, paroxetine, bupropion, duloxetine, and other CYP450 2D6 inhibitors may increase TCA concentrations
- Fluvoxamine, a CYP450 1A2 inhibitor, can decrease the conversion of imipramine to desmethylimipramine (desipramine) and increase imipramine plasma concentrations
- Cimetidine may increase plasma concentrations of TCAs and cause anticholinergic symptoms

- Phenothiazines or haloperidol may raise TCA blood concentrations
- May alter effects of antihypertensive drugs; may inhibit hypotensive effects of clonidine
- Use with sympathomimetic agents may increase sympathetic activity
- Methylphenidate may inhibit metabolism of TCAs
- Activation and agitation, especially following switching or adding antidepressants, may represent the induction of a bipolar state, especially a mixed dysphoric bipolar II condition sometimes associated with suicidal ideation, and require the addition of lithium, a mood stabilizer or an atypical antipsychotic, and/or discontinuation of imipramine

 ### Other Warnings/ Precautions

- Add or initiate other antidepressants with caution for up to 2 weeks after discontinuing imipramine
- Generally, do not use with MAO inhibitors, including 14 days after MAOIs are stopped; do not start an MAOI until 2 weeks after discontinuing imipramine, but see Pearls
- Use with caution in patients with history of seizure, urinary retention, narrow angle-closure glaucoma, hyperthyroidism
- TCAs can increase QTc interval, especially at toxic doses, which can be attained not only by overdose but also by combining with drugs that inhibit its metabolism via CYP450 2D6, potentially causing torsade de pointes-type arrhythmia or sudden death
- Because TCAs can prolong QTc interval, use with caution in patients who have bradycardia or who are taking drugs that can induce bradycardia (e.g., beta blockers, calcium channel blockers, clonidine, digitalis)
- Because TCAs can prolong QTc interval, use with caution in patients who have hypokalemia and/or hypomagnesemia or who are taking drugs that can induce hypokalemia and/or magnesemia (e.g., diuretics, stimulant laxatives, intravenous amphotericin B, glucocorticoids, tetracosactide)
- When treating children, carefully weigh the risks and benefits of pharmacological treatment against the risks and benefits of nontreatment with antidepressants and make sure to document this in the patient's chart
- Distribute the brochures provided by the FDA and the drug companies
- Warn patients and their caregivers about the possibility of activating side effects and advise them to report such symptoms immediately
- Monitor patients for activation of suicidal ideation, especially children and adolescents

Do Not Use

- If patient is recovering from myocardial infarction
- If patient is taking agents capable of significantly prolonging QTc interval (e.g., pimozide, thioridazine, selected antiarrhythmics, moxifloxacin, sparfloxacin)
- If there is a history of QTc prolongation or cardiac arrhythmia, recent acute myocardial infarction, uncompensated heart failure
- If patient is taking drugs that inhibit TCA metabolism, including CYP450 2D6 inhibitors, except by an expert
- If there is reduced CYP450 2D6 function, such as patients who are poor 2D6 metabolizers, except by an expert and at low doses
- If there is a proven allergy to imipramine, desipramine, or lofepramine

SPECIAL POPULATIONS

Renal Impairment
- Cautious use; may need lower dose

Hepatic Impairment
- Cautious use; may need lower dose

Cardiac Impairment
- TCAs have been reported to cause arrhythmias, prolongation of conduction time, orthostatic hypotension, sinus tachycardia, and heart failure, especially in the diseased heart
- Myocardial infarction and stroke have been reported with TCAs
- TCAs produce QTc prolongation, which may be enhanced by the existence of

bradycardia, hypokalemia, congenital or acquired long QTc interval, which should be evaluated prior to administering imipramine
- Use with caution if treating concomitantly with a medication likely to produce prolonged bradycardia, hypokalemia, slowing of intracardiac conduction, or prolongation of the QTc interval
- Avoid TCAs in patients with a known history of QTc prolongation, recent acute myocardial infarction, and uncompensated heart failure
- TCAs may cause a sustained increase in heart rate in patients with ischemic heart disease and may worsen (decrease) heart rate variability, an independent risk of mortality in cardiac populations
- Since SSRIs may improve (increase) heart rate variability in patients following a myocardial infarct and may improve survival as well as mood in patients with acute angina or following a myocardial infarction, these are more appropriate agents for cardiac population than tricyclic/tetracyclic antidepressants
- ✳ Risk/benefit ratio may not justify use of TCAs in cardiac impairment

Elderly
- May be more sensitive to anticholinergic, cardiovascular, hypotensive, and sedative effects
- Initial 30–40 mg/day; maximum dose 100 mg/day

 ### Children and Adolescents
- Carefully weigh the risks and benefits of pharmacological treatment against the risks and benefits of nontreatment with antidepressants and make sure to document this in the patient's chart
- Monitor patients face-to-face regularly, particularly during the first several weeks of treatment
- Use with caution, observing for activation of known or unknown bipolar disorder and/or suicidal ideation, and inform parents or guardian of this risk so they can help observe child or adolescent patients
- Used age 6 and older for enuresis; age 12 and older for other disorders

- Several studies show lack of efficacy of TCAs for depression
- May be used to treat hyperactive/impulsive behaviors
- Some cases of sudden death have occurred in children taking TCAs
- Adolescents: initial 30–40 mg/day; maximum 100 mg/day
- Children: initial 1.5 mg/kg/day; maximum 5 mg/kg/day
- Functional enuresis: 50 mg/day (age 6–12) or 75 mg/day (over 12)

 ### Pregnancy
- Risk Category D [positive evidence of risk to human fetus; potential benefits may still justify its use during pregnancy]
- Crosses the placenta
- Should be used only if potential benefits outweigh potential risks
- Adverse effects have been reported in infants whose mothers took a TCA (lethargy, withdrawal symptoms, fetal malformations)
- Evaluate for treatment with an antidepressant with a better risk/benefit ratio

Breast Feeding
- Some drug is found in mother's breast milk
- ✳ Recommended either to discontinue drug or bottle feed
- Immediate postpartum period is a high-risk time for depression, especially in women who have had prior depressive episodes, so drug may need to be reinstituted late in the third trimester or shortly after childbirth to prevent a recurrence during the postpartum period
- Must weigh benefits of breast feeding with risks and benefits of antidepressant treatment versus non-treatment to both the infant and the mother
- For many patients this may mean continuing treatment during breast feeding

THE ART OF PSYCHOPHARMACOLOGY

Potential Advantages
- Patients with insomnia
- Severe or treatment-resistant depression
- Patients with enuresis

Potential Disadvantages
- Pediatric and geriatric patients
- Patients concerned with weight gain
- Cardiac patients

Primary Target Symptoms
- Depressed mood
- Chronic pain

Pearls
- Was once one of the most widely prescribed agents for depression
- ✳ Probably the most preferred TCA for treating enuresis in children
- ✳ Preference of some prescribers for imipramine over other TCAs for the treatment of enuresis is based more upon art and anecdote and empiric clinical experience than comparative clinical trials with other TCAs
- Tricyclic antidepressants are no longer generally considered a first-line treatment option for depression because of their side effect profile
- TCAs may aggravate psychotic symptoms
- Alcohol should be avoided because of additive CNS effects
- Underweight patients may be more susceptible to adverse cardiovascular effects
- Children, patients with inadequate hydration, and patients with cardiac disease may be more susceptible to TCA-induced cardiotoxicity than healthy adults
- For the expert only: although generally prohibited, a heroic but potentially dangerous treatment for severely treatment-resistant patients is to give a tricyclic/tetracyclic antidepressant other than clomipramine simultaneously with an MAO inhibitor for patients who fail to respond to numerous other antidepressants
- If this option is elected, start the MAOI with the tricyclic/tetracyclic antidepressant simultaneously at low doses after appropriate drug washout, then alternately increase doses of these agents every few days to a week as tolerated
- Although very strict dietary and concomitant drug restrictions must be observed to prevent hypertensive crises and serotonin syndrome, the most common side effects of MAOI/tricyclic or tetracyclic combinations may be weight gain and orthostatic hypotension
- Patients on TCAs should be aware that they may experience symptoms such as photosensitivity or blue-green urine
- SSRIs may be more effective than TCAs in women, and TCAs may be more effective than SSRIs in men
- Since tricyclic/tetracyclic antidepressants are substrates for CYP450 2D6, and 7% of the population (especially Caucasians) may have a genetic variant leading to reduced activity of 2D6, such patients may not safely tolerate normal doses of tricyclic/tetracyclic antidepressants and may require dose reduction
- Phenotypic testing may be necessary to detect this genetic variant prior to dosing with a tricyclic/tetracyclic antidepressant, especially in vulnerable populations such as children, elderly, cardiac populations, and those on concomitant medications
- Patients who seem to have extraordinarily severe side effects at normal or low doses may have this phenotypic CYP450 2D6 variant and require low doses or switching to another antidepressant not metabolized by 2D6

Suggested Reading

Anderson IM. Meta-analytical studies on new antidepressants. Br Med Bull 2001; 57:161–178.

Anderson IM. Selective serotonin reuptake inhibitors versus tricyclic antidepressants: a meta-analysis of efficacy and tolerability. J Aff Disorders 2000;58:19–36.

Preskorn SH. Comparison of the tolerability of bupropion, fluoxetine, imipramine, nefazodone, paroxetine, sertraline, and venlafaxine. J Clin Psychiatry 1995;56(Suppl 6):12–21.

Workman EA, Short DD. Atypical antidepressants versus imipramine in the treatment of major depression: a meta-analysis. J Clin Psychiatry 1993;54:5–12.

ISOCARBOXAZID

Brands • Marplan
see index for additional brand names

Generic? Not in U.S.

 Class
• Monoamine oxidase inhibitor (MAOI)

Commonly Prescribed For
(bold for FDA approved)
• **Depression**
• Treatment-resistant depression
• Treatment-resistant panic disorder
• Treatment-resistant social anxiety disorder

 How The Drug Works
• Irreversibly blocks monoamine oxidase (MAO) from breaking down norepinephrine, serotonin, and dopamine
• This presumably boosts noradrenergic, serotonergic, and dopaminergic neurotransmission

How Long Until It Works
• Onset of therapeutic actions usually not immediate, but often delayed 2 to 4 weeks
• If it is not working within 6 to 8 weeks, it may require a dosage increase or it may not work at all
• May continue to work for many years to prevent relapse of symptoms

If It Works
• The goal of treatment is complete remission of current symptoms as well as prevention of future relapses
• Treatment most often reduces or even eliminates symptoms, but not a cure since symptoms can recur after medicine stopped
• Continue treatment until all symptoms are gone (remission)
• Once symptoms gone, continue treating for 1 year for the first episode of depression
• For second and subsequent episodes of depression, treatment may need to be indefinite
• Use in anxiety disorders may also need to be indefinite

If It Doesn't Work
• Many patients only have a partial response where some symptoms are improved but others persist (especially insomnia, fatigue, and problems concentrating)
• Other patients may be nonresponders, sometimes called treatment-resistant or treatment-refractory
• Some patients who have an initial response may relapse even though they continue treatment, sometimes called "poop-out"
• Consider increasing dose, switching to another agent or adding an appropriate augmenting agent
• Consider psychotherapy
• Consider evaluation for another diagnosis or for a comorbid condition (e.g., medical illness, substance abuse, etc.)
• Some patients may experience apparent lack of consistent efficacy due to activation of latent or underlying bipolar disorder, and require antidepressant discontinuation and a switch to a mood stabilizer

 Best Augmenting Combos for Partial Response or Treatment-Resistance
✻ Augmentation of MAOIs has not been systematically studied, and this is something for the expert, to be done with caution and with careful monitoring
✻ A stimulant such as d-amphetamine or methylphenidate (with caution; may activate bipolar disorder and suicidal ideation; may elevate blood pressure)
• Lithium
• Mood stabilizing anticonvulsants
• Atypical antipsychotics (with special caution for those agents with monoamine reuptake blocking properties, such as ziprasidone and zotepine)

Tests
• Patients should be monitored for changes in blood pressure
• Patients receiving high doses or long-term treatment should have hepatic function evaluated periodically
✻ Since MAO inhibitors are frequently associated with weight gain, before starting treatment, weigh all patients and determine if the patient is already overweight (BMI 25.0–29.9) or obese (BMI ≥30)

- Before giving a drug that can cause weight gain to an overweight or obese patient, consider determining whether the patient already has pre-diabetes (fasting plasma glucose 100–125 mg/dl), diabetes (fasting plasma glucose >126 mg/dl), or dyslipidemia (increased total cholesterol, LDL cholesterol and triglycerides; decreased HDL cholesterol), and treat or refer such patients for treatment, including nutrition and weight management, physical activity counseling, smoking cessation, and medical management
- ✱ Monitor weight and BMI during treatment
- ✱ While giving a drug to a patient who has gained >5% of initial weight, consider evaluating for the presence of pre-diabetes, diabetes, or dyslipidemia, or consider switching to a different antidepressant

SIDE EFFECTS

How Drug Causes Side Effects

- Theoretically due to increases in monoamines in parts of the brain and body and at receptors other than those that cause therapeutic actions (e.g., unwanted actions of serotonin in sleep centers causing insomnia, unwanted actions of norepinephrine on vascular smooth muscle causing hypertension, etc.)
- Side effects are generally immediate, but immediate side effects often disappear in time

Notable Side Effects

- Dizziness, sedation, headache, sleep disturbances, fatigue, weakness, tremor, movement problems, blurred vision, increased sweating
- Constipation, dry mouth, nausea, change in appetite, weight gain
- Sexual dysfunction
- Orthostatic hypotension (dose-related); syncope may develop at high doses

Life Threatening or Dangerous Side Effects

- Hypertensive crisis (especially when MAOIs are used with certain tyramine-containing foods or prohibited drugs)
- Induction of mania

- Rare activation of suicidal ideation and behavior (suicidality)
- Seizures
- Hepatotoxicity

Weight Gain

- Many experience and/or can be significant in amount

Sedation

- Many experience and/or can be significant in amount
- Can also cause activation

What To Do About Side Effects

- Wait
- Wait
- Wait
- Lower the dose
- Take at night if daytime sedation
- Switch after appropriate washout to an SSRI or newer antidepressant

Best Augmenting Agents for Side Effects

- Trazodone (with caution) for insomnia
- Benzodiazepines for insomnia
- ✱ Single oral or sublingual dose of a calcium channel blocker (e.g., nifedipine) for urgent treatment of hypertension due to drug interaction or dietary tyramine
- Many side effects cannot be improved with an augmenting agent

DOSING AND USE

Usual Dosage Range

- 40–60 mg/day

Dosage Forms

- Tablet 10 mg

How to Dose

- Initial 10 mg twice a day; increase by 10 mg/day every 2–4 days; dosed 2–4 times/day; maximum dose 60 mg/day

Dosing Tips

- Orthostatic hypotension, especially at high doses, may require splitting into 3 or 4 daily doses
- Patients receiving high doses may need to be evaluated periodically for effects on the liver
- Little evidence to support efficacy of isocarboxazid at doses below 30 mg/day

Overdose

- Dizziness, sedation, ataxia, headache, insomnia, restlessness, anxiety, irritability; cardiovascular effects, confusion, respiratory depression, or coma may also occur

Long-Term Use

- May require periodic evaluation of hepatic function
- MAOIs may lose some efficacy long-term

Habit Forming

- Some patients have developed dependence to MAOIs

How to Stop

- Generally no need to taper, as drug wears off slowly over 2–3 weeks

Pharmacokinetics

- Clinical duration of action may be up to 21 days due to irreversible enzyme inhibition

 Drug Interactions

- Tramadol may increase the risk of seizures in patients taking an MAO inhibitor
- Can cause a fatal "serotonin syndrome" when combined with drugs that block serotonin reuptake (e.g., SSRIs, SNRIs, sibutramine, tramadol, etc.), so do not use with a serotonin reuptake inhibitor or for up to 5 weeks after stopping the serotonin reuptake inhibitor
- Hypertensive crisis with headache, intracranial bleeding, and death may result from combining MAO inhibitors with sympathomimetic drugs (e.g., amphetamines, methylphenidate, cocaine, dopamine, epinephrine, norepinephrine, and related compounds methyldopa, levodopa, L-tryptophan, L-tyrosine, and phenylalanine)
- Excitation, seizures, delirium, hyperpyrexia, circulatory collapse, coma, and death may result from combining MAO inhibitors with mepiridine or dextromethorphan
- Do not combine with another MAO inhibitor, alcohol, buspirone, bupropion, or guanethidine
- Adverse drug reactions can results from combining MAO inhibitors with tricyclic/tetracyclic antidepressants and related compounds, including carbamazepine, cyclobenzaprine, and mirtazapine, and should be avoided except by experts to treat difficult cases (see Pearls)
- MAO inhibitors in combination with spinal anesthesia may cause combined hypotensive effects
- Combination of MAOIs and CNS depressants may enhance sedation and hypotension

 Other Warnings/ Precautions

- Use requires low tyramine diet
- Patients taking MAO inhibitors should avoid high protein food that has undergone protein breakdown by aging, fermentation, pickling, smoking, or bacterial contamination
- Patients taking MAO inhibitors should avoid cheeses (especially aged varieties), pickled herring, beer, wine, liver, yeast extract, dry sausage, hard salami, pepperoni, Lebanon bologna, pods of broad beans (fava beans), yogurt, and excessive use of caffeine and chocolate
- Patient and prescriber must be vigilant to potential interactions with any drug, including antihypertensives and over-the-counter cough/cold preparations
- Over-the-counter medications to avoid include cough and cold preparations, including those containing dextromethorphan, nasal decongestants (tablets, drops, or spray), hay-fever medications, sinus medications, asthma inhalant medications, anti-appetite medications, weight reducing preparations, "pep" pills

- Use cautiously in patients receiving reserpine, anesthetics, disulfiram, metrizamide, anticholinergic agents
- Isocarboxazid is not recommended for use in patients who cannot be monitored closely
- When treating children, carefully weigh the risks and benefits of pharmacological treatment against the risks and benefits of nontreatment with antidepressants and make sure to document this in the patient's chart
- Distribute the brochures provided by the FDA and the drug companies
- Warn patients and their caregivers about the possibility of activating side effects and advise them to report such symptoms immediately
- Monitor patients for activation of suicidal ideation, especially children and adolescents

Do Not Use

- If patient is taking meperidine (pethidine)
- If patient is taking a sympathomimetic agent or taking guanethidine
- If patient is taking another MAOI
- If patient is taking any agent that can inhibit serotonin reuptake (e.g., SSRIs, sibutramine, tramadol, milnacipran, duloxetine, venlafaxine, clomipramine, etc.)
- If patient is taking diuretics, dextromethorphan, buspirone, bupropion
- If patient has pheochromocytoma
- If patient has cardiovascular or cerebrovascular disease
- If patient has frequent or severe headaches
- If patient is undergoing elective surgery and requires general anesthesia
- If patient has a history of liver disease or abnormal liver function tests
- If patient is taking a prohibited drug
- If patient is not compliant with a low-tyramine diet
- If there is a proven allergy to isocarboxazid

SPECIAL POPULATIONS

Renal Impairment

- Use with caution – drug may accumulate in plasma
- May require lower than usual adult dose

Hepatic Impairment

- Not for use in hepatic impairment

Cardiac Impairment

- Contraindicated in patients with congestive heart failure or hypertension
- Any other cardiac impairment may require lower than usual adult dose
- Patients with angina pectoris or coronary artery disease should limit their exertion

Elderly

- Initial dose lower than usual adult dose
- Elderly patients may have greater sensitivity to adverse effects

 Children and Adolescents

- Not recommended for use under age 16
- Carefully weigh the risks and benefits of pharmacological treatment against the risks and benefits of nontreatment with antidepressants and make sure to document this in the patient's chart
- Distribute the brochures provided by the FDA and the drug companies
- Warn patients and their caregivers about the possibility of activating side effects and advise them to report such symptoms immediately
- Use with caution, observing for activation of known or unknown bipolar disorder and/or suicidal ideation, and inform parents or guardian of this risk so they can help observe child or adolescent patients

Pregnancy

- Risk Category C [some animal studies show adverse effects, no controlled studies in humans]
- Not generally recommended for use during pregnancy, especially during first trimester
- Should evaluate patient for treatment with an antidepressant with a better risk/benefit ratio

Breast Feeding

- Some drug is found in mother's breast milk
- Immediate postpartum period is a high-risk time for depression, especially in women who have had prior depressive episodes, so drug may need to be reinstituted late in the third trimester or shortly after

childbirth to prevent a recurrence during the postpartum period
- Should evaluate patient for treatment with an antidepressant with a better risk/benefit ratio

THE ART OF PSYCHOPHARMACOLOGY

Potential Advantages
- Atypical depression
- Severe depression
- Treatment-resistant depression or anxiety disorders

Potential Disadvantages
- Requires compliance to dietary restrictions, concomitant drug restrictions
- Patients with cardiac problems or hypertension
- Multiple daily doses

Primary Target Symptoms
- Depressed mood
- Somatic symptoms
- Sleep and eating disturbances
- Psychomotor retardation
- Morbid preoccupation

 Pearls
- MAOIs are generally reserved for second-line use after SSRIs, SNRIs, and combinations of newer antidepressants have failed
- Despite little utilization, some patients respond to isocarboxazid who do not respond to other antidepressants including other MAOIs
- Patient should be advised not to take any prescription or over-the-counter drugs without consulting their doctor because of possible drug interactions with the MAOI
- Headache is often the first symptom of hypertensive crisis
- Foods generally to avoid as they are usually high in tyramine content: dry sausage, pickled herring, liver, broad bean pods, sauerkraut, cheese, yogurt, alcoholic beverages, nonalcoholic beer and wine, chocolate, caffeine, meat and fish
- The rigid dietary restrictions may reduce compliance

- Mood disorders can be associated with eating disorders (especially in adolescent females), and isocarboxazid can be used to treat both depression and bulimia
- MAOIs are a viable second-line treatment option in depression, but are not frequently used
- ✳ Myths about the danger of dietary tyramine can be exaggerated, but prohibitions against concomitant drugs often not followed closely enough
- Orthostatic hypotension, insomnia, and sexual dysfunction are often the most troublesome common side effects
- ✳ MAOIs should be for the expert, especially if combining with agents of potential risk (e.g., stimulants, trazodone, TCAs)
- ✳ MAOIs should not be neglected as therapeutic agents for the treatment-resistant
- Although generally prohibited, a heroic but potentially dangerous treatment for severely treatment-resistant patients is for an expert to give a tricyclic/tetracyclic antidepressant other than clomipramine simultaneously with an MAO inhibitor for patients who fail to respond to numerous other antidepressants
- Use of MAOIs with clomipramine is always prohibited because of the risk of serotonin syndrome and death
- Amoxapine may be the preferred trycyclic/tetracyclic antidepressant to combine with an MAOI in heroic cases due to its theoretically protective 5HT2A antagonist properties
- If this option is elected, start the MAOI with the tricyclic/tetracyclic antidepressant simultaneously at low doses after appropriate drug washout, then alternately increase doses of these agents every few days to a week as tolerated
- Although very strict dietary and concomitant drug restrictions must be observed to prevent hypertensive crises and serotonin syndrome, the most common side effects of MAOI and tricyclic/tetracyclic combinations may be weight gain and orthostatic hypotension

Suggested Reading

Kennedy SH. Continuation and maintenance treatments in major depression: the neglected role of monoamine oxidase inhibitors. J Psychiatry Neurosci 1997;22:127–31.

Lippman SB, Nash K. Monoamine oxidase inhibitor update. Potential adverse food and drug interactions. Drug Saf 1990;5:195–204.

Larsen JK, Rafaelsen OJ. Long-term treatment of depression with isocarboxazide. Acta Psychiatr Scand 1980;62(5):456–63.

LOFEPRAMINE

THERAPEUTICS

Brands • Deprimyl
• Gamanil
see index for additional brand names

Generic? Yes

Class
• Tricyclic antidepressant (TCA)
• Predominantly a norepinephrine/
noradrenaline reuptake inhibitor

Commonly Prescribed For
(bold for FDA approved)
• Major depressive disorder
• Anxiety
• Insomnia
• Neuropathic pain/chronic pain
• Treatment-resistant depression

How The Drug Works
• Boosts neurotransmitter
norepinephrine/noradrenaline
• Blocks norepinephrine reuptake pump
(norepinephrine transporter), presumably
increasing noradrenergic
neurotransmission
• Since dopamine is inactivated by
norepinephrine reuptake in frontal cortex,
which largely lacks dopamine transporters,
lofepramine can increase dopamine
neurotransmission in this part of the brain
• A more potent inhibitor of norepinephrine
reuptake pump than serotonin reuptake
pump (serotonin transporter)
• At high doses may also boost
neurotransmitter serotonin and presumably
increase serotonergic neurotransmission

How Long Until It Works
• May have immediate effects in treating
insomnia or anxiety
• Onset of therapeutic actions usually not
immediate, but often delayed 2 to 4 weeks
• If it is not working within 6 to 8 weeks for
depression, it may require a dosage
increase or it may not work at all
• May continue to work for many years to
prevent relapse of symptoms

If It Works
• The goal of treatment of depression is
complete remission of current symptoms
as well as prevention of future relapses
• The goal of treatment of chronic
neuropathic pain is to reduce symptoms as
much as possible, especially in
combination with other treatments
• Treatment of depression most often
reduces or even eliminates symptoms, but
not a cure since symptoms can recur after
medicine stopped
• Treatment of chronic neuropathic pain may
reduce symptoms, but rarely eliminates
them completely, and is not a cure since
symptoms can recur after medicine is
stopped
• Continue treatment of depression until all
symptoms are gone (remission)
• Once symptoms of depression are gone,
continue treating for 1 year for the first
episode of depression
• For second and subsequent episodes of
depression, treatment may need to be
indefinite
• Use in anxiety disorders and chronic pain
may also need to be indefinite, but long-
term treatment is not well studied in these
conditions

If It Doesn't Work
• Many depressed patients only have a
partial response where some symptoms
are improved but others persist (especially
insomnia, fatigue, and problems
concentrating)
• Other depressed patients may be
nonresponders, sometimes called
treatment-resistant or treatment-refractory
• Consider increasing dose, switching to
another agent or adding an appropriate
augmenting agent
• Consider psychotherapy
• Consider evaluation for another diagnosis
or for a comorbid condition (e.g, medical
illness, substance abuse, etc.)
• Some patients may experience apparent
lack of consistent efficacy due to activation
of latent or underlying bipolar disorder, and
require antidepressant discontinuation and
a switch to a mood stabilizer

Best Augmenting Combos for Partial Response or Treatment-Resistance

- Lithium, buspirone, thyroid hormone (for depression)
- Gabapentin, tiagabine, other anticonvulsants, even opiates if done by experts while monitoring carefully in difficult cases (for chronic pain)

Tests

- None for healthy individuals
- ✻ Since tricyclic and tetracyclic antidepressants are frequently associated with weight gain, before starting treatment, weigh all patients and determine if the patient is already overweight (BMI 25.0–29.9) or obese (BMI ≥30)
- Before giving a drug that can cause weight gain to an overweight or obese patient, consider determining whether the patient already has pre-diabetes (fasting plasma glucose 100–125 mg/dl), diabetes (fasting plasma glucose >126 mg/dl), or dyslipidemia (increased total cholesterol, LDL cholesterol and triglycerides; decreased HDL cholesterol), and treat or refer such patients for treatment, including nutrition and weight management, physical activity counseling, smoking cessation, and medical management
- ✻ Monitor weight and BMI during treatment
- ✻ While giving a drug to a patient who has gained >5% of initial weight, consider evaluating for the presence of pre-diabetes, diabetes, or dyslipidemia, or consider switching to a different antidepressant
- EKGs may be useful for selected patients (e.g., those with personal or family history of QTc prolongation; cardiac arrhythmia; recent myocardial infarction; uncompensated heart failure; or taking agents that prolong QTc interval such as pimozide, thioridazine, selected antiarrhythmics, moxifloxacin, sparfloxacin, etc.)
- Patients at risk for electrolyte disturbances (e.g., patients on diuretic therapy) should have baseline and periodic serum potassium and magnesium measurements

SIDE EFFECTS

How Drug Causes Side Effects

- Anticholinergic activity may explain sedative effects, dry mouth, constipation, and blurred vision
- Sedative effects and weight gain may be due to antihistamine properties
- Blockade of alpha adrenergic 1 receptors may explain dizziness, sedation, and hypotension
- Cardiac arrhythmias and seizures, especially in overdose, may be caused by blockade of ion channels

Notable Side Effects

- Blurred vision, constipation, urinary retention, increased appetite, dry mouth, nausea, diarrhea, heartburn, unusual taste in mouth, weight gain
- Fatigue, weakness, dizziness, sedation, headache, anxiety, nervousness, restlessness
- Sexual dysfunction, sweating

Life Threatening or Dangerous Side Effects

- Paralytic ileus, hyperthermia (TCAs + anticholinergic agents)
- Lowered seizure threshold and rare seizures
- Orthostatic hypotension, sudden death, arrhythmias, tachycardia
- QTc prolongation
- Hepatic failure, extrapyramidal symptoms
- Increased intraocular pressure
- Rare induction of mania
- Rare activation of suicidal ideation and behavior (suicidality)

Weight Gain

unusual   not unusual   common   problematic

- Many experience and/or can be significant in amount
- Can increase appetite and carbohydrate craving

Sedation

unusual   not unusual   common   problematic

- Many experience and/or can be significant in amount

- Tolerance to sedative effect may develop with long-term use

What To Do About Side Effects
- Wait
- Wait
- Wait
- Lower the dose
- Switch to an SSRI or newer antidepressant

Best Augmenting Agents for Side Effects
- Many side effects cannot be improved with an augmenting agent

DOSING AND USE

Usual Dosage Range
- 140–210 mg/day

Dosage Forms
- Tablet 70 mg multiscored
- Liquid 70 mg/5mL

How to Dose
- Initial 70 mg/day once daily or in divided doses; gradually increase daily dose to achieve desired therapeutic effects; dose at bedtime for daytime sedation and in morning for insomnia; maximum dose 280 mg/day for inpatients, 210 mg/day for outpatients

 Dosing Tips
- If given in a single dose, should generally be administered at bedtime because of its sedative properties
- If given in split doses, largest dose should generally be given at bedtime because of its sedative properties
- If patients experience nightmares, split dose and do not give large dose at bedtime
- Unusual dose compared to most TCAs
- Patients treated for chronic pain may only require lower doses
- If intolerable anxiety, insomnia, agitation, akathisia, or activation occur either upon dosing initiation or discontinuation, consider the possibility of activated bipolar disorder, and switch to a mood stabilizer or an atypical antipsychotic

Overdose
- Death may occur; convulsions, cardiac dysrhythmias, severe hypotension, CNS depression, coma, changes in ECG

Long-Term Use
- Safe

Habit Forming
- No

How to Stop
- Taper to avoid withdrawal effects
- Even with gradual dose reduction some withdrawal symptoms may appear within the first 2 weeks
- Many patients tolerate 50% dose reduction for 3 days, then another 50% reduction for 3 days, then discontinuation
- If withdrawal symptoms emerge during discontinuation, raise dose to stop symptoms and then restart withdrawal much more slowly

Pharmacokinetics
- Substrate for CYP450 2D6
- Half-life of parent compound approximately 1.5–6 hours
- ✳ Major metabolite is the antidepressant desipramine, with a half-life of approximately 24 hours

 Drug Interactions
- Tramadol increases the risk of seizures in patients taking TCAs
- Use of TCAs with anticholinergic drugs may result in paralytic ileus or hyperthermia
- Fluoxetine, paroxetine, bupropion, duloxetine, and other CYP450 2D6 inhibitors may increase TCA concentrations
- Cimetidine may increase plasma concentrations of TCAs and cause anticholinergic symptoms
- Phenothiazines or haloperidol may raise TCA blood concentrations
- May alter effects of antihypertensive drugs; may inhibit hypotensive effects of clonidine
- Use with sympathomimetic agents may increase sympathetic activity
- Methylphenidate may inhibit metabolism of TCAs
- Activation and agitation, especially following switching or adding

antidepressants, may represent the induction of a bipolar state, especially a mixed dysphoric bipolar II condition sometimes associated with suicidal ideation, and require the addition of lithium, a mood stabilizer or an atypical antipsychotic, and/or discontinuation of lofepramine

 Other Warnings/ Precautions

- Add or initiate other antidepressants with caution for up to 2 weeks after discontinuing lofepramine
- Generally, do not use with MAO inhibitors, including 14 days after MAOIs are stopped; do not start an MAOI until 2 weeks after discontinuing lofepramine, but see Pearls
- Use with caution in patients with history of seizure, urinary retention, narrow angle-closure glaucoma, hyperthyroidism
- TCAs can increase QTc interval, especially at toxic doses, which can be attained not only by overdose but also by combining with drugs that inhibit its metabolism via CYP450 2D6, potentially causing torsade de pointes-type arrhythmia or sudden death
- Because TCAs can prolong QTc interval, use with caution in patients who have bradycardia or who are taking drugs that can induce bradycardia (e.g., beta blockers, calcium channel blockers, clonidine, digitalis)
- Because TCAs can prolong QTc interval, use with caution in patients who have hypokalemia and/or hypomagnesemia or who are taking drugs that can induce hypokalemia and/or magnesemia (e.g., diuretics, stimulant laxatives, intravenous amphotericin B, glucocorticoids, tetracosactide)
- When treating children, carefully weigh the risks and benefits of pharmacological treatment against the risks and benefits of nontreatment with antidepressants and make sure to document this in the patient's chart
- Distribute the brochures provided by the FDA and the drug companies
- Warn patients and their caregivers about the possibility of activating side effects and advise them to report such symptoms immediately

- Monitor patients for activation of suicidal ideation, especially children and adolescents

Do Not Use

- If patient is recovering from myocardial infarction
- If patient is taking agents capable of significantly prolonging QTc interval (e.g., pimozide, thioridazine, selected antiarrhythmics, moxifloxacin, sparfloxacin)
- If there is a history of QTc prolongation or cardiac arrhythmia, recent acute myocardial infarction, uncompensated heart failure
- If patient is taking drugs that inhibit TCA metabolism, including CYP450 2D6 inhibitors, except by an expert
- If there is reduced CYP450 2D6 function, such as patients who are poor 2D6 metabolizers, except by an expert and at low doses
- If there is a proven allergy to lofepramine, desipramine, or imipramine

SPECIAL POPULATIONS

Renal Impairment
- Use with caution

Hepatic Impairment
- Use with caution

Cardiac Impairment
- TCAs have been reported to cause arrhythmias, prolongation of conduction time, orthostatic hypotension, sinus tachycardia, and heart failure, especially in the diseased heart
- Myocardial infarction and stroke have been reported with TCAs
- TCAs produce QTc prolongation, which may be enhanced by the existence of bradycardia, hypokalemia, congenital or acquired long QTc interval, which should be evaluated prior to administering lofepramine
- Use with caution if treating concomitantly with a medication likely to produce prolonged bradycardia, hypokalemia, slowing of intracardiac conduction, or prolongation of the QTc interval

- Avoid TCAs in patients with a known history of QTc prolongation, recent acute myocardial infarction, and uncompensated heart failure
- TCAs may cause a sustained increase in heart rate in patients with ischemic heart disease and may worsen (decrease) heart rate variability, an independent risk of mortality in cardiac populations
- Since SSRIs may improve (increase) heart rate variability in patients following a myocardial infarct and may improve survival as well as mood in patients with acute angina or following a myocardial infarction, these are more appropriate agents for cardiac population than tricyclic/tetracyclic antidepressants
- ✳ Risk/benefit ratio may not justify use of TCAs in cardiac impairment

Elderly

- May be more sensitive to anticholinergic, cardiovascular, hypotensive, and sedative effects

Children and Adolescents

- Carefully weigh the risks and benefits of pharmacological treatment against the risks and benefits of nontreatment with antidepressants and make sure to document this in the patient's chart
- Monitor patients face-to-face regularly, particularly during the first several weeks of treatment
- Use with caution, observing for activation of known or unknown bipolar disorder and/or suicidal ideation, and inform parents or guardian of this risk so they can help observe child or adolescent patients
- Not recommended for use under age 18
- Several studies show lack of efficacy of TCAs for depression
- May be used to treat enuresis or hyperactive/impulsive behaviors
- Some cases of sudden death have occurred in children taking TCAs

Pregnancy

- Risk Category C [some animal studies show adverse effects, no controlled studies in humans]
- Crosses the placenta

- Adverse effects have been reported in infants whose mothers took a TCA (lethargy, withdrawal symptoms, fetal malformations)
- Not generally recommended for use during pregnancy, especially during first trimester
- Must weigh the risk of treatment (first trimester fetal development, third trimester newborn delivery) to the child against the risk of no treatment (recurrence of depression, maternal health, infant bonding) to the mother and child
- For many patients this may mean continuing treatment during pregnancy

Breast Feeding

- Some drug is found in mother's breast milk
- ✳ Recommended either to discontinue drug or bottle feed
- Immediate postpartum period is a high-risk time for depression, especially in women who have had prior depressive episodes, so drug may need to be reinstituted late in the third trimester or shortly after childbirth to prevent a recurrence during the postpartum period
- Must weigh benefits of breast feeding with risks and benefits of antidepressant treatment versus non-treatment to both the infant and the mother
- For many patients this may mean continuing treatment during breast feeding

THE ART OF PSYCHOPHARMACOLOGY

Potential Advantages

- Patients with insomnia
- Severe or treatment-resistant depression
- Anxious depression

Potential Disadvantages

- Pediatric and geriatric patients
- Patients concerned with weight gain
- Cardiac patients

Primary Target Symptoms

- Depressed mood

Pearls

- Tricyclic antidepressants are often a first-line treatment option for chronic pain

105

- Tricyclic antidepressants are no longer generally considered a first-line option for depression because of their side effect profile
- Tricyclic antidepressants continue to be useful for severe or treatment-resistant depression
- Noradrenergic reuptake inhibitors such as lofepramine can be used as a second-line treatment for smoking cessation, cocaine dependence, and attention deficit disorder
- ✳ Lofepramine is a short acting prodrug of the TCA desipramine
- ✳ Fewer anticholinergic side effects, particularly sedation, than some other tricyclics
- Once a popular TCA in the UK, but not widely marketed throughout the world
- TCAs may aggravate psychotic symptoms
- Alcohol should be avoided because of additive CNS effects
- Underweight patients may be more susceptible to adverse cardiovascular effects
- Children, patients with inadequate hydration, and patients with cardiac disease may be more susceptible to TCA-induced cardiotoxicity than healthy adults
- For the expert only: although generally prohibited, a heroic treatment (but potentially dangerous) for severely treatment-resistant patients is to give a tricyclic/tetracyclic antidepressant other than clomipramine simultaneously with an MAO inhibitor for patients who fail to respond to numerous other antidepressants
- If this option is elected, start the MAOI with the tricyclic/tetracyclic antidepressant simultaneously at low doses after appropriate drug washout, then alternately increase doses of these agents every few days to a week as tolerated
- Although very strict dietary and concomitant drug restrictions must be observed to prevent hypertensive crises and serotonin syndrome, the most common side effects of MAOI/tricyclic or tetracyclic combinations may be weight gain and orthostatic hypotension
- Patients on TCAs should be aware that they may experience symptoms such as photosensitivity or blue-green urine
- SSRIs may be more effective than TCAs in women, and TCAs may be more effective than SSRIs in men
- Since tricyclic/tetracyclic antidepressants are substrates for CYP450 2D6, and 7% of the population (especially Caucasians) may have a genetic variant leading to reduced activity of 2D6, such patients may not safely tolerate normal doses of tricyclic/tetracyclic antidepressants and may require dose reduction
- Phenotypic testing may be necessary to detect this genetic variant prior to dosing with a tricyclic/tetracyclic antidepressant, especially in vulnerable populations such as children, elderly, cardiac populations, and those on concomitant medications
- Patients who seem to have extraordinarily severe side effects at normal or low doses may have this phenotypic CYP450 2D6 variant and require low doses or switching to another antidepressant not metabolized by 2D6

Suggested Reading

Anderson IM. Meta-analytical studies on new antidepressants. Br Med Bull. 2001; 57:161–178.

Anderson IM. Selective serotonin reuptake inhibitors versus tricyclic antidepressants: a meta-analysis of efficacy and tolerability. J Aff Disorders. 2000;58:19–36.

Kerihuel JC, Dreyfus JF. Meta-analyses of the efficacy and tolerability of the tricyclic antidepressant lofepramine. J Int Med Res. 1991;19:183–201.

Lancaster SG, Gonzales JP. Lofepramine. A review of its pharmacodynamic and pharmacokinetic properties, and therapeutic efficacy in depressive illness. Drugs. 1989; 37:123–40.

Brands • Ludiomil
see index for additional brand names

Generic? Yes

Class

- Tricyclic antidepressant (TCA), sometimes classified as a tetracyclic antidepressant (tetra)
- Predominantly a norepinephrine/noradrenaline reuptake inhibitor

Commonly Prescribed For
(bold for FDA approved)
- **Depression**
- Anxiety
- Insomnia
- Neuropathic pain/chronic pain
- Treatment-resistant depression

How The Drug Works

- Boosts neurotransmitter norepinephrine/noradrenaline
- Blocks norepinephrine reuptake pump (norepinephrine transporter), presumably increasing noradrenergic neurotransmission
- Since dopamine is inactivated by norepinephrine reuptake in frontal cortex, which largely lacks dopamine transporters, maprotiline can thus increase dopamine neurotransmission in this part of the brain
- A more potent inhibitor of norepinephrine reuptake pump than serotonin reuptake pump (serotonin transporter)
- At high doses may also boost neurotransmitter serotonin and presumably increase serotonergic neurotransmission

How Long Until It Works

- Onset of therapeutic actions usually not immediate, but often delayed 2 to 4 weeks
- If it is not working within 6 to 8 weeks for depression, it may require a dosage increase or it may not work at all
- May continue to work for many years to prevent relapse of symptoms

If It Works

- The goal of treatment of depression is complete remission of current symptoms as well as prevention of future relapses
- The goal of treatment of chronic neuropathic pain is to reduce symptoms as much as possible, especially in combination with other treatments
- Treatment of depression most often reduces or even eliminates symptoms, but not a cure since symptoms can recur after medicine stopped
- Treatment of chronic neuropathic pain may reduce symptoms, but rarely eliminates them completely, and is not a cure since symptoms can recur after medicine is stopped
- Continue treatment of depression until all symptoms are gone (remission)
- Once symptoms of depression are gone, continue treating for 1 year for the first episode of depression
- For second and subsequent episodes of depression, treatment may need to be indefinite
- Use in anxiety disorders and chronic pain may also need to be indefinite, but long-term treatment is not well-studied in these conditions

If It Doesn't Work

- Many depressed patients only have a partial response where some symptoms are improved but others persist (especially insomnia, fatigue, and problems concentrating)
- Other depressed patients may be nonresponders, sometimes called treatment-resistant or treatment-refractory
- Consider increasing dose, switching to another agent or adding an appropriate augmenting agent
- Consider psychotherapy
- Consider evaluation for another diagnosis or for a comorbid condition (e.g., medical illness, substance abuse, etc.)
- Some patients may experience apparent lack of consistent efficacy due to activation of latent or underlying bipolar disorder, and require antidepressant discontinuation and a switch to a mood stabilizer

Best Augmenting Combos for Partial Response or Treatment-Resistance

• Lithium, buspirone, thyroid hormone (for depression)
• Gabapentin, tiagabine, other anticonvulsants, even opiates if done by experts while monitoring carefully in difficult cases (for chronic pain)

Tests

• None for healthy individuals
✳ Since tricyclic and tetracyclic antidepressants are frequently associated with weight gain, before starting treatment, weigh all patients and determine if the patient is already overweight (BMI 25.0–29.9) or obese (BMI ≥30)
• Before giving a drug that can cause weight gain to an overweight or obese patient, consider determining whether the patient already has pre-diabetes (fasting plasma glucose 100–125 mg/dl), diabetes (fasting plasma glucose >126 mg/dl), or dyslipidemia (increased total cholesterol, LDL cholesterol and triglycerides; decreased HDL cholesterol), and treat or refer such patients for treatment, including nutrition and weight management, physical activity counseling, smoking cessation, and medical management
✳ Monitor weight and BMI during treatment
✳ While giving a drug to a patient who has gained >5% of initial weight, consider evaluating for the presence of pre-diabetes, diabetes, or dyslipidemia, or consider switching to a different antidepressant
• EKGs may be useful for selected patients (e.g., those with personal or family history of QTc prolongation; cardiac arrhythmia; recent myocardial infarction; uncompensated heart failure; or taking agents that prolong QTc interval such as pimozide, thioridazine, selected antiarrhythmics, moxifloxacin, sparfloxacin, etc.)
• Patients at risk for electrolyte disturbances (e.g., patients on diuretic therapy) should have baseline and periodic serum potassium and magnesium measurements

SIDE EFFECTS

How Drug Causes Side Effects

• Anticholinergic activity may explain sedative effects, dry mouth, constipation, and blurred vision
• Sedative effects and weight gain may be due to antihistamine properties
• Blockade of alpha adrenergic 1 receptors may explain dizziness, sedation, and hypotension
• Cardiac arrhythmias and seizures, especially in overdose, may be caused by blockade of ion channels

Notable Side Effects

• Blurred vision, constipation, urinary retention, increased appetite, dry mouth, nausea, diarrhea, heartburn, unusual taste in mouth, weight gain
• Fatigue, weakness, dizziness, sedation, headache, anxiety, nervousness, restlessness
• Sexual dysfunction (impotence, change in libido)
• Sweating, rash, itching

Life Threatening or Dangerous Side Effects

• Paralytic ileus, hyperthermia (TCAs/ tetracyclics + anticholinergic agents)
• Lowered seizure threshold and rare seizures
• Orthostatic hypotension, sudden death, arrhythmias, tachycardia
• QTc prolongation
• Hepatic failure, extrapyramidal symptoms
• Increased intraocular pressure
• Rare induction of mania
• Rare activation of suicidal ideation and behavior (suicidality)

Weight Gain

unusual · not unusual · common · problematic

• Many experience and/or can be significant in amount
• Can increase appetite and carbohydrate craving

Sedation

unusual · not unusual · common · problematic

• Many experience and/or can be significant in amount
• Tolerance to sedative effect may develop with long-term use

What To Do About Side Effects
• Wait
• Wait
• Wait
• Lower the dose
• Switch to an SSRI or newer antidepressant

Best Augmenting Agents for Side Effects
• Many side effects cannot be improved with an augmenting agent

DOSING AND USE

Usual Dosage Range
• 75–150 mg/day (for depression)
• 50–150 mg/day (for chronic pain)

Dosage Forms
• Tablet 25 mg, 50 mg, 75 mg

How to Dose
• Initial 25 mg/day at bedtime; increase by 25 mg every 3–7 days
• 75 mg/day; after 2 weeks increase dose gradually by 25 mg/day; maximum dose generally 225 mg/day

 Dosing Tips
• If given in a single dose, should generally be administered at bedtime because of its sedative properties
• If given in split doses, largest dose should generally be given at bedtime because of its sedative properties
• If patients experience nightmares, split dose and do not give large dose at bedtime
• Patients treated for chronic pain may only require lower doses
* Risk of seizures increases with dose, especially with maprotiline above 200 mg/day
• If intolerable anxiety, insomnia, agitation, akathisia, or activation occur either upon dosing initiation or discontinuation, consider the possibility of activated bipolar

disorder, and switch to a mood stabilizer or an atypical antipsychotic

Overdose
• Death may occur; convulsions, cardiac dysrhythmias, severe hypotension, CNS depression, coma, changes in ECG

Long-Term Use
• Safe

Habit Forming
• No

How to Stop
• Taper to avoid withdrawal effects
• Even with gradual dose reduction some withdrawal symptoms may appear within the first 2 weeks
• Many patients tolerate 50% dose reduction for 3 days, then another 50% reduction for 3 days, then discontinuation
• If withdrawal symptoms emerge during discontinuation, raise dose to stop symptoms and then restart withdrawal much more slowly

Pharmacokinetics
• Substrate for CYP450 2D6
• Mean half-life approximately 51 hours
• Peak plasma concentration 8–24 hours

 Drug Interactions
• Tramadol increases the risk of seizures in patients taking TCAs
• Use of TCAs/tetracyclics with anticholinergic drugs may result in paralytic ileus or hyperthermia
• Fluoxetine, paroxetine, bupropion, duloxetine, and other CYP450 2D6 inhibitors may increase TCA/tetracyclic concentrations
• Cimetidine may increase plasma concentrations of TCAs/tetracyclics and cause anticholinergic symptoms
• Phenothiazines or haloperidol may raise TCA/tetracyclic blood concentrations
• May alter effects of antihypertensive drugs; may inhibit hypotensive effects of clonidine
• Use with sympathomimetic agents may increase sympathetic activity
• Methylphenidate may inhibit metabolism of TCAs/tetracyclics

- Activation and agitation, especially following switching or adding antidepressants, may represent the induction of a bipolar state, especially a mixed dysphoric bipolar II condition sometimes associated with suicidal ideation, and require the addition of lithium, a mood stabilizer or an atypical antipsychotic, and/or discontinuation of maprotiline

 Other Warnings/ Precautions
- Add or initiate other antidepressants with caution for up to 2 weeks after discontinuing maprotiline
- Generally, do not use with MAO inhibitors, including 14 days after MAOIs are stopped; do not start an MAOI until 2 weeks after discontinuing maprotiline, but see Pearls
- Use with caution in patients with history of seizures, urinary retention, narrow angle-closure glaucoma, hyperthyroidism
- TCAs/tetracyclics can increase QTc interval, especially at toxic doses, which can be attained not only by overdose but also by combining with drugs that inhibit TCA/tetracyclic metabolism via CYP450 2D6, potentially causing torsade de pointes-type arrhythmia or sudden death
- Because TCAs/tetracyclics can prolong QTc interval, use with caution in patients who have bradycardia or who are taking drugs that can induce bradycardia (e.g., beta blockers, calcium channel blockers, clonidine, digitalis)
- Because TCAs/tetracyclics can prolong QTc interval, use with caution in patients who have hypokalemia and/or hypomagnesemia or who are taking drugs that can induce hypokalemia and/or magnesemia (e.g., diuretics, stimulant laxatives, intravenous amphotericin B, glucocorticoids, tetracosactide)
- When treating children, carefully weigh the risks and benefits of pharmacological treatment against the risks and benefits of nontreatment with antidepressants and make sure to document this in the patient's chart
- Distribute the brochures provided by the FDA and the drug companies
- Warn patients and their caregivers about the possibility of activating side effects and advise them to report such symptoms immediately
- Monitor patients for activation of suicidal ideation, especially children and adolescents

Do Not Use
- If patient is recovering from myocardial infarction
- If patient is taking agents capable of significantly prolonging QTc interval (e.g., pimozide, thioridazine, selected antiarrhythmics, moxifloxacin, sparfloxacin)
- If there is a history of QTc prolongation or cardiac arrhythmia, recent acute myocardial infarction, uncompensated heart failure
- If patient is taking drugs that inhibit TCA/tetracyclic metabolism, including CYP450 2D6 inhibitors, except by an expert
- If there is reduced CYP450 2D6 function, such as patients who are poor 2D6 metabolizers, except by an expert and at low doses
- If there is a proven allergy to maprotiline

SPECIAL POPULATIONS

Renal Impairment
- Use with caution

Hepatic Impairment
- Use with caution

Cardiac Impairment
- TCAs/tetracyclics have been reported to cause arrhythmias, prolongation of conduction time, orthostatic hypotension, sinus tachycardia, and heart failure, especially in the diseased heart
- Myocardial infarction and stroke have been reported with TCAs/tetracyclics
- TCAs/tetracyclics produce QTc prolongation, which may be enhanced by the existence of bradycardia, hypokalemia, congenital or acquired long QTc interval, which should be evaluated prior to administering maprotiline
- Use with caution if treating concomitantly with a medication likely to produce prolonged bradycardia, hypokalemia, slowing of intracardiac conduction, or prolongation of the QTc interval

- Avoid TCAs/tetracyclics in patients with a known history of QTc prolongation, recent acute myocardial infarction, and uncompensated heart failure
- TCAs/tetracyclics may cause a sustained increase in heart rate in patients with ischemic heart disease and may worsen (decrease) heart rate variability, an independent risk of mortality in cardiac populations
- Since SSRIs may improve (increase) heart rate variability in patients following a myocardial infarct and may improve survival as well as mood in patients with acute angina or following a myocardial infarction, these are more appropriate agents for cardiac population than tricyclic/tetracyclic antidepressants
* Risk/benefit ratio may not justify use of TCAs/tetracyclics in cardiac impairment

Elderly
- May be more sensitive to anticholinergic, cardiovascular, hypotensive, and sedative effects
- Usual dose generally 50–75 mg/day

Children and Adolescents
- Carefully weigh the risks and benefits of pharmacological treatment against the risks and benefits of nontreatment with antidepressants and make sure to document this in the patient's chart
- Monitor patients face-to-face regularly, particularly during the first several weeks of treatment
- Use with caution, observing for activation of known or unknown bipolar disorder and/or suicidal ideation, and inform parents or guardian of this risk so they can help observe child or adolescent patients
- Not recommended for use under age 18
- Several studies show lack of efficacy of TCAs/tetracyclics for depression
- May be used to treat enuresis or hyperactive/impulsive behaviors
- Some cases of sudden death have occurred in children taking TCAs/tetracyclics
- Maximum dose for children and adolescents is 75 mg/day

Pregnancy
- Risk Category B [animal studies do not show adverse effects, no controlled studies in humans]
- Adverse effects have been reported in infants whose mothers took a TCA/tetracyclic (lethargy, withdrawal symptoms, fetal malformations)
- Must weigh the risk of treatment (first trimester fetal development, third trimester newborn delivery) to the child against the risk of no treatment (recurrence of depression, maternal health, infant bonding) to the mother and child
- For many patients this may mean continuing treatment during pregnancy

Breast Feeding
- Some drug is found in mother's breast milk
* Recommended either to discontinue drug or bottle feed
- Immediate postpartum period is a high-risk time for depression, especially in women who have had prior depressive episodes, so drug may need to be reinstituted late in the third trimester or shortly after childbirth to prevent a recurrence during the postpartum period
- Must weigh benefits of breast feeding with risks and benefits of antidepressant treatment versus non-treatment to both the infant and the mother
- For many patients this may mean continuing treatment during breast feeding

THE ART OF PSYCHOPHARMACOLOGY

Potential Advantages
- Patients with insomnia
- Severe or treatment-resistant depression

Potential Disadvantages
- Pediatric and geriatric patients
- Patients concerned with weight gain
- Cardiac patients
- Patients with seizure disorders

Primary Target Symptoms
- Depressed mood
- Chronic pain

Pearls

- Tricyclic/tetracyclic antidepressants are often a first-line treatment option for chronic pain
- Tricyclic/tetracyclic antidepressants are no longer generally considered a first-line treatment option for depression because of their side effect profile
- Tricyclic/tetracyclic antidepressants continue to be useful for severe or treatment-resistant depression
- ✳ May have somewhat increased risk of seizures compared to some other TCAs, especially at higher doses
- TCAs/tetracyclics may aggravate psychotic symptoms
- Alcohol should be avoided because of additive CNS effects
- Underweight patients may be more susceptible to adverse cardiovascular effects
- Children, patients with inadequate hydration, and patients with cardiac disease may be more susceptible to TCA/tetracyclic-induced cardiotoxicity than healthy adults
- For the expert only: a heroic treatment (but potentially dangerous) for severely treatment-resistant patients is to give simultaneously with monoamine oxidase inhibitors for patients who fail to respond to numerous other antidepressants
- If this option is elected, start the MAOI with the tricyclic/tetracyclic antidepressant simultaneously at low doses after appropriate drug washout, then alternately increase doses of these agents every few days to a week as tolerated

- Although very strict dietary and concomitant drug restrictions must be observed to prevent hypertensive crises and serotonin syndrome, the most common side effects of MAOI/ tricyclic or tetracyclic combinations may be weight gain and orthostatic hypotension
- Patients on tricyclics/tetracyclics should be aware that they may experience symptoms such as photosensitivity or blue-green urine
- SSRIs may be more effective than TCAs/tetracyclics in women, and TCAs/tetracyclics may be more effective than SSRIs in men
- ✳ May have a more rapid onset of action than some other TCAs/tetracyclics
- Since tricyclic/tetracyclic antidepressants are substrates for CYP450 2D6, and 7% of the population (especially Caucasians) may have a genetic variant leading to reduced activity of 2D6, such patients may not safely tolerate normal doses of tricyclic/tetracyclic antidepressants and may require dose reduction
- Phenotypic testing may be necessary to detect this genetic variant prior to dosing with a tricyclic/tetracyclic antidepressant, especially in vulnerable populations such as children, elderly, cardiac populations, and those on concomitant medications
- Patients who seem to have extraordinarily severe side effects at normal or low doses may have this phenotypic CYP450 2D6 variant and require low doses or switching to another antidepressant not metabolized by 2D6

Suggested Reading

Anderson IM. Meta-analytical studies on new antidepressants. Br Med Bull. 2001; 57:161–178.

Anderson IM. Selective serotonin reuptake inhibitors versus tricyclic antidepressants: a meta-analysis of efficacy and tolerability. J Aff Disorders. 2000;58:19–36.

Kane JM, Lieberman J. The efficacy of amoxapine, maprotiline, and trazodone in comparison to imipramine and amitriptyline: a review of the literature. Psychopharmacol Bull. 1984;20:240–9.

MILNACIPRAN

THERAPEUTICS

Brands • Toledomin
• Ixel
see index for additional brand names

Generic? No

Class

• SNRI (dual serotonin and norepinephrine reuptake inhibitor); antidepressant; chronic pain treatment

Commonly Prescribed For
(bold for FDA approved)
• Major depressive disorder
• Fibromyalgia
• Neuropathic pain/chronic pain

How The Drug Works

• Boosts neurotransmitters serotonin, norepinephrine/noradrenaline, and dopamine
• Blocks serotonin reuptake pump (serotonin transporter), presumably increasing serotonergic neurotransmission
• Blocks norepinephrine reuptake pump (norepinephrine transporter), presumably increasing noradrenergic neurotransmission
• Presumably desensitizes both serotonin 1A receptors and beta adrenergic receptors
✳ Weak noncompetitive NMDA-receptor antagonist (high doses), which may contribute to actions in chronic pain
• Since dopamine is inactivated by norepinephrine reuptake in frontal cortex, which largely lacks dopamine transporters, milnacipran can increase dopamine neurotransmission in this part of the brain

How Long Until It Works

• Onset of therapeutic actions usually not immediate, but often delayed 2 to 4 weeks
• If it is not working within 6 to 8 weeks, it may require a dosage increase or it may not work at all
• May continue to work for many years to prevent relapse of symptoms in depression

If It Works

• The goal of treatment of depression is complete remission of current symptoms as well as prevention of future relapses
• The goal of treatment of fibromyalgia and chronic neuropathic pain is to reduce symptoms as much as possible, especially in combination with other treatments
• Treatment of depression most often reduces or even eliminates symptoms, but is not a cure since symptoms can recur after medicine stopped
• Treatment of fibromyalgia and chronic neuropathic pain may reduce symptoms, but rarely eliminates them completely, and is not a cure since symptoms can recur after medicine is stopped
• Continue treatment of depression until all symptoms are gone (remission)
• Once symptoms of depression are gone, continue treating for 1 year for the first episode of depression
• For second and subsequent episodes of depression, treatment may need to be indefinite
• Use in fibromyalgia and chronic neuropathic pain may also need to be indefinite, but long-term treatment is not well-studied in these conditions

If It Doesn't Work

• Many depressed patients only have a partial response where some symptoms are improved but others persist (especially insomnia, fatigue, and problems concentrating)
• Other depressed patients may be nonresponders, sometimes called treatment-resistant or treatment-refractory
• Some depressed patients who have an initial response may relapse even though they continue treatment, sometimes called "poop-out"
• Consider increasing dose, switching to another agent or adding an appropriate augmenting agent
• Consider psychotherapy
• Consider evaluation for another diagnosis or for a comorbid condition (e.g., medical illness, substance abuse, etc.)
• Some patients may experience apparent lack of consistent efficacy due to activation of latent or underlying bipolar disorder, and require antidepressant discontinuation and switch to a mood stabilizer

Best Augmenting Combos for Partial Response or Treatment-Resistance

- Augmentation experience is limited compared to other antidepressants
- Benzodiazepines can reduce insomnia and anxiety
- Adding other agents to milnacipran for treating depression could follow the same practice for augmenting SSRIs or other SNRIs if done by experts while monitoring carefully in difficult cases
- Although no controlled studies and little clinical experience, adding other agents for treating fibromyalgia and chronic neuropathic pain could theoretically include gabapentin, tiagabine, other anticonvulsants, or even opiates if done by experts while monitoring carefully in difficult cases
- Mirtazapine, bupropion, reboxetine, atomoxetine (use combinations of antidepressants with caution as this may activate bipolar disorder and suicidal ideation)
- Modafinil, especially for fatigue, sleepiness, and lack of concentration
- Mood stabilizers or atypical antipsychotics for bipolar depression, psychotic depression or treatment-resistant depression
- Hypnotics or trazodone for insomnia
- Classically, lithium, buspirone, or thyroid hormone

Tests

- Check blood pressure before initiating treatment and regularly during treatment

SIDE EFFECTS

How Drug Causes Side Effects

- Theoretically due to increases in serotonin and norepinephrine concentrations at receptors in parts of the brain and body other than those that cause therapeutic actions (e.g., unwanted actions of serotonin in sleep centers causing insomnia, unwanted actions of norepinephrine on acetylcholine release causing urinary retention or constipation)
- Most side effects are immediate but often go away with time

Notable Side Effects

- Most side effects increase with higher doses, at least transiently
- Headache, nervousness, insomnia, sedation
- Nausea, diarrhea, decreased appetite
- Sexual dysfunction (abnormal ejaculation/orgasm, impotence)
- Asthenia, sweating
- SIADH (syndrome of inappropriate antidiuretic hormone secretion)
- Dose-dependent increased blood pressure
- Dry mouth, constipation
- Dysuria, urological complaints, urinary hesitancy, urinary retention
- Increase in heart rate
- Palpitations

Life Threatening or Dangerous Side Effects

- Rare induction of mania
- Rare activation of suicidal ideation and behavior (suicidality)
- Rare seizures

Weight Gain

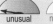

unusual   not unusual   common   problematic

- Reported but not expected

Sedation

unusual   not unusual   **common**   problematic

- Many experience and/or can be significant in amount

What To Do About Side Effects

- Wait
- Wait
- Wait
- Lower the dose
- In a few weeks, switch or add other drugs

Best Augmenting Agents for Side Effects

- For urinary hesitancy, give an alpha 1 blocker such as tamsulosin or naftopidil
- Often best to try another antidepressant monotherapy prior to resorting to augmentation strategies to treat side effects
- Trazodone or a hypnotic for insomnia

- Bupropion, sildenafil, vardenafil, or tadalafil for sexual dysfunction
- Benzodiazepines for anxiety, agitation
- Mirtazapine for insomnia, agitation, and gastrointestinal side effects
- Many side effects are dose-dependent (i.e., they increase as dose increases, or they reemerge until tolerance re-develops)
- Many side effects are time-dependent (i.e., they start immediately upon dosing and upon each dose increase, but go away with time)
- Activation and agitation may represent the induction of a bipolar state, especially a mixed dysphoric bipolar II condition sometimes associated with suicidal ideation, and require the addition of lithium, a mood stabilizer or an atypical antipsychotic, and/or discontinuation of milnacipran

DOSING AND USE

Usual Dosage Range
- 30–200 mg/day in 2 doses

Dosage Forms
- Capsule 25 mg, 50 mg (France, other European countries, and worldwide markets)
- Capsule 15 mg, 25 mg, 50 mg (Japan)

How to Dose
- Should be administered in 2 divided doses
- Begin at 25 mg twice daily and increase as necessary and as tolerated up to 100 mg twice daily; maximum dose 300 mg/day

 Dosing Tips

✳ Once daily dosing has far less consistent efficacy, so only give as twice daily
- Higher doses (>200 mg/day) not consistently effective in all studies of depression
- Nevertheless, some patients respond better to higher doses (200–300 mg/day) than to lower doses
- Different doses in different countries
- Different doses in different indications and different populations

- Preferred dose for depression may be 50 mg twice daily to 100 mg twice daily in France
- Preferred dose for depression in the elderly may be 15 mg twice daily to 25 mg twice daily in Japan
- Preferred dosing for depression in other adults may be 25 mg twice daily to 50 mg twice daily in Japan
- Preferred dose for fibromyalgia may be 100 mg twice daily
✳ Thus, clinicians must be aware that titration of twice daily dosing across a 10-fold range (30 mg – 300 mg total daily dose) can optimize milnacipran's efficacy in broad clinical use
- Patients with agitation or anxiety may require slower titration to optimize tolerability
- Higher doses usually well tolerated in fibromyalgia patients
- No pharmacokinetic drug interactions (not an inhibitor of CYP450 2D6 or 3A4)
- As milnacipran is a more potent norepinephrine reuptake inhibitor than a serotonin reuptake inhibitor, some patients may require dosing at the higher end of the dosing range to obtain robust dual SNRI actions
- At high doses, NMDA glutamate antagonist actions may be a factor

Overdose
- Vomiting, hypertension, sedation, tachycardia
- The emetic effect of high doses of milnacipran may reduce the risk of serious adverse effects

Long-Term Use
- Safe

Habit Forming
- No

How to Stop
- Taper is prudent, but usually not necessary

Pharmacokinetics
- Half-life 8 hours
- No active metabolite

Drug Interactions

- Tramadol increases the risk of seizures in patients taking an antidepressant
- Can cause a fatal "serotonin syndrome" when combined with MAO inhibitors, so do not use with MAO inhibitors or for at least 14 days after MAOIs are stopped
- Do not start an MAO inhibitor for at least 2 weeks after discontinuing milnacipran
- Switching from or addition of other norepinephrine reuptake inhibitors should be done with caution, as the additive pro-noradrenergic effects may enhance therapeutic actions in depression, but also enhance noradrenergically-mediated side effects
- Few known adverse pharmacokinetic drug interactions

Other Warnings/ Precautions

- Use with caution in patients with history of seizures
- Use with caution in patients with bipolar disorder unless treated with concomitant mood stabilizing agent
- When treating children, carefully weigh the risks and benefits of pharmacological treatment against the risks and benefits of nontreatment with antidepressants and make sure to document this in the patient's chart
- Distribute the brochures provided by the FDA and the drug companies
- Warn patients and their caregivers about the possibility of activating side effects and advise them to report such symptoms immediately
- Monitor patients for activation of suicidal ideation, especially children and adolescents

Do Not Use

- If patient has uncontrolled narrow angle-closure glaucoma
- If patient is taking an MAO inhibitor
- If there is a proven allergy to milnacipran

Renal Impairment

- Should receive lower doses; amount of dose adjustment related to degree of impairment

Hepatic Impairment

- No dose adjustment necessary

Cardiac Impairment

- Drug should be used with caution

Elderly

- Some patients may tolerate lower doses better

Children and Adolescents

- Carefully weigh the risks and benefits of pharmacological treatment against the risks and benefits of nontreatment with antidepressants and make sure to document this in the patient's chart
- Monitor patients face-to-face regularly, particularly during the first several weeks of treatment
- Use with caution, observing for activation of known or unknown bipolar disorder and/or suicidal ideation, and inform parents or guardian of this risk so they can help observe child or adolescent patients
- Not well-studied

Pregnancy

- Not generally recommended for use during pregnancy, especially during first trimester
- Nonetheless, continuous treatment during pregnancy may be necessary and has not been proven to be harmful to the fetus
- Must weigh the risk of treatment (first trimester fetal development, third trimester newborn delivery) to the child against the risk of no treatment (recurrence of depression, maternal health, infant bonding) to the mother and child
- For many patients this may mean continuing treatment during pregnancy
- Neonates exposed to SSRIs or SNRIs late in the third trimester have developed complications requiring prolonged hospitalization, respiratory support, and tube feeding; reported symptoms are consistent with either a direct toxic effect

of SSRIs and SNRIs or, possibly, a drug discontinuation syndrome, and include respiratory distress, cyanosis, apnea, seizures, temperature instability, feeding difficulty, vomiting, hypoglycemia, hypotonia, hypertonia, hyperreflexia, tremor, jitteriness, irritability, and constant crying

Breast Feeding

- Unknown if milnacipran is secreted in human breast milk, but all psychotropics assumed to be secreted in breast milk
- Immediate postpartum period is a high-risk time for depression, especially in women who have had prior depressive episodes, so drug may need to be reinstituted late in the third trimester or shortly after childbirth to prevent a recurrence during the postpartum period
- Must weigh benefits of breast feeding with risks and benefits of antidepressant treatment versus non-treatment to both the infant and the mother
- For many patients, this may mean continuing treatment during breast feeding

THE ART OF PSYCHOPHARMACOLOGY

Potential Advantages

- Patients with retarded depression
- Patients with hypersomnia
- Patients with atypical depression
- Patients with depression may have higher remission rates on SNRIs than on SSRIs
- Depressed patients with somatic symptoms, fatigue, and pain
- Fibromyalgia, chronic pain syndrome

Potential Disadvantages

- Patients with urologic disorders, prostate disorders
- Patients with borderline or uncontrolled hypertension
- Patients with agitation and anxiety (short-term)

Primary Target Symptoms

- Depressed mood

- Energy, motivation, and interest
- Sleep disturbance
- Physical symptoms
- Pain

 Pearls

- Not studied in stress urinary incontinence
- Not well studied in ADHD or anxiety disorders, but may be effective
- ✳ Has greater potency for norepinephrine reuptake blockade than for serotonin reuptake blockade, but this is of unclear clinical significance as a differentiating feature from other SNRIs, although it might contribute to its therapeutic activity in fibromyalgia and chronic pain
- ✳ Onset of action in fibromyalgia may be somewhat faster than depression (i.e., 2 weeks rather than 2–8 weeks)
- Therapeutic actions in fibromyalgia are partial, with symptom reduction but not necessarily remission of painful symptoms in many patients
- ✳ Potent noradrenergic actions may account for possibly higher incidence of sweating and urinary hesitancy than other SNRIs
- Urinary hesitancy more common in men than women and in older men than in younger men
- Alpha 1 antagonists such as tamsulosin or naftopidil can reverse urinary hesitancy or retention
- Alpha 1 antagonists given prophylactically may prevent urinary hesitancy or retention in patients at higher risk, such as elderly men with borderline urine flow
- May be better tolerated than tricyclic or tetracyclic antidepressants in the treatment of fibromyalgia or other chronic pain syndromes
- No pharmacokinetic interactions or elevations in plasma drug levels of tricyclic or tetracyclic antidepressants when adding or switching to or from milnacipran

Suggested Reading

Bisserbe JC. Clinical utility of milnacipran in comparison with other antidepressants. Int Clin Psychopharmacol 2002;17 Suppl 1:S43–50.

Montgomery SA, Prost JF, Solles A, Briley M. Efficacy and tolerability of milnacipran: an overview. Int Clin Psychopharmacol 1996;11 Suppl 4:47–51.

Puozzo C, Panconi E, Deprez D. Pharmacology and pharmacokinetics of milnacipran. Int Clin Psychopharmacol 2002;17 Suppl 1:S25–35.

Spencer CM, Wilde MI. Milnacipran. A review of its use in depression. Drugs 1998; 56:405–27.

MIRTAZAPINE

THERAPEUTICS

Brands • Remeron
see index for additional brand names

Generic? Yes

Class
- Alpha 2 antagonist; NaSSA (noradrenaline and specific serotonergic agent); dual serotonin and norepinephrine agent; antidepressant

Commonly Prescribed For
(bold for FDA approved)
- **Major depressive disorder**
- Panic disorder
- Generalized anxiety disorder
- Posttraumatic stress disorder

How The Drug Works
- Boost neurotransmitters serotonin and norepinephrine/noradrenaline
- Blocks alpha 2 adrenergic presynaptic receptor, thereby increasing norepinephrine neurotransmission
- Blocks alpha 2 adrenergic presynaptic receptor on serotonin neurons (heteroreceptors), thereby increasing serotonin neurotransmission
- This is a novel mechanism independent of norepinephrine and serotonin reuptake blockade
- Blocks 5HT2A, 5HT2C, and 5HT3 serotonin receptors
- Blocks H1 histamine receptors

How Long Until It Works
✳ Actions on insomnia and anxiety can start shortly after initiation of dosing
- Onset of therapeutic actions in depression, however, is usually not immediate, but often delayed 2 to 4 weeks
- If it is not working within 6 to 8 weeks for depression, it may require a dosage increase or it may not work at all
- May continue to work for many years to prevent relapse of symptoms

If It Works
- The goal of treatment is complete remission of current symptoms as well as prevention of future relapses
- Treatment most often reduces or even eliminates symptoms, but not a cure since symptoms can recur after medicine stopped
- Continue treatment until all symptoms are gone (remission)
- Once symptoms gone, continue treating for 1 year for the first episode of depression
- For second and subsequent episodes of depression, treatment may need to be indefinite
- Use in anxiety disorders may also need to be indefinite

If It Doesn't Work
- Many patients only have a partial response where some symptoms are improved but others persist (especially insomnia, fatigue, and problems concentrating)
- Other patients may be nonresponders, sometimes called treatment-resistant or treatment-refractory
- Consider increasing dose, switching to another agent or adding an appropriate augmenting agent
- Consider psychotherapy
- Consider evaluation for another diagnosis or for a comorbid condition (e.g., medical illness, substance abuse, etc.)
- Some patients may experience apparent lack of consistent efficacy due to activation of latent or underlying bipolar disorder, and require antidepressant discontinuation and a switch to a mood stabilizer

Best Augmenting Combos for Partial Response or Treatment-Resistance
- SSRIs, bupropion, reboxetine, atomoxetine (use combinations of antidepressants with caution as this may activate bipolar disorder and suicidal ideation)
✳ Venlafaxine ("California rocket fuel"; a potentially powerful dual serotonin and norepinephrine combination, but observe for activation of bipolar disorder and suicidal ideation)
- Modafinil, especially for fatigue, sleepiness, and lack of concentration

- Mood stabilizers or atypical antipsychotics for bipolar depression, psychotic depression or treatment-resistant depression
- Benzodiazepines
- Hypnotics or trazodone for insomnia

Tests

- None for healthy individuals
- May need liver function tests for those with hepatic abnormalities before initiating treatment
- May need to monitor blood count during treatment for those with blood dyscrasias, leucopenia, or granulocytopenia
- Since some antidepressants such as mirtazapine can be associated with significant weight gain, before starting treatment, weigh all patients and determine if the patient is already overweight (BMI>25.0–29.9) or obese (BMI>30)
- Before giving a drug that can cause weight gain to an overweight or obese patient, consider determining whether the patient already has pre-diabetes (fasting plasma glucose 100–125 mg/dl), diabetes (fasting plasma glucose >126 mg/dl), or dyslipidemia (increased total cholesterol, LDL cholesterol and triglycerides; decreased HDL cholesterol), and treat or refer such patients for treatment, including nutrition and weight management, physical activity counseling, smoking cessation, and medical management
- ✳ Monitor weight and BMI during treatment
- ✳ While giving a drug to a patient who has gained >5% of initial weight, consider evaluating for the presence of pre-diabetes, diabetes, or dyslipidemia, or consider switching to a different antipsychotic

SIDE EFFECTS

How Drug Causes Side Effects

- Most side effects are immediate but often go away with time
- ✳ Histamine 1 receptor antagonism may explain sedative effects
- ✳ Histamine 1 receptor antagonism plus 5HT2C antagonism may explain some aspects of weight gain

Notable Side Effects

- Dry mouth, constipation, increased appetite, weight gain
- Sedation, dizziness, abnormal dreams, confusion
- Flu-like symptoms (may indicate low white blood cell or granulocyte count)
- Change in urinary function
- Hypotension

 ### Life Threatening or Dangerous Side Effects

- Rare seizures
- Rare induction of mania
- Rare activation of suicidal ideation and behavior (suicidality)

Weight Gain

unusual   not unusual   common   problematic

- Many experience and/or can be significant in amount

Sedation

unusual   not unusual   common   problematic

- Many experience and/or can be significant in amount

What To Do About Side Effects

- Wait
- Wait
- Wait
- Switch to another drug

Best Augmenting Agents for Side Effects

- Often best to try another antidepressant monotherapy prior to resorting to augmentation strategies to treat side effects
- Many side effects are dose-dependent (i.e., they increase as dose increases, or they reemerge until tolerance re-develops)
- Many side effects are time-dependent (i.e., they start immediately upon dosing and upon each dose increase, but go away with time)
- Trazodone or a hypnotic for insomnia
- Many side effects cannot be improved with an augmenting agent
- Activation and agitation may represent the induction of a bipolar state, especially a

mixed dysphoric bipolar II condition sometimes associated with suicidal ideation, and require the addition of lithium, a mood stabilizer or an atypical antipsychotic, and/or discontinuation of mirtazapine

DOSING AND USE

Usual Dosage Range
- 15–45 mg at night

Dosage Forms
- Tablet 15 mg scored, 30 mg scored, 45 mg
- SolTab disintegrating tablet 15 mg, 30 mg, 45 mg

How to Dose
- Initial 15 mg/day in the evening; increase every 1–2 weeks until desired efficacy is reached; maximum generally 45 mg/day

 Dosing Tips
- Sedation may not worsen as dose increases
- ✳ Breaking a 15 mg tablet in half and administering 7.5 mg dose may actually increase sedation
- Some patients require more than 45 mg daily, including up to 90 mg in difficult patients who tolerate these doses
- If intolerable anxiety, insomnia, agitation, akathisia, or activation occur either upon dosing initiation or discontinuation, consider the possibility of activated bipolar disorder and switch to a mood stabilizer or an atypical antipsychotic

Overdose
- Rarely lethal; all fatalities have involved other medications; symptoms include sedation, disorientation, memory impairment, rapid heartbeat

Long-Term Use
- Safe

Habit Forming
- Not expected

How to Stop
- Taper is prudent to avoid withdrawal effects, but tolerance, dependence, and withdrawal effects not reliably reported

Pharmacokinetics
- Half-life 20–40 hours

 Drug Interactions
- Tramadol increases the risk of seizures in patients taking an antidepressant
- No significant pharmacokinetic drug interactions
- Can cause a fatal "serotonin syndrome" when combined with MAO inhibitors, so do not use with MAO inhibitors or for at least 14 days after MAOIs are stopped
- Do not start an MAO inhibitor for at least 2 weeks after discontinuing mirtazapine

 Other Warnings/ Precautions
- Drug may lower white blood cell count (rare; may not be increased compared to other antidepressants but controlled studies lacking; not a common problem reported in post marketing surveillance)
- Drug may increase cholesterol
- May cause photosensitivity
- Avoid alcohol, which may increase sedation and cognitive and motor effects
- Use with caution in patients with history of seizures
- Use with caution in patients with bipolar disorder unless treated with concomitant mood stabilizing agent
- When treating children, carefully weigh the risks and benefits of pharmacological treatment against the risks and benefits of nontreatment with antidepressants and make sure to document this in the patient's chart
- Distribute the brochures provided by the FDA and the drug companies
- Warn patients and their caregivers about the possibility of activating side effects and advise them to report such symptoms immediately
- Monitor patients for activation of suicidal ideation, especially children and adolescents

Do Not Use

- If patient is taking an MAO inhibitor
- If there is a proven allergy to mirtazapine

SPECIAL POPULATIONS

Renal Impairment

- Drug should be used with caution

Hepatic Impairment

- Drug should be used with caution
- May require lower dose

Cardiac Impairment

- Drug should be used with caution
- The potential risk of hypotension should be considered

Elderly

- Some patients may tolerate lower doses better

Children and Adolescents

- Carefully weigh the risks and benefits of pharmacological treatment against the risks and benefits of nontreatment with antidepressants and make sure to document this in the patient's chart
- Monitor patients face-to-face regularly, particularly during the first several weeks of treatment
- Use with caution, observing for activation of known or unknown bipolar disorder and/or suicidal ideation, and inform parents or guardian of this risk so they can help observe child or adolescent patients
- Safety and efficacy have not been established

Pregnancy

- Risk Category C [some animal studies show adverse effects; no controlled studies in humans]
- Not generally recommended for use during pregnancy, especially during first trimester
- Must weigh the risk of treatment (first trimester fetal development, third trimester newborn delivery) to the child against the risk of no treatment (recurrence of depression, maternal health, infant bonding) to the mother and child
- For many patients this may mean continuing treatment during pregnancy

Breast Feeding

- Unknown if mirtazapine is secreted in human breast milk, but all psychotropics assumed to be secreted in breast milk
- If child becomes irritable or sedated, breast feeding or drug may need to be discontinued
- Immediate postpartum period is a high-risk time for depression, especially in women who have had prior depressive episodes, so drug may need to be reinstituted late in the third trimester or shortly after childbirth to prevent a recurrence during the postpartum period
- Must weigh benefits of breast feeding with risks and benefits of antidepressant treatment versus non-treatment to both the infant and the mother
- For many patients, this may mean continuing treatment during breast feeding

THE ART OF PSYCHOPHARMACOLOGY

Potential Advantages

- Patients particularly concerned about sexual side effects
- Patients with symptoms of anxiety
- Patients on concomitant medications
- As an augmenting agent to boost the efficacy of other antidepressants

Potential Disadvantages

- Patients particularly concerned about gaining weight
- Patients with low energy

Primary Target Symptoms

- Depressed mood
- Sleep disturbance
- Anxiety

Pearls

- ✳ Adding alpha 2 antagonism to agents that block serotonin and/or norepinephrine reuptake may be synergistic for severe depression
- Adding mirtazapine to venlafaxine or SSRIs may reverse drug-induced anxiety and insomnia

- Adding mirtazapine's 5HT3 antagonism to venlafaxine or SSRIs may reverse drug-induced nausea, diarrhea, stomach cramps, and gastrointestinal side effects
- SSRIs, venlafaxine, bupropion, phentermine, or stimulants may mitigate mirtazapine-induced weight gain
- If weight gain has not occurred by week 6 of treatment, it is less likely for there to be significant weight gain
- Has been demonstrated to have an earlier onset of action than SSRIs
- ✳ Does not affect the CYP450 system, and so may be preferable in patients requiring concomitant medications
- Preliminary evidence suggests efficacy as an augmenting agent to haloperidol in treating negative symptoms of schizophrenia
- Anecdotal reports of efficacy in recurrent brief depression
- Weight gain as a result of mirtazapine treatment is more likely in women than in men, and before menopause rather than after
- ✳ May cause sexual dysfunction only infrequently
- Patients can have carryover sedation and intoxicated-like feeling if particularly sensitive to sedative side effects when initiating dosing
- Rarely, patients may complain of visual "trails" or after-images on mirtazapine

Suggested Reading

Anttila SA, Leinonen EV. A review of the pharmacological and clinical profile of mirtazapine. CNS Drug Rev 2001;7(3):249–64.

Benkert O, Muller M, Szegedi A. An overview of the clinical efficacy of mirtazapine. Hum Psychopharmacol. 2002;17 Suppl 1:S23–6.

Falkai P. Mirtazapine: other indications. J Clin Psychiatry 1999;60(suppl 17):36–40.

Fawcett J, Barkin RL. A meta-analysis of eight randomized, double-blind, controlled clinical trials of mirtazapine for the treatment of patients with major depression and symptoms of anxiety. J Clin Psychiatry. 1998; 59:123–127.

Masand PS, Gupta S. Long-term side effects of newer-generation antidepressants: SSRIS, venlafaxine, nefazodone, bupropion, and mirtazapine. Ann Clin Psychiatry 2002; 14:175–82.

MOCLOBEMIDE

Brands • Aurorix
• Arima
• Manerix
see index for additional brand names

Generic? No

Class
• Reversible inhibitor of monoamine oxidase A (MAO-A) (RIMA)

Commonly Prescribed For
(bold for FDA approved)
• Depression
• Social anxiety disorder

 How The Drug Works
• Reversibly blocks MAO-A from breaking down norepinephrine, dopamine, and serotonin
• This presumably boosts noradrenergic, serotonergic, and dopaminergic neurotransmission
• MAO-A inhibition predominates unless significant concentrations of monoamines build up (e.g., due to dietary tyramine), in which case MAO-A inhibition is theoretically reversed

How Long Until It Works
• Onset of therapeutic actions usually not immediate, but often delayed 2 to 4 weeks
• If it is not working within 6 to 8 weeks, it may require a dosage increase or it may not work at all
• May continue to work for many years to prevent relapse of symptoms

If It Works
• The goal of treatment is complete remission of current symptoms as well as prevention of future relapses
• Treatment most often reduces or even eliminates symptoms, but not a cure since symptoms can recur after medicine stopped
• Continue treatment until all symptoms are gone (remission)
• Once symptoms gone, continue treating for 1 year for the first episode of depression

• For second and subsequent episodes of depression, treatment may need to be indefinite
• Use in anxiety disorders may also need to be indefinite

If It Doesn't Work
• Many patients only have a partial response where some symptoms are improved but others persist (especially insomnia, fatigue, and problems concentrating)
• Other patients may be nonresponders, sometimes called treatment-resistant or treatment-refractory
• Consider increasing dose, switching to another agent or adding an appropriate augmenting agent
• Consider psychotherapy
• Consider evaluation for another diagnosis or for a comorbid condition (e.g., medical illness, substance abuse, etc.)
• Some patients may experience apparent lack of consistent efficacy due to activation of latent or underlying bipolar disorder, and require antidepressant discontinuation and a switch to a mood stabilizer

 Best Augmenting Combos for Partial Response or Treatment-Resistance
✳ Augmentation of MAOIs has not been systematically studied, and this is something for the expert, to be done with caution and with careful monitoring, but may be somewhat less risky with moclobemide than with other MAO inhibitors
✳ A stimulant such as d-amphetamine or methylphenidate (with caution; may activate bipolar disorder and suicidal ideation)
• Lithium
• Mood stabilizing anticonvulsants
• Atypical antipsychotics (with special caution for those agents with monoamine reuptake blocking properties, such as ziprasidone and zotepine)

Tests
• Patients should be monitored for changes in blood pressure

SIDE EFFECTS

How Drug Causes Side Effects
- Theoretically due to increases in monoamines in parts of the brain and body and at receptors other than those that cause therapeutic actions (e.g., unwanted actions of serotonin in sleep centers causing insomnia, unwanted actions of norepinephrine on vascular smooth muscle causing changes in blood pressure)
- Side effects are generally immediate, but immediate side effects often disappear in time

Notable Side Effects
- Insomnia, dizziness, agitation, anxiety, restlessness
- Dry mouth, diarrhea, constipation, nausea, vomiting
- Galactorrhea
- Rare hypertension

 Life Threatening or Dangerous Side Effects
- Hypertensive crisis (especially when MAOIs are used with certain tyramine containing foods – reduced risk compared to irreversible MAOIs)
- Induction of mania
- Rare activation of suicidal ideation and behavior (suicidality)
- Seizures

Weight Gain

unusual / not unusual / common / problematic
- Reported but not expected

Sedation

unusual / not unusual / common / problematic
- Occurs in significant minority

What To Do About Side Effects
- Wait
- Wait
- Wait
- Lower the dose
- Switch to an SSRI or newer antidepressant

Best Augmenting Agents for Side Effects
- Trazodone (with caution) for insomnia
- Benzodiazepines for insomnia
- ✳ Single oral or sublingual dose of a calcium channel blocker (e.g., nifedipine) for urgent treatment of hypertension due to drug interaction or dietary tyramine
- Many side effects cannot be improved with an augmenting agent

DOSING AND USE

Usual Dosage Range
- 300–600 mg/day

Dosage Forms
- Tablet 100 mg scored, 150 mg scored

How to Dose
- Initial 300 mg/day in 3 divided doses after a meal; increase dose gradually; maximum dose generally 600 mg/day; minimum dose generally 150 mg/day

 Dosing Tips
- ✳ At higher doses, moclobemide also inhibits MAO-B and thereby loses its selectivity for MAO-A, with uncertain clinical consequences
- ✳ Taking moclobemide after meals as opposed to before may minimize the chances of interactions with tyramine
- May be less toxic in overdose than tricyclic antidepressants and older MAOIs
- Clinical duration of action may be longer than biological half-life and allow twice daily dosing in some patients, or even once daily dosing, especially at lower doses

Overdose
- Agitation, aggression, behavioral disturbances, gastrointestinal irritation

Long-Term Use
- MAOIs may lose efficacy long-term

Habit Forming
- Some patients have developed dependence to MAOIs

How to Stop
- Taper not generally necessary

Pharmacokinetics

- Partially metabolized by CYP450 2C19 and 2D6
- Inactive metabolites
- Elimination half-life approximately 1–4 hours
- Clinical duration of action at least 24 hours

 Drug Interactions

- Tramadol may increase the risk of seizures in patients taking an MAO inhibitor
- Can cause a fatal "serotonin syndrome" when combined with drugs that block serotonin reuptake (e.g., SSRIs, SNRIs, sibutramine, tramadol, etc.), so do not use with a serotonin reuptake inhibitor or for up to 5 weeks after stopping the serotonin reuptake inhibitor
- Hypertensive crisis with headache, intracranial bleeding, and death may result from combining MAO inhibitors with sympathomimetic drugs (e.g., amphetamines, methylphenidate, cocaine, dopamine, epinephrine, norepinephrine, and related compounds methyldopa, levodopa, L-tryptophan, L-tyrosine, and phenylalanine)
- Excitation, seizures, delirium, hyperpyrexia, circulatory collapse, coma, and death may result from combining MAO inhibitors with mepiridine or dextromethorphan
- Do not combine with another MAO inhibitor, alcohol, buspirone, bupropion, or guanethidine
- Adverse drug reactions can result from combining MAO inhibitors with tricyclic/tetracyclic antidepressants and related compounds, including carbamazepine, cyclobenzaprine, and mirtazapine, and should be avoided except by experts to treat difficult cases
- MAO inhibitors in combination with spinal anesthesia may cause combined hypotensive effects
- Combination of MAOIs and CNS depressants may enhance sedation and hypotension
- Cimetidine may increase plasma concentrations of moclobemide
- Moclobemide may enhance the effects of non-steroidal anti-inflammatory drugs such as ibuprofen
- Risk of hypertensive crisis may be increased if moclobemide is used concurrently with levodopa or other dopaminergic agents

 Other Warnings/ Precautions

- Use still requires low tyramine diet, although more tyramine may be tolerated with moclobemide than with other MAO inhibitors before eliciting a hypertensive reaction
- Patients taking MAO inhibitors should avoid high protein food that has undergone protein breakdown by aging, fermentation, pickling, smoking, or bacterial contamination
- Patients taking MAO inhibitors should avoid cheeses (especially aged varieties), pickled herring, beer, wine, liver, yeast extract, dry sausage, hard salami, pepperoni, Lebanon bologna, pods of broad beans (fava beans), yogurt, and excessive use of caffeine and chocolate
- Patient and prescriber must be vigilant to potential interactions with any drug, including antihypertensives and over-the-counter cough/cold preparations
- Over-the-counter medications to avoid include cough and cold preparations, including those containing dextromethorphan, nasal decongestants (tablets, drops, or spray), hay-fever medications, sinus medications, asthma inhalant medications, anti-appetite medications, weight reducing preparations, "pep" pills
- Use cautiously in hypertensive patients
- Moclobemide is not recommended for use in patients who cannot be monitored closely
- When treating children, carefully weigh the risks and benefits of pharmacological treatment against the risks and benefits of nontreatment with antidepressants and make sure to document this in the patient's chart
- Distribute the brochures provided by the FDA and the drug companies
- Warn patients and their caregivers about the possibility of activating side effects and advise them to report such symptoms immediately

- Monitor patients for activation of suicidal ideation, especially children and adolescents

Do Not Use

- If patient is taking meperidine (pethidine)
- If patient is taking a sympathomimetic agent or taking guanethidine
- If patient is taking another MAOI
- If patient is taking any agent that can inhibit serotonin reuptake (e.g., SSRIs, sibutramine, tramadol, milnacipran, duloxetine, venlafaxine, clomipramine, etc.)
- If patient is in an acute confusional state
- If patient has pheochromocytoma or thyrotoxicosis
- If patient has frequent or severe headaches
- If patient is undergoing elective surgery and requires general anesthesia
- If there is a proven allergy to moclobemide

SPECIAL POPULATIONS

Renal Impairment

- Use with caution

Hepatic Impairment

- Plasma concentrations are increased
- May require one-half to one-third of usual adult dose

Cardiac Impairment

- Cardiac impairment may require lower than usual adult dose
- Patients with angina pectoris or coronary artery disease should limit their exertion

Elderly

- Elderly patients may have greater sensitivity to adverse effects

 ### Children and Adolescents

- Not recommended for use under age 18
- Carefully weigh the risks and benefits of pharmacological treatment against the risks and benefits of nontreatment with antidepressants and make sure to document this in the patient's chart
- Monitor patients face-to-face regularly, particularly during the first several weeks of treatment
- Use with caution, observing for activation of known or unknown bipolar disorder

and/or suicidal ideation, and inform parents or guardian of this risk so they can help observe child or adolescent patients

 ### Pregnancy

- Not generally recommended for use during pregnancy, especially during first trimester
- Should evaluate patient for treatment with an antidepressant with a better risk/benefit ratio

Breast Feeding

- Some drug is found in mother's breast milk
- Effects on infant are unknown
- Immediate postpartum period is a high-risk time for depression, especially in women who have had prior depressive episodes, so drug may need to be reinstituted late in the third trimester or shortly after childbirth to prevent a recurrence during the postpartum period
- Should evaluate patient for treatment with an antidepressant with a better risk/benefit ratio

THE ART OF PSYCHOPHARMACOLOGY

Potential Advantages

- Atypical depression
- Severe depression
- Treatment-resistant depression or anxiety disorders

Potential Disadvantages

- Patients noncompliant with dietary restrictions, concomitant drug restrictions, and twice daily dosing after meals

Primary Target Symptoms

- Depressed mood

 ### Pearls

- MAOIs are generally reserved for second-line use after SSRIs, SNRIs, and combinations of newer antidepressants have failed
- Patient should be advised not to take any prescription or over-the-counter drugs without consulting their doctor because of possible drug interactions with the MAOI

- Headache is often the first symptom of hypertensive crisis
- Moclobemide has a much reduced risk of interactions with tyramine than nonselective MAOIs
- Especially at higher doses of moclobemide, foods with high tyramine need to be avoided: dry sausage, pickled herring, liver, broad bean pods, sauerkraut, cheese, yogurt, alcoholic beverages, nonalcoholic beer and wine, chocolate, caffeine, meat and fish
- The rigid dietary restrictions may reduce compliance
* May be a safer alternative to classical irreversible nonselective MAO-A and MAO-B inhibitors with less propensity for tyramine and drug interactions and hepatotoxicity (although not entirely free of interactions)
- May not be as effective at low doses, and may have more side effects at higher doses
- Moclobemide's profile at higher doses may be more similar to classical MAOIs
- MAOIs are a viable second-line treatment option in depression, but are not frequently used
* Myths about the danger of dietary tyramine can be exaggerated, but prohibitions against concomitant drugs often not followed closely enough
- Orthostatic hypotension, insomnia, and sexual dysfunction are often the most troublesome common side effects
* MAOIs should be for the expert, especially if combining with agents of potential risk (e.g., stimulants, trazodone, TCAs)
* MAOIs should not be neglected as therapeutic agents for the treatment-resistant
- Although generally prohibited, a heroic but potentially dangerous treatment for severely treatment-resistant patients is for an expert to give a tricyclic/tetracyclic antidepressant other than clomipramine simultaneously with an MAO inhibitor for patients who fail to respond to numerous other antidepressants
- Use of MAOIs with clomipramine is always prohibited because of the risk of serotonin syndrome and death
- Amoxapine may be the preferred trycyclic/tetracyclic antidepressant to combine with an MAOI in heroic cases due to its theoretically protective 5HT2A antagonist properties
- If this option is elected, start the MAOI with the tricyclic/tetracyclic antidepressant simultaneously at low doses after appropriate drug washout, then alternately increase doses of these agents every few days to a week as tolerated
- Although very strict dietary and concomitant drug restrictions must be observed to prevent hypertensive crises and serotonin syndrome, the most common side effects of MAOI and tricyclic/tetracyclic combinations may be weight gain and orthostatic hypotension

Suggested Reading

Amrein R, Martin JR, Cameron AM. Moclobemide in patients with dementia and depression. Adv Neurol 1999;80:509–19.

Fulton B, Benfield P. Moclobemide. An update of its pharmacological properties and therapeutic use. Drugs 1996;52:450–74.

Kennedy SH. Continuation and maintenance treatments in major depression: the neglected role of monoamine oxidase inhibitors. J Psychiatry Neurosci 1997;22:127–31.

Lippman SB, Nash K. Monoamine oxidase inhibitor update. Potential adverse food and drug interactions. Drug Saf 1990;5:195–204

Nutt D, Montgomery SA. Moclobemide in the treatment of social phobia. Int Clin Psychopharmacol 1996;11 (Suppl 3):77–82.

NEFAZODONE

THERAPEUTICS

Brands • Dutonin
see index for additional brand names

Generic? Yes

Class
• SARI (serotonin 2 antagonist/reuptake inhibitor); antidepressant

Commonly Prescribed For
(bold for FDA approved)
• **Depression**
• **Relapse prevention in MDD**
• Panic disorder
• Posttraumatic stress disorder

How The Drug Works
• Blocks serotonin 2A receptors potently
• Blocks serotonin reuptake pump (serotonin transporter) and norepinephrine reuptake pump (norepinephrine transporter) less potently

How Long Until It Works
• Can improve insomnia and anxiety early after initiating dosing
• Onset of therapeutic actions usually not immediate, but often delayed 2 to 4 weeks
• If it is not working within 6 to 8 weeks for depression, it may require a dosage increase or it may not work at all
• May continue to work for many years to prevent relapse of symptoms

If It Works
• The goal of treatment is complete remission of current symptoms as well as prevention of future relapses
• Treatment most often reduces or even eliminates symptoms, but not a cure since symptoms can recur after medicine stopped
• Continue treatment until all symptoms are gone (remission)
• Once symptoms gone, continue treating for 1 year for the first episode of depression
• For second and subsequent episodes of depression, treatment may need to be indefinite
• Use in anxiety disorders may also need to be indefinite

If It Doesn't Work
• Many patients only have a partial response where some symptoms are improved but others persist (especially insomnia, fatigue, and problems concentrating)
• Other patients may be nonresponders, sometimes called treatment-resistant or treatment-refractory
• Some patients who have an initial response may relapse even though they continue treatment, sometimes called "poop-out"
• Consider increasing dose, switching to another agent or adding an appropriate augmenting agent
• Consider psychotherapy, especially cognitive-behavioral psychotherapies, which have been specifically shown to enhance nefazodone's antidepressant actions
• Consider evaluation for another diagnosis or for a comorbid condition (e.g., medical illness, substance abuse, etc.)
• Some patients may experience apparent lack of consistent efficacy due to activation of latent or underlying bipolar disorder, and require antidepressant discontinuation and a switch to a mood stabilizer

Best Augmenting Combos for Partial Response or Treatment-Resistance
✳ Venlafaxine and escitalopram may be the best tolerated when switching or augmenting with a serotonin reuptake inhibitor, as neither is a potent CYP450 2D6 inhibitor (use combinations of antidepressants with caution as this may activate bipolar disorder and suicidal ideation)
• Modafinil, especially for fatigue, sleepiness, and lack of concentration
• Mood stabilizers or atypical antipsychotics for bipolar depression, psychotic depression or treatment-resistant depression
• Benzodiazepines for anxiety, but give alprazolam cautiously with nefazodone as alprazolam levels can be much higher in the presence of nefazodone
• Classically, lithium, buspirone, or thyroid hormone

Tests

✻ Liver function testing is not required but is often prudent given the small but finite risk of serious hepatoxicity

✻ However, to date no clinical strategy, including routine liver function tests, has been identified to reduce the risk of irreversible liver failure

SIDE EFFECTS

How Drug Causes Side Effects

• Blockade of alpha adrenergic 1 receptors may explain dizziness, sedation, and hypotension

• A metabolite of nefazodone, mCPP (meta-chloro-phenyl-piperazine), can cause side effects if its levels rise significantly

✻ If CYP450 2D6 is absent (7% of Caucasians lack CYP450 2D6) or inhibited (concomitant treatment with CYP450 2D6 inhibitors such as fluoxetine or paroxetine), increased levels of mCPP can form, leading to stimulation of 5HT2C receptors and causing dizziness, insomnia, and agitation

• Most side effects are immediate but often go away with time

Notable Side Effects

• Nausea, dry mouth, constipation, dyspepsia, increased appetite

• Headache, dizziness, vision changes, sedation, insomnia, agitation, confusion, memory impairment

• Ataxia, paresthesia, asthenia

• Cough increased

• Rare postural hypotension

Life Threatening or Dangerous Side Effects

• Rare seizures

• Rare induction of mania

• Rare activation of suicidal ideation and behavior (suicidality)

• Rare priapism (no causal relationship established)

• Hepatic failure requiring liver transplant and/or fatal

Weight Gain

unusual   not unusual   common   problematic

• Reported but not expected

Sedation

unusual   not unusual   common   problematic

• Many experience and/or can be significant in amount

What To Do About Side Effects

• Wait

• Wait

• Wait

• Take once-daily at night to reduce daytime sedation

• Lower the dose and try titrating again more slowly as tolerated

• Switch to another agent

Best Augmenting Agents for Side Effects

• Often best to try another antidepressant monotherapy prior to resorting to augmentation strategies to treat side effects

• Many side effects cannot be improved with an augmenting agent

• Many side effects are dose-dependent (i.e., they increase as dose increases, or they reemerge until tolerance re-develops)

• Many side effects are time-dependent (i.e., they start immediately upon dosing and upon each dose increase, but go away with time)

• Activation and agitation may represent the induction of a bipolar state, especially a mixed dysphoric bipolar II condition sometimes associated with suicidal ideation, and require the addition of lithium, a mood stabilizer or an atypical antipsychotic, and/or discontinuation of nefazodone

DOSING AND USE

Usual Dosage Range

• 300–600 mg/day

Dosage Forms

• Tablet 50 mg, 100 mg scored, 150 mg scored, 200 mg, 250 mg

How to Dose
- Initial dose 100 mg twice a day; increase by 100–200 mg/day each week until desired efficacy is reached; maximum dose 600 mg twice a day

 Dosing Tips
- Take care switching from or adding to SSRIs (especially fluoxetine or paroxetine) because of side effects due to the drug interaction
- Do not underdose the elderly
- Normally twice daily dosing, especially when initiating treatment
- Patients may tolerate all dosing once daily at night once titrated
- Often much more effective at 400–600 mg/day than at lower doses if tolerated
- Slow titration can enhance tolerability when initiating dosing

Overdose
- Rarely lethal; sedation, nausea, vomiting, low blood pressure

Long-Term Use
- Safe

Habit Forming
- No

How to Stop
- Taper is prudent to avoid withdrawal effects, but problems in withdrawal not common

Pharmacokinetics
- Half-life of parent compound is 2–4 hours
- Half-life of active mebatolites up to 12 hours
- Inhibits CYP450 3A4

 Drug Interactions
- Tramadol increases the risk of seizures in patients taking an antidepressant
- May interact with SSRIs such as paroxetine, fluoxetine, and others that inhibit CYP450 2D6
- ✳ Since a metabolite of nefazodone, mCPP, is a substrate of CYP450 2D6, combination of 2D6 inhibitors with nefazodone will raise mCPP levels, leading to stimulation of 5HT2C receptors and causing dizziness and agitation
- Can cause a fatal "serotonin syndrome" when combined with MAO inhibitors, so do not use with MAO inhibitors or for at least 14 days after MAOIs are stopped
- Do not start an MAO inhibitor for at least 2 weeks after discontinuing nefazodone
- Via CYP450 3A4 inhibition, nefazodone may increase the half-life of alprazolam and triazolam, so their dosing may need to be reduced by half or more
- Via CYP450 3A4, nefazodone may increase plasma concentrations of buspirone, so buspirone dose may need to be reduced
- Via CYP450 3A4 inhibition, nefazodone could theoretically increase concentrations of certain cholesterol lowering HMG CoA reductase inhibitors, especially simvastatin, atorvastatin, and lovastatin, but not pravastatin or fluvastatin, which would increase the risk of rhabdomyolysis; thus, coadministration of nefazodone with certain HMG CoA reductase inhibitors should proceed with caution
- Via CYP450 3A4 inhibition, nefazodone could theoretically increase the concentrations of pimozide, and cause QTc prolongation and dangerous cardiac arrhythmias
- Nefazodone may reduce clearance of haloperidol, so haloperidol dose may need to be reduced
- It is recommended to discontinue nefazodone prior to elective surgery because of the potential for interaction with general anesthetics

 Other Warnings/ Precautions
- ✳ Hepatotoxicity, sometimes requiring liver transplant and/or fatal, has occurred with nefazodone use. Risk may be one in every 250,000 to 300,000 patient years. Patients should be advised to report symptoms such as jaundice, dark urine, loss of appetite, nausea, and abdominal pain to prescriber immediately. If patient develops signs of hepatocellular injury, such as increased serum AST or serum ALPT levels >3 times the upper limit of normal, nefazodone treatment should be discontinued.

✳ No risk factor yet predicts who will develop irreversible liver failure with nefazodone and no clinical strategy, including routine monitoring of liver function tests, is known to reduce the risk of liver failure
- Use with caution in patients with history of seizures
- Use with caution in patients with bipolar disorder unless treated with concomitant mood stabilizing agent
- When treating children, carefully weigh the risks and benefits of pharmacological treatment against the risks and benefits of nontreatment with antidepressants and make sure to document this in the patient's chart
- Distribute the brochures provided by the FDA and the drug companies
- Warn patients and their caregivers about the possibility of activating side effects and advise them to report such symptoms immediately
- Monitor patients for activation of suicidal ideation, especially children and adolescents

Do Not Use
- If patient is taking an MAO inhibitor
- If patient has acute hepatic impairment or elevated baseline serum transaminases
- If patient was previously withdrawn from nefazodone treatment due to hepatic injury
- If patient is taking pimozide, as nefazodone could raise pimozide levels and increase QTc interval, perhaps causing dangerous arrhythmia
- If patient is taking carbamazepine, as this agent can dramatically reduce nefazodone levels and thus interfere with its antidepressant actions
- If there is a proven allergy to nefazodone

SPECIAL POPULATIONS

Renal Impairment
- No dose adjustment necessary

Hepatic Impairment
- Contraindicated in patients with known hepatic impairment

Cardiac Impairment
- Use in patients with cardiac impairment has not been studied, so use with caution because of risk of orthostatic hypotension

Elderly
- Recommended to initiate treatment at half the usual adult dose, but to follow the same titration schedule as with younger patients, including same ultimate dose

Children and Adolescents
- Carefully weigh the risks and benefits of pharmacological treatment against the risks and benefits of nontreatment with antidepressants and make sure to document this in the patient's chart
- Monitor patients face-to-face regularly, particularly during the first several weeks of treatment
- Use with caution, observing for activation of known or unknown bipolar disorder and/or suicidal ideation, and inform parents or guardian of this risk so they can help observe child or adolescent patients
- Safety and efficacy have not been established
- Preliminary research indicates efficacy and tolerability of nefazodone in children and adolescents with depression

Pregnancy
- Risk Category C [some animal studies show adverse effects; no controlled studies in humans]
- Not generally recommended for use during pregnancy, especially during first trimester
- Must weigh the risk of treatment (first trimester fetal development, third trimester newborn delivery) to the child against the risk of no treatment (recurrence of depression, maternal health, infant bonding) to the mother and child
- For many patients this may mean continuing treatment during pregnancy

Breast Feeding
- Unknown if nefazodone is secreted in human breast milk, but all psychotropics assumed to be secreted in breast milk
- Trace amounts may be present in nursing children whose mothers are on nefazodone

- If child becomes irritable or sedated, breast feeding or drug may need to be discontinued
- Immediate postpartum period is a high-risk time for depression, especially in women who have had prior depressive episodes, so drug may need to be reinstituted late in the third trimester or shortly after childbirth to prevent a recurrence during the postpartum period
- Must weigh benefits of breast feeding with risks and benefits of antidepressant treatment versus non-treatment to both the infant and the mother
- For many patients, this may mean continuing treatment during breast feeding

THE ART OF PSYCHOPHARMACOLOGY

Potential Advantages
- Depressed patients with anxiety or insomnia who do not respond to other antidepressants
- Patients with SSRI-induced sexual dysfunction

Potential Disadvantages
- Patients who have difficulty with a long titration period or twice-daily dosing

- Patients with hepatic impairment

Primary Target Symptoms
- Depressed mood
- Sleep disturbance
- Anxiety

 Pearls

- Preliminary data for efficacy in panic disorder and PTSD
- Fluoxetine and paroxetine may not be tolerated when switching or augmenting
- For elderly patients with early dementia and agitated depression, consider nefazodone in the morning and additional trazodone at night
- Anecdotal reports suggest that nefazodone may be effective in treating PMDD
- ✳ Studies suggest that cognitive-behavioral psychotherapy enhances the efficacy of nefazodone in chronic depression
- ✳ Risk of hepatotoxicity makes this agent a second-line choice and has led to its withdrawal from some markets, including the withdrawal of Serzone from the U.S. market
- Rarely, patients may complain of visual "trails" or after-images on nefazodone

 Suggested Reading

DeVane CL, Grothe DR, Smith SL. Pharmacology of antidepressants: focus on nefazodone. J Clin Psychiatry 2002; 63(1):10–7.

Dunner DL, Laird LK, Zajecka J, Bailey L, Sussman N, Seabolt JL. Six-year perspectives on the safety and tolerability of nefazodone. J Clin Psychiatry 2002;63(1):32–41.

Khouzam HR. The antidepressant nefazodone. A review of its pharmacology, clinical efficacy, adverse effects, dosage, and administration. Journal of Psychosocial Nursing and Mental Health Services 2000;38:20–25.

Masand PS, Gupta S. Long-term side effects of newer-generation antidepressants: SSRIS, venlafaxine, nefazodone, bupropion, and mirtazapine. Ann Clin Psychiatry 2002; 14:175–82.

Schatzberg AF, Prather MR, Keller MB, Rush AJ, Laird LK, Wright CW. Clinical use of nefazodone in major depression: a 6-year perspective. J Clin Psychiatry 2002; 63(1):18–31.

NORTRIPTYLINE

Brands • Pamelor
see index for additional brand names

Generic? Yes

Class
- Tricyclic antidepressant (TCA)
- Predominantly a norepinephrine/
  noradrenaline reuptake inhibitor

Commonly Prescribed For
(bold for FDA approved)
- **Major depressive disorder**
- Anxiety
- Insomnia
- Neuropathic pain/chronic pain
- Treatment-resistant depression

How The Drug Works
- Boosts neurotransmitter norepinephrine/
  noradrenaline
- Blocks norepinephrine reuptake pump
  (norepinephrine transporter), presumably
  increasing noradrenergic neurotransmission
- Since dopamine is inactivated by
  norepinephrine reuptake in frontal cortex,
  which largely lacks dopamine transporters,
  nortriptyline can increase dopamine
  neurotransmission in this part of the brain
- A more potent inhibitor of norepinephrine
  reuptake pump than serotonin reuptake
  pump (serotonin transporter)
- At high doses may also boost
  neurotransmitter serotonin and presumably
  increase serotonergic neurotransmission

How Long Until It Works
- May have immediate effects in treating
  insomnia or anxiety
- Onset of therapeutic actions usually not
  immediate, but often delayed 2 to 4 weeks
- If it is not working within 6 to 8 weeks for
  depression, it may require a dosage
  increase or it may not work at all
- May continue to work for many years to
  prevent relapse of symptoms

If It Works
- The goal of treatment of depression is
  complete remission of current symptoms
  as well as prevention of future relapses

- The goal of treatment of chronic
  neuropathic pain is to reduce symptoms as
  much as possible, especially in
  combination with other treatments
- Treatment of depression most often
  reduces or even eliminates symptoms, but
  not a cure since symptoms can recur after
  medicine stopped
- Treatment of chronic neuropathic pain may
  reduce symptoms, but rarely eliminates
  them completely, and is not a cure since
  symptoms can recur after medicine is
  stopped
- Continue treatment of depression until all
  symptoms are gone (remission)
- Once symptoms of depression are gone,
  continue treating for 1 year for the first
  episode of depression
- For second and subsequent episodes of
  depression, treatment may need to be
  indefinite
- Use in anxiety disorders and chronic pain
  may also need to be indefinite, but long-
  term treatment is not well studied in these
  conditions

If It Doesn't Work
- Many depressed patients only have a
  partial response where some symptoms
  are improved but others persist (especially
  insomnia, fatigue, and problems
  concentrating)
- Other depressed patients may be
  nonresponders, sometimes called
  treatment-resistant or treatment-refractory
- Consider increasing dose, switching to
  another agent or adding an appropriate
  augmenting agent
- Consider psychotherapy
- Consider evaluation for another diagnosis
  or for a comorbid condition (e.g., medical
  illness, substance abuse, etc.)
- Some patients may experience apparent
  lack of consistent efficacy due to activation
  of latent or underlying bipolar disorder, and
  require antidepressant discontinuation and
  a switch to a mood stabilizer

 ## Best Augmenting Combos
for Partial Response or
Treatment-Resistance
- Lithium, buspirone, thyroid hormone (for
  depression)
- Gabapentin, tiagabine, other
  anticonvulsants, even opiates if done by

experts while monitoring carefully in difficult cases (for chronic pain)

Tests

✳ None for healthy individuals, although monitoring of plasma drug levels is available

✳ Since tricyclic and tetracyclic antidepressants are frequently associated with weight gain, before starting treatment, weigh all patients and determine if the patient is already overweight (BMI 25.0–29.9) or obese (BMI ≥30)

• Before giving a drug that can cause weight gain to an overweight or obese patient, consider determining whether the patient already has pre-diabetes (fasting plasma glucose 100–125 mg/dl), diabetes (fasting plasma glucose >126 mg/dl), or dyslipidemia (increased total cholesterol, LDL cholesterol and triglycerides; decreased HDL cholesterol), and treat or refer such patients for treatment, including nutrition and weight management, physical activity counseling, smoking cessation, and medical management

✳ Monitor weight and BMI during treatment

✳ While giving a drug to a patient who has gained >5% of initial weight, consider evaluating for the presence of pre-diabetes, diabetes, or dyslipidemia, or consider switching to a different antidepressant

• EKGs may be useful for selected patients (e.g., those with personal or family history of QTc prolongation; cardiac arrhythmia; recent myocardial infarction; uncompensated heart failure; or taking agents that prolong QTc interval such as pimozide, thioridazine, selected antiarrhythmics, moxifloxacin, sparfloxacin, etc.)

• Patients at risk for electrolyte disturbances (e.g., patients on diuretic therapy) should have baseline and periodic serum potassium and magnesium measurements

SIDE EFFECTS

How Drug Causes Side Effects

• Anticholinergic activity may explain sedative effects, dry mouth, constipation, and blurred vision

• Sedative effects and weight gain may be due to antihistamine properties

• Blockade of alpha adrenergic 1 receptors may explain dizziness, sedation, and hypotension

• Cardiac arrhythmias and seizures, especially in overdose, may be caused by blockade of ion channels

Notable Side Effects

• Blurred vision, constipation, urinary retention, increased appetite, dry mouth, nausea, diarrhea, heartburn, unusual taste in mouth, weight gain

• Fatigue, weakness, dizziness, sedation, headache, anxiety, nervousness, restlessness

• Sexual dysfunction (impotence, change in libido)

• Sweating, rash, itching

 ### Life Threatening or Dangerous Side Effects

• Paralytic ileus, hyperthermia (TCAs + anticholinergic agents)

• Lowered seizure threshold and rare seizures

• Orthostatic hypotension, sudden death, arrhythmias, tachycardia

• QTc prolongation

• Hepatic failure, extrapyramidal symptoms

• Increased intraocular pressure

• Rare induction of mania

• Rare activation of suicidal ideation and behavior (suicidality)

Weight Gain

unusual not unusual common problematic

• Many experience and/or can be significant in amount

• Can increase appetite and carbohydrate craving

Sedation

unusual not unusual common problematic

• Many experience and/or can be significant in amount

• Tolerance to sedative effect may develop with long-term use

What To Do About Side Effects

• Wait

• Wait

• Wait

- Lower the dose
- Switch to an SSRI or newer antidepressant

Best Augmenting Agents for Side Effects
- Many side effects cannot be improved with an augmenting agent

DOSING AND USE

Usual Dosage Range
- 75–150 mg/day once daily or in up to 4 divided doses (for depression)
- 50–150 mg/day (for chronic pain)

Dosage Forms
- Capsule 10 mg, 25 mg, 50 mg, 75 mg
- Liquid 10 mg/5mL

How to Dose
- Initial 10–25 mg/day at bedtime; increase by 25 mg every 3–7 days; can be dosed once daily or in divided doses; maximum dose 300 mg/day
- When treating nicotine dependence, nortriptyline should be initiated 10–28 days before cessation of smoking to achieve steady drug states

 Dosing Tips
- If given in a single dose, should generally be administered at bedtime because of its sedative properties
- If given in split doses, largest dose should generally be given at bedtime because of its sedative properties
- If patients experience nightmares, split dose and do not give large dose at bedtime
- Patients treated for chronic pain may only require lower doses
- Risk of seizure increases with dose
- ✳ Monitoring plasma levels of nortriptyline is recommended in patients who do not respond to the usual dose or whose treatment is regarded as urgent
- Some formulations of nortriptyline contain sodium bisulphate, which may cause allergic reactions in some patients, perhaps more frequently in asthmatics
- If intolerable anxiety, insomnia, agitation, akathisia, or activation occur either upon dosing initiation or discontinuation,

consider the possibility of activated bipolar disorder, and switch to a mood stabilizer or an atypical antipsychotic

Overdose
- Death may occur; CNS depression, convulsions, cardiac dysrhythmias, severe hypotension, ECG changes, coma

Long-Term Use
- Safe

Habit Forming
- No

How to Stop
- Taper to avoid withdrawal effects
- Even with gradual dose reduction some withdrawal symptoms may appear within the first two weeks
- Many patients tolerate 50% dose reduction for 3 days, then another 50% reduction for 3 days, then discontinuation
- If withdrawal symptoms emerge during discontinuation, raise dose to stop symptoms and then restart withdrawal much more slowly

Pharmacokinetics
- Substrate for CYP450 2D6
- Nortriptyline is the active metabolite of amitriptyline, formed by demethylation via CYP450 1A2
- Half-life approximately 36 hours

 Drug Interactions
- Tramadol increases the risk of seizures in patients taking TCAs
- Use of TCAs with anticholinergic drugs may result in paralytic ileus or hyperthermia
- Fluoxetine, paroxetine, bupropion, duloxetine and other CYP450 2D6 inhibitors may increase TCA concentrations and cause side effects including dangerous arrhythmias
- Cimetidine may increase plasma concentrations of TCAs and cause anticholinergic symptoms
- Phenothiazines or haloperidol may raise TCA blood concentrations
- May alter effects of antihypertensive drugs; may inhibit hypotensive effects of clonidine

- Use of TCAs with sympathomimetic agents may increase sympathetic activity
- Methylphenidate may inhibit metabolism of TCAs
- Nortriptyline may raise plasma levels of dicumarol
- Activation and agitation, especially following switching or adding antidepressants, may represent the induction of a bipolar state, especially a mixed dysphoric bipolar II condition sometimes associated with suicidal ideation, and require the addition of lithium, a mood stabilizer or an atypical antipsychotic, and/or discontinuation of nortriptyline

 Other Warnings/ Precautions

- Add or initiate other antidepressants with caution for up to 2 weeks after discontinuing nortriptyline
- Generally, do not use with MAO inhibitors, including 14 days after MAOIs are stopped; do not start an MAOI until 2 weeks after discontinuing nortriptyline, but see Pearls
- Use with caution in patients with history of seizures, urinary retention, narrow angle-closure glaucoma, hyperthyroidism
- TCAs can increase QTc interval, especially at toxic doses, which can be attained not only by overdose but also by combining with drugs that inhibit TCA metabolism via CYP450 2D6, potentially causing torsade de pointes-type arrhythmia or sudden death
- Because TCAs can prolong QTc interval, use with caution in patients who have bradycardia or who are taking drugs that can induce bradycardia (e.g., beta blockers, calcium channel blockers, clonidine, digitalis)
- Because TCAs can prolong QTc interval, use with caution in patients who have hypokalemia and/or hypomagnesemia or who are taking drugs that can induce hypokalemia and/or magnesemia (e.g., diuretics, stimulant laxatives, intravenous amphotericin B, glucocorticoids, tetracosactide)
- When treating children, carefully weigh the risks and benefits of pharmacological treatment against the risks and benefits of nontreatment with antidepressants and

make sure to document this in the patient's chart
- Distribute the brochures provided by the FDA and the drug companies
- Warn patients and their caregivers about the possibility of activating side effects and advise them to report such symptoms immediately
- Monitor patients for activation of suicidal ideation, especially children and adolescents

Do Not Use
- If patient is recovering from myocardial infarction
- If patient is taking agents capable of significantly prolonging QTc interval (e.g., pimozide, thioridazine, selected antiarrhythmics, moxifloxacin, sparfloxacin)
- If there is a history of QTc prolongation or cardiac arrhythmia, recent acute myocardial infarction, uncompensated heart failure
- If patient is taking drugs that inhibit TCA metabolism, including CYP450 2D6 inhibitors, except by an expert
- If there is reduced CYP450 2D6 function, such as patients who are poor 2D6 metabolizers, except by an expert and at low doses
- If there is a proven allergy to nortriptyline or amitriptyline

SPECIAL POPULATIONS

Renal Impairment
- Use with caution; may need to lower dose
- May need to monitor plasma levels

Hepatic Impairment
- Use with caution
- May need to monitor plasma levels
- May require a lower dose with slower titration

Cardiac Impairment
- TCAs have been reported to cause arrhythmias, prolongation of conduction time, orthostatic hypotension, sinus tachycardia, and heart failure, especially in the diseased heart
- Myocardial infarction and stroke have been reported with TCAs

- TCAs produce QTc prolongation, which may be enhanced by the existence of bradycardia, hypokalemia, congenital or acquired long QTc interval, which should be evaluated prior to administering nortriptyline
- Use with caution if treating concomitantly with a medication likely to produce prolonged bradycardia, hypokalemia, slowing of intracardiac conduction, or prolongation of the QTc interval
- Avoid TCAs in patients with a known history of QTc prolongation, recent acute myocardial infarction, and uncompensated heart failure
- TCAs may cause a sustained increase in heart rate in patients with ischemic heart disease and may worsen (decrease) heart rate variability, an independent risk of mortality in cardiac populations
- Since SSRIs may improve (increase) heart rate variability in patients following a myocardial infarct and may improve survival as well as mood in patients with acute angina or following a myocardial infarction, these are more appropriate agents for cardiac population than tricyclic/tetracyclic antidepressants
- ⁎ Risk/benefit ratio may not justify use of TCAs in cardiac impairment

Elderly

- May be more sensitive to anticholinergic, cardiovascular, hypotensive, and sedative effects
- May require lower dose; it may be useful to monitor plasma levels in elderly patients

Children and Adolescents

- Carefully weigh the risks and benefits of pharmacological treatment against the risks and benefits of nontreatment with antidepressants and make sure to document this in the patient's chart
- Monitor patients face-to-face regularly, particularly during the first several weeks of treatment
- Use with caution, observing for activation of known or unknown bipolar disorder and/or suicidal ideation, and inform parents or guardian of this risk so they can help observe child or adolescent patients
- Not recommended for use under age 12

- Not intended for use under age 6
- Several studies show lack of efficacy of TCAs for depression
- May be used to treat enuresis or hyperactive/impulsive behaviors
- Some cases of sudden death have occurred in children taking TCAs
- Plasma levels may need to be monitored
- Dose in children generally less than 50 mg/day
- May be useful to monitor plasma levels in children and adolescents

 Pregnancy

- Risk Category D [positive evidence of risk to human fetus; potential benefits may still justify its use during pregnancy]
- Crosses the placenta
- Should be used only if potential benefits outweigh potential risks
- Adverse effects have been reported in infants whose mothers took a TCA (lethargy, withdrawal symptoms, fetal malformations)
- Evaluate for treatment with an antidepressant with a better risk/benefit ratio

Breast Feeding

- Some drug is found in mother's breast milk
- ⁎ Recommended either to discontinue drug or bottle feed
- Immediate postpartum period is a high-risk time for depression, especially in women who have had prior depressive episodes, so drug may need to be reinstituted late in the third trimester or shortly after childbirth to prevent a recurrence during the postpartum period
- Must weigh benefits of breast feeding with risks and benefits of antidepressant treatment versus non-treatment to both the infant and the mother
- For many patients this may mean continuing treatment during breast feeding

THE ART OF PSYCHOPHARMACOLOGY

Potential Advantages

- Patients with insomnia
- Severe or treatment-resistant depression
- Patients for whom therapeutic drug monitoring is desirable

Potential Disadvantages
- Pediatric and geriatric patients
- Patients concerned with weight gain
- Cardiac patients

Primary Target Symptoms
- Depressed mood
- Chronic pain

 Pearls

- Tricyclic antidepressants are often a first-line treatment option for chronic pain
- Tricyclic antidepressants are no longer generally considered a first-line option for depression because of their side effect profile
- Tricyclic antidepressants continue to be useful for severe or treatment-resistant depression
- Noradrenergic reuptake inhibitors such as nortriptyline can be used as a second-line treatment for smoking cessation, cocaine dependence, and attention deficit disorder
- TCAs may aggravate psychotic symptoms
- Alcohol should be avoided because of additive CNS effects
- Underweight patients may be more susceptible to adverse cardiovascular effects
- Children, patients with inadequate hydration, and patients with cardiac disease may be more susceptible to TCA-induced cardiotoxicity than healthy adults
- For the expert only: although generally prohibited, a heroic but potentially dangerous treatment for severely treatment-resistant patients is for an expert to give a tricyclic/tetracyclic antidepressant other than clomipramine simultaneously with an MAO inhibitor for patients who fail to respond to numerous other antidepressants
- If this option is elected, start the MAOI with the tricyclic/tetracyclic antidepressant simultaneously at low doses after

appropriate drug washout, then alternately increase doses of these agents every few days to a week as tolerated
- Although very strict dietary and concomitant drug restrictions must be observed to prevent hypertensive crises and serotonin syndrome, the most common side effects of MAOI and tricyclic/tetracyclic antidepressant combinations may be weight gain and orthostatic hypotension
- Patients on TCAs should be aware that they may experience symptoms such as photosensitivity or blue-green urine
- SSRIs may be more effective than TCAs in women, and TCAs may be more effective than SSRIs in men
- Not recommended for first-line use in children with ADHD because of the availability of safer treatments with better documented efficacy and because of nortriptyline's potential for sudden death in children
- ✳ Nortriptyline is one of the few TCAs where monitoring of plasma drug levels has been well studied
- Since tricyclic/tetracyclic antidepressants are substrates for CYP450 2D6, and 7% of the population (especially Caucasians) may have a genetic variant leading to reduced activity of 2D6, such patients may not safely tolerate normal doses of tricyclic/tetracyclic antidepressants and may require dose reduction
- Phenotypic testing may be necessary to detect this genetic variant prior to dosing with a tricyclic/tetracyclic antidepressant, especially in vulnerable populations such as children, elderly, cardiac populations, and those on concomitant medications
- Patients who seem to have extraordinarily severe side effects at normal or low doses may have this phenotypic CYP450 2D6 variant and require low doses or switching to another antidepressant not metabolized by 2D6

Suggested Reading

Anderson IM. Meta-analytical studies on new antidepressants. Br Med Bull 2001; 57:161–178.

Anderson IM. Selective serotonin reuptake inhibitors versus tricyclic antidepressants: a meta-analysis of efficacy and tolerability. J Aff Disorders 2000;58:19–36.

Hughes JR, Stead LF, Lancaster T. Antidepressants for smoking cessation. Cochrane Database Syst Rev 2000;4:CD000031.

Wilens TE, Biederman J, Baldessarini RJ, Geller B, Schleifer D, Spencer TJ, Birmajer B, Goldblatt A. Cardiovascular effects of therapeutic doses of tricyclic antidepressants in children and adolescents. J Am Acad Child Adolesc Psychiatry 1996;35(11):1491–501.

PAROXETINE

THERAPEUTICS

Brands
- Paxil
- Paxil CR

see index for additional brand names

Generic? Yes (not for paroxetine CR)

Class
- SSRI (selective serotonin reuptake inhibitor); often classified as an antidepressant, but it is not just an antidepressant

Commonly Prescribed For
(bold for FDA approved)
- **Major depressive disorder (paroxetine and paroxetine CR)**
- **Obsessive-compulsive disorder (OCD)**
- **Panic disorder (paroxetine and paroxetine CR)**
- **Social anxiety disorder (social phobia) (paroxetine and paroxetine CR)**
- **Posttraumatic stress disorder (PTSD)**
- **Generalized anxiety disorder (GAD)**
- **Premenstrual dysphoric disorder (PMDD) (paroxetine CR)**

How The Drug Works
- Boosts neurotransmitter serotonin
- Blocks serotonin reuptake pump (serotonin transporter)
- Desensitizes serotonin receptors, especially serotonin 1A autoreceptors
- Presumably increases serotonergic neurotransmission
- Paroxetine also has mild anticholinergic actions
- Paroxetine may have mild norepinephrine reuptake blocking actions

How Long Until It Works
* Some patients may experience relief of insomnia or anxiety early after initiation of treatment
- Onset of therapeutic actions usually not immediate, but often delayed 2 to 4 weeks
- If it is not working within 6 to 8 weeks for depression, it may require a dosage increase or it may not work at all
- By contrast, for generalized anxiety, onset of response and increases in remission rates may still occur after 8 weeks of treatment and for up to 6 months after initiating dosing
- May continue to work for many years to prevent relapse of symptoms

If It Works
- The goal of treatment is complete remission of current symptoms as well as prevention of future relapses
- Treatment most often reduces or even eliminates symptoms, but not a cure since symptoms can recur after medicine stopped
- Continue treatment until all symptoms are gone (remission) or significantly reduced (e.g., OCD, PTSD)
- Once symptoms are gone, continue treating for 1 year for the first episode of depression
- For second and subsequent episodes of depression, treatment may need to be indefinite
- Use in anxiety disorders may also need to be indefinite

If It Doesn't Work
- Many patients only have a partial response where some symptoms are improved but others persist (especially insomnia, fatigue, and problems concentrating in depression)
- Other patients may be nonresponders, sometimes called treatment-resistant or treatment-refractory
- Some patients who have an initial response may relapse even though they continue treatment, sometimes called "poop-out"
- Consider increasing dose, switching to another agent or adding an appropriate augmenting agent
- Consider psychotherapy
- Consider evaluation for another diagnosis or for a comorbid condition (e.g., medical illness, substance abuse, etc.)
- Some patients may experience apparent lack of consistent efficacy due to activation of latent or underlying bipolar disorder, and require antidepressant discontinuation and a switch to a mood stabilizer

Best Augmenting Combos for Partial Response or Treatment-Resistance
- Trazodone, especially for insomnia
- Bupropion, mirtazapine, reboxetine, or atomoxetine (add with caution and at lower

doses since paroxetine could theoretically raise atomoxetine levels); use combinations of antidepressants with caution as this may activate bipolar disorder and suicidal ideation
- Modafinil, especially for fatigue, sleepiness, and lack of concentration
- Mood stabilizers or atypical antipsychotics for bipolar depression, psychotic depression, treatment-resistant depression, or treatment-resistant anxiety disorders
- Benzodiazepines
- If all else fails for anxiety disorders, consider gabapentin or tiagabine
- Hypnotics for insomnia
- Classically, lithium, buspirone, or thyroid hormone

Tests
- None for healthy individuals

SIDE EFFECTS

How Drug Causes Side Effects
- Theoretically due to increases in serotonin concentrations at serotonin receptors in parts of the brain and body other than those that cause therapeutic actions (e.g., unwanted actions of serotonin in sleep centers causing insomnia, unwanted actions of serotonin in the gut causing diarrhea, etc.)
- Increasing serotonin can cause diminished dopamine release and might contribute to emotional flattening, cognitive slowing, and apathy in some patients
- Most side effects are immediate but often go away with time, in contrast to most therapeutic effects which are delayed and are enhanced over time
- * Paroxetine's weak antimuscarinic properties can cause constipation, dry mouth, sedation

Notable Side Effects
- Sexual dysfunction (men: delayed ejaculation, erectile dysfunction; men and women: decreased sexual desire, anorgasmia)
- Gastrointestinal (decreased appetite, nausea, diarrhea, constipation, dry mouth)
- Mostly central nervous system (insomnia but also sedation, agitation, tremors, headache, dizziness)

- Note: patients with diagnosed or undiagnosed bipolar or psychotic disorders may be more vulnerable to CNS-activating actions of SSRIs
- Autonomic (sweating)
- Bruising and rare bleeding
- Rare hyponatremia (mostly in elderly patients and generally reversible on discontinuation of paroxetine)

Life Threatening or Dangerous Side Effects
- Rare seizures
- Rare induction of mania
- Rare activation of suicidal ideation and behavior (suicidality)

Weight Gain

unusual / not unusual / common / problematic
- Occurs in significant minority

Sedation

unusual / not unusual / common / problematic
- Many experience and/or can be significant in amount
- Generally transient

What To Do About Side Effects
- Wait
- Wait
- Wait
- If paroxetine is sedating, take at night to reduce daytime drowsiness
- Reduce dose to 5–10 mg (12.5 mg for CR) until side effects abate, then increase as tolerated, usually to at least 20 mg (25 mg CR)
- In a few weeks, switch or add other drugs

Best Augmenting Agents for Side Effects
- Often best to try another SSRI or another antidepressant monotherapy prior to resorting to augmentation strategies to treat side effects
- Trazodone or a hypnotic for insomnia
- Bupropion, sildenafil, vardenafil, or tadalafil for sexual dysfunction
- Bupropion for emotional flattening, cognitive slowing, or apathy

- Mirtazapine for insomnia, agitation, and gastrointestinal side effects
- Benzodiazepines for jitteriness and anxiety, especially at initiation of treatment and especially for anxious patients
- Many side effects are dose-dependent (i.e., they increase as dose increases, or they reemerge until tolerance re-develops)
- Many side effects are time-dependent (i.e., they start immediately upon dosing and upon each dose increase, but go away with time)
- Activation and agitation may represent the induction of a bipolar state, especially a mixed dysphoric bipolar II condition sometimes associated with suicidal ideation, and require the addition of lithium, a mood stabilizer or an atypical antipsychotic, and/or discontinuation of paroxetine

DOSING AND USE

Usual Dosage Range
- Depression: 20–50 mg (25–62.5 mg CR)

Dosage Forms
- Tablets 10 mg scored, 20 mg scored, 30 mg, 40 mg
- Controlled release tablets 12.5 mg, 25 mg
- Liquid 10 mg/5mL – 250 mL bottle

How to Dose
- Depression: initial 20 mg (25 mg CR); usually wait a few weeks to assess drug effects before increasing dose, but can increase by 10 mg/day (12.5 mg/day CR) once a week; maximum generally 50 mg/day (62.5 mg/day CR); single dose
- Panic disorder: initial 10 mg/day (12.5 mg/day CR); usually wait a few weeks to assess drug effects before increasing dose, but can increase by 10 mg/day (12.5 mg/day CR) once a week; maximum generally 60 mg/day (75 mg/day CR); single dose
- Social anxiety disorder: initial 20 mg/day (25 mg/day CR); usually wait a few weeks to assess drug effects before increasing dose, but can increase by 10 mg/day (12.5 mg/day CR) once a week; maximum 60 mg/day (75 mg/day CR); single dose
- Other anxiety disorders: initial 20 mg/day (25 mg/day CR); usually wait a few weeks

to assess drug effects before increasing dose, but can increase by 10 mg/day (12.5 mg/day CR) once a week; maximum 60 mg/day (75 mg/day CR); single dose

 Dosing Tips
- 20 mg tablet is scored, so to save costs, give 10 mg as half of 20 mg tablet, since 10 mg and 20 mg tablets cost about the same in many markets
- Given once daily, often at bedtime, but any time of day tolerated
- 20 mg/day (25 mg/day CR) is often sufficient for patients with social anxiety disorder and depression
- Other anxiety disorders, as well as difficult cases in general, may require higher dosing
- Occasional patients are dosed above 60 mg/day (75 mg/day CR), but this is for experts and requires caution
- If intolerable anxiety, insomnia, agitation, akathisia, or activation occur either upon dosing initiation or discontinuation, consider the possibility of activated bipolar disorder and switch to a mood stabilizer or an atypical antipsychotic
- Liquid formulation easiest for doses below 10 mg when used for cases that are very intolerant to paroxetine or especially for very slow down-titration during discontinuation for patients with withdrawal symptoms
- Paroxetine CR tablets not scored, so chewing or cutting in half can destroy controlled release properties
- Unlike other SSRIs and antidepressants where dosage increments can be double and triple the starting dose, paroxetine's dosing increments are in 50% increments (i.e., 20, 30, 40; or 25, 37.5, 50 CR)
- Paroxetine inhibits its own metabolism and thus plasma concentrations can double when oral doses increase by 50%; plasma concentrations can increase 2–7 fold when oral doses are doubled
- ✳ Main advantage of CR is reduced side effects, especially nausea and perhaps sedation, sexual dysfunction, and withdrawal
- ✳ For patients with severe problems discontinuing paroxetine, dosing may need to be tapered over many months (i.e.,

reduce dose by 1% every 3 days by crushing tablet and suspending or dissolving in 100 mL of fruit juice and then disposing of 1 mL while drinking the rest; 3–7 days later, dispose of 2 mL, and so on). This is both a form of very slow biological tapering and a form of behavioral desensitization

- For some patients with severe problems discontinuing paroxetine, it may be useful to add an SSRI with a long half-life, especially fluoxetine, prior to taper of paroxetine; while maintaining fluoxetine dosing, first slowly taper paroxetine and then taper fluoxetine
- Be sure to differentiate between re-emergence of symptoms requiring re-institution of treatment and withdrawal symptoms

Overdose
- Rarely lethal in monotherapy overdose; vomiting, sedation, heart rhythm disturbances, dilated pupils, dry mouth

Long-Term Use
- Safe

Habit Forming
- No

How to Stop
- Taper to avoid withdrawal effects (dizziness, nausea, stomach cramps, sweating, tingling, dysesthesias)
- Many patients tolerate 50% dose reduction for 3 days, then another 50% reduction for 3 days, then discontinuation
- If withdrawal symptoms emerge during discontinuation, raise dose to stop symptoms and then restart withdrawal much more slowly
- ✻ Withdrawal effects can be more common or more severe with paroxetine than with some other SSRIs
- Paroxetine's withdrawal effects may be related in part to the fact that it inhibits its own metabolism
- Thus, when paroxetine is withdrawn, the rate of its decline can be faster as it stops inhibiting its metabolism
- Controlled release paroxetine may slow the rate of decline and thus reduce withdrawal reactions in some patients

- Re-adaptation of cholinergic receptors after prolonged blockade may contribute to withdrawal effects of paroxetine

Pharmacokinetics
- Inactive metabolites
- Half-life approximately 24 hours
- Inhibits CYP450 2D6

 Drug Interactions
- Tramadol increases the risk of seizures in patients taking an antidepressant
- Can increase tricyclic antidepressant levels; use with caution with tricyclic antidepressants or when switching from a TCA to paroxetine
- Can cause a fatal "serotonin syndrome" when combined with MAO inhibitors, so do not use it with MAO inhibitors or for at least 14 days after MAOIs are stopped
- Do not start an MAO inhibitor for at least 2 weeks after discontinuing paroxetine
- May displace highly protein bound drugs (e.g., warfarin)
- There are reports of elevated theophylline levels associated with paroxetine treatment, so it is recommended that theophylline levels be monitored when these drugs are administered together
- May increase anticholinergic effects of procyclidine and other drugs with anticholinergic properties
- Can rarely cause weakness, hyperreflexia, and incoordination when combined with sumatriptan or possibly with other triptans, requiring careful monitoring of patient
- Via CYP450 2D6 inhibition, paroxetine could theoretically interfere with the analgesic actions of codeine, and increase the plasma levels of some beta blockers and of atomoxetine
- Via CYP450 2D6 inhibition, paroxetine could theoretically increase concentrations of thioridazine and cause dangerous cardiac arrhythmias
- Paroxetine increases pimozide levels, and pimozide prolongs QT interval, so concomitant use of pimozide and paroxetine is contraindicated

Other Warnings/ Precautions

- Add or initiate other antidepressants with caution for up to 2 weeks after discontinuing paroxetine
- Use with caution in patients with history of seizures
- Use with caution in patients with bipolar disorder unless treated with concomitant mood stabilizing agent
- When treating children, carefully weigh the risks and benefits of pharmacological treatment against the risks and benefits of nontreatment with antidepressants and make sure to document this in the patient's chart
- Distribute the brochures provided by the FDA and the drug companies
- Warn patients and their caregivers about the possibility of activating side effects and advise them to report such symptoms immediately
- Monitor patients for activation of suicidal ideation, especially children and adolescents

Do Not Use

- If patient is taking an MAO inhibitor
- If patient is taking thioridazine
- If patient is taking pimozide
- If there is a proven allergy to paroxetine

SPECIAL POPULATIONS

Renal Impairment

- Lower dose [initial 10 mg/day (12.5 mg CR), maximum 40 mg/day (50 mg/day CR)]

Hepatic Impairment

- Lower dose [initial 10 mg/day (12.5 mg CR), maximum 40 mg/day (50 mg/day CR)]

Cardiac Impairment

- Preliminary research suggests that paroxetine is safe in these patients
- Treating depression with SSRIs in patients with acute angina or following myocardial infarction may reduce cardiac events and improve survival as well as mood

Elderly

- Lower dose [initial 10 mg/day (12.5 mg CR), maximum 40 mg/day (50 mg/day CR)]

 Children and Adolescents

- Carefully weigh the risks and benefits of pharmacological treatment against the risks and benefits of nontreatment with antidepressants and make sure to document this in the patient's chart
- Monitor patients face-to-face regularly, particularly during the first several weeks of treatment
- Use with caution, observing for activation of known or unknown bipolar disorder and/or suicidal ideation, and inform parents or guardian of this risk so they can help observe child or adolescent patients
- Not specifically approved, but preliminary evidence suggests efficacy in children and adolescents with OCD, social phobia, or depression

 Pregnancy

- Risk Category D [positive evidence of risk to human fetus; potential benefits may still justify its use during pregnancy]
- Not generally recommended for use during pregnancy, especially during first trimester
- Epidemiological data have shown an increased risk of cardiovascular malformations (primarily ventricular and atrial septal defects) in infants born to women who took paroxetine during the first trimester
- Unless the benefits of paroxetine to the mother justify continuing treatment, consider discontinuing paroxetine or switching to another antidepressant
- Paroxetine use late in pregnancy may be associated with higher risk of neonatal complications, including respiratory distress
- At delivery there may be more bleeding in the mother and transient irritability or sedation in the newborn
- Must weigh the risk of treatment (first trimester fetal development, third trimester newborn delivery) to the child against the risk of no treatment (recurrence of

depression, maternal health, infant bonding) to the mother and child
- For many patients this may mean continuing treatment during pregnancy
- Neonates exposed to SSRIs or SNRIs late in the third trimester have developed complications requiring prolonged hospitalization, respiratory support, and tube feeding; reported symptoms are consistent with either a direct toxic effect of SSRIs and SNRIs or, possibly, a drug discontinuation syndrome, and include respiratory distress, cyanosis, apnea, seizures, temperature instability, feeding difficulty, vomiting, hypoglycemia, hypotonia, hypertonia, hyperreflexia, tremor, jitteriness, irritability, and constant crying

Breast Feeding
- Some drug is found in mother's breast milk
- Trace amounts may be present in nursing children whose mothers are on paroxetine
- If child becomes irritable or sedated, breast feeding or drug may need to be discontinued
- Immediate postpartum period is a high-risk time for depression, especially in women who have had prior depressive episodes, so drug may need to be reinstituted late in the third trimester or shortly after childbirth to prevent a recurrence during the postpartum period
- Must weigh benefits of breast feeding with risks and benefits of antidepressant treatment versus non-treatment to both the infant and the mother
- For many patients, this may mean continuing treatment during breast feeding

THE ART OF PSYCHOPHARMACOLOGY

Potential Advantages
- Patients with anxiety disorders and insomnia
- Patients with mixed anxiety/depression

Potential Disadvantages
- Patients with hypersomnia
- Alzheimer/cognitive disorders
- Patients with psychomotor retardation, fatigue, and low energy

Primary Target Symptoms
- Depressed mood
- Anxiety
- Sleep disturbance, especially insomnia
- Panic attacks, avoidant behavior, re-experiencing, hyperarousal

 Pearls

✳ Often a preferred treatment of anxious depression as well as major depressive disorder comorbid with anxiety disorders
✳ Withdrawal effects may be more likely than for some other SSRIs when discontinued (especially akathisia, restlessness, gastrointestinal symptoms, dizziness, tingling, dysesthesias, nausea, stomach cramps, restlessness)
- Inhibits own metabolism, so dosing is not linear
✳ Paroxetine has mild anticholinergic actions that can enhance the rapid onset of anxiolytic and hypnotic efficacy but also cause mild anticholinergic side effects
- Can cause cognitive and affective "flattening"
- May be less activating than other SSRIs
- Paroxetine is a potent CYP450 2D6 inhibitor
- SSRIs may be less effective in women over 50, especially if they are not taking estrogen
- SSRIs may be useful for hot flushes in perimenopausal women
- Some anecdotal reports suggest greater weight gain and sexual dysfunction than some other SSRIs, but the clinical significance of this is unknown
- For sexual dysfunction, can augment with bupropion, sildenafil, tadalafil, or switch to a non-SSRI such as bupropion or mirtazapine
- Some postmenopausal women's depression will respond better to paroxetine plus estrogen augmentation than to paroxetine alone
- Nonresponse to paroxetine in elderly may require consideration of mild cognitive impairment or Alzheimer disease
- CR formulation may enhance tolerability, especially for nausea
- Can be better tolerated than some SSRIs for patients with anxiety and insomnia and can reduce these symptoms early in dosing

Suggested Reading

Bourin M, Chue P, Guillon Y. Paroxetine: a review. CNS Drug Rev. 2001;7:25–47.

Edwards JG, Anderson I. Systematic review and guide to selection of selective serotonin reuptake inhibitors. Drugs. 1999;57:507–533.

Green B. Focus on paroxetine. Curr Med Res Opin. 2003;19:13–21.

Wagstaff AJ, Cheer SM, Matheson AJ, Ormrod D, Goa KL. Paroxetine: an update of its use in psychiatric disorders in adults. Drugs. 2002;62:655–703.

THERAPEUTICS

Brands • Nardil
• Nardelzine
see index for additional brand names

Generic? Yes

Class
• Monoamine oxidase inhibitor (MAOI)

Commonly Prescribed For
(bold for FDA approved)
• **Depressed patients characterized as "atypical", "nonendogenous", or "neurotic"**
• Treatment-resistant depression
• Treatment-resistant panic disorder
• Treatment-resistant social anxiety disorder

How The Drug Works
• Irreversibly blocks monoamine oxidase (MAO) from breaking down norepinephrine, serotonin, and dopamine
• This presumably boosts noradrenergic, serotonergic, and dopaminergic neurotransmission

How Long Until It Works
• Onset of therapeutic actions usually not immediate, but often delayed 2 to 4 weeks
• If it is not working within 6 to 8 weeks, it may require a dosage increase or it may not work at all
• May continue to work for many years to prevent relapse of symptoms

If It Works
• The goal of treatment is complete remission of current symptoms as well as prevention of future relapses
• Treatment most often reduces or even eliminates symptoms, but not a cure since symptoms can recur after medicine stopped
• Continue treatment until all symptoms are gone (remission)
• Once symptoms gone, continue treating for 1 year for the first episode of depression
• For second and subsequent episodes of depression, treatment may need to be indefinite

• Use in anxiety disorders may also need to be indefinite

If It Doesn't Work
• Many patients only have a partial response where some symptoms are improved but others persist (especially insomnia, fatigue, and problems concentrating)
• Other patients may be nonresponders, sometimes called treatment-resistant or treatment-refractory
• Some patients who have an initial response may relapse even though they continue treatment, sometimes called "poop-out"
• Consider increasing dose, switching to another agent, or adding an appropriate augmenting agent
• Consider psychotherapy
• Consider evaluation for another diagnosis or for a comorbid condition (e.g., medical illness, substance abuse, etc.)
• Some patients may experience apparent lack of consistent efficacy due to activation of latent or underlying bipolar disorder, and require antidepressant discontinuation and a switch to a mood stabilizer

Best Augmenting Combos for Partial Response or Treatment-Resistance

✱ Augmentation of MAOIs has not been systematically studied, and this is something for the expert, to be done with caution and with careful monitoring
✱ A stimulant such as d-amphetamine or methylphenidate (with caution; may activate bipolar disorder and suicidal ideation; may elevate blood pressure)
• Lithium
• Mood stabilizing anticonvulsants
• Atypical antipsychotics (with special caution for those agents with monoamine reuptake blocking properties, such as ziprasidone and zotepine)

Tests
• Patients should be monitored for changes in blood pressure
• Patients receiving high doses or long-term treatment should have hepatic function evaluated periodically
✱ Since MAO inhibitors are frequently associated with weight gain, before starting treatment, weigh all patients and determine

if the patient is already overweight
(BMI 25.0–29.9) or obese (BMI ≥30)
- Before giving a drug that can cause weight
gain to an overweight or obese patient,
consider determining whether the patient
already has pre-diabetes (fasting plasma
glucose 100–125 mg/dl), diabetes (fasting
plasma glucose >126 mg/dl), or
dyslipidemia (increased total cholesterol,
LDL cholesterol and triglycerides;
decreased HDL cholesterol), and treat or
refer such patients for treatment, including
nutrition and weight management, physical
activity counseling, smoking cessation, and
medical management
* Monitor weight and BMI during treatment
* While giving a drug to a patient who has
gained >5% of initial weight, consider
evaluating for the presence of pre-diabetes,
diabetes, or dyslipidemia, or consider
switching to a different antidepressant

SIDE EFFECTS

How Drug Causes Side Effects
- Theoretically due to increases in
monoamines in parts of the brain and body
and at receptors other than those that
cause therapeutic actions (e.g., unwanted
actions of serotonin in sleep centers
causing insomnia, unwanted actions of
norepinephrine on vascular smooth muscle
causing changes in blood pressure, etc.)
- Side effects are generally immediate, but
immediate side effects often disappear in
time

Notable Side Effects
- Dizziness, sedation, headache, sleep
disturbances, fatigue, weakness, tremor,
movement problems, blurred vision,
increased sweating
- Constipation, dry mouth, nausea, change in
appetite, weight gain
- Sexual dysfunction
- Orthostatic hypotension (dose-related);
syncope may develop at high doses

Life Threatening or Dangerous Side Effects
- Hypertensive crisis (especially when MAOIs
are used with certain tyramine-containing
foods or prohibited drugs)

- Induction of mania
- Rare activation of suicidal ideation and
behavior (suicidality)
- Seizures
- Hepatotoxicity

Weight Gain

unusual not unusual common problematic
- Many experience and/or can be significant
in amount

Sedation

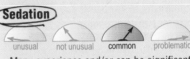

unusual not unusual common problematic
- Many experience and/or can be significant
in amount
- Can also cause activation

What To Do About Side Effects
- Wait
- Wait
- Wait
- Lower the dose
- Take at night if daytime sedation
- Switch after appropriate washout to an
SSRI or newer antidepressant

Best Augmenting Agents for Side Effects
- Trazodone (with caution) for insomnia
- Benzodiazepines for insomnia
* Single oral or sublingual dose of a
calcium channel blocker (e.g., nifedipine)
for urgent treatment of hypertension due to
drug interaction or dietary tyramine
- Many side effects cannot be improved with
an augmenting agent

DOSING AND USE

Usual Dosage Range
- 45–75 mg/day

Dosage Forms
- Tablet 15 mg

How to Dose
- Initial 45 mg/day in 3 divided doses;
increase to 60–90 mg/day; after desired
therapeutic effect is achieved lower dose as
far as possible

Dosing Tips

- Once dosing is stabilized, some patients may tolerate once or twice daily dosing rather than 3-times-a-day dosing
- Orthostatic hypotension, especially at high doses, may require splitting into 4 daily doses
- Patients receiving high doses may need to be evaluated periodically for effects on the liver
- Little evidence to support efficacy of phenelzine below doses of 45 mg/day

Overdose

- Death may occur; dizziness, ataxia, sedation, headache, insomnia, restlessness, anxiety, irritability, cardiovascular effects, confusion, respiratory depression, coma

Long-Term Use

- May require periodic evaluation of hepatic function
- MAOIs may lose efficacy long-term

Habit Forming

- Some patients have developed dependence to MAOIs

How to Stop

- Generally no need to taper, as the drug wears off slowly over 2–3 weeks

Pharmacokinetics

- Clinical duration of action may be up to 21 days due to irreversible enzyme inhibition

Drug Interactions

- Tramadol may increase the risk of seizures in patients taking an MAO inhibitor
- Can cause a fatal "serotonin syndrome" when combined with drugs that block serotonin reuptake (e.g., SSRIs, SNRIs, sibutramine, tramadol, etc.), so do not use with a serotonin reuptake inhibitor or for up to 5 weeks after stopping the serotonin reuptake inhibitor
- Hypertensive crisis with headache, intracranial bleeding, and death may result from combining MAO inhibitors with sympathomimetic drugs (e.g., amphetamines, methylphenidate, cocaine, dopamine, epinephrine, norepinephrine, and related compounds methyldopa, levodopa, L-tryptophan, L-tyrosine, and phenylalanine)
- Excitation, seizures, delirium, hyperpyrexia, circulatory collapse, coma, and death may result from combining MAO inhibitors with mepiridine or dextromethorphan
- Do not combine with another MAO inhibitor, alcohol, buspirone, bupropion, or guanethidine
- Adverse drug reactions can result from combining MAO inhibitors with tricyclic/tetracyclic antidepressants and related compounds, including carbamazepine, cyclobenzaprine, and mirtazapine, and should be avoided except by experts to treat difficult cases
- MAO inhibitors in combination with spinal anesthesia may cause combined hypotensive effects
- Combination of MAOIs and CNS depressants may enhance sedation and hypotension

Other Warnings/ Precautions

- Use requires low tyramine diet
- Patients taking MAO inhibitors should avoid high protein food that has undergone protein breakdown by aging, fermentation, pickling, smoking, or bacterial contamination
- Patients taking MAO inhibitors should avoid cheeses (especially aged varieties), pickled herring, beer, wine, liver, yeast extract, dry sausage, hard salami, pepperoni, Lebanon bologna, pods of broad beans (fava beans), yogurt, and excessive use of caffeine and chocolate
- Patient and prescriber must be vigilant to potential interactions with any drug, including antihypertensives and over-the-counter cough/cold preparations
- Over-the-counter medications to avoid include cough and cold preparations, including those containing dextromethorphan, nasal decongestants (tablets, drops, or spray), hay-fever medications, sinus medications, asthma inhalant medications, anti-appetite medications, weight reducing preparations, "pep" pills

- Hypoglycemia may occur in diabetic patients receiving insulin or oral antidiabetic agents
- Use cautiously in patients receiving reserpine, anesthetics, disulfiram, metrizamide, anticholinergic agents
- Phenelzine is not recommended for use in patients who cannot be monitored closely
- When treating children, carefully weigh the risks and benefits of pharmacological treatment against the risks and benefits of nontreatment with antidepressants and make sure to document this in the patient's chart
- Distribute the brochures provided by the FDA and the drug companies
- Warn patients and their caregivers about the possibility of activating side effects and advise them to report such symptoms immediately
- Monitor patients for activation of suicidal ideation, especially children and adolescents

Do Not Use
- If patient is taking meperidine (pethidine)
- If patient is taking a sympathomimetic agent or taking guanethidine
- If patient is taking another MAOI
- If patient is taking any agent that can inhibit serotonin reuptake (e.g., SSRIs, sibutramine, tramadol, milnacipran, duloxetine, venlafaxine, clomipramine, etc.)
- If patient is taking diuretics, dextromethorphan, buspirone, bupropion
- If patient has pheochromocytoma
- If patient has cardiovascular or cerebrovascular disease
- If patient has frequent or severe headaches
- If patient is undergoing elective surgery and requires general anesthesia
- If patient has a history of liver disease or abnormal liver function tests
- If patient is taking a prohibited drug
- If patient is not compliant with a low-tyramine diet
- If there is a proven allergy to phenelzine

Renal Impairment
- Use with caution – drug may accumulate in plasma

- May require lower than usual adult dose

Hepatic Impairment
- Phenelzine should not be used

Cardiac Impairment
- Contraindicated in patients with congestive heart failure or hypertension
- Any other cardiac impairment may require lower than usual adult dose
- Patients with angina pectoris or coronary artery disease should limit their exertion

Elderly
- Initial dose 7.5 mg/day; increase every few days by 7.5–15 mg/day
- Elderly patients may have greater sensitivity to adverse effects

 Children and Adolescents
- Not recommended for use under age 16
- Carefully weigh the risks and benefits of pharmacological treatment against the risks and benefits of nontreatment with antidepressants and make sure to document this in the patient's chart
- Monitor patients face-to-face regularly, particularly during the first several weeks of treatment
- Use with caution, observing for activation of known or unknown bipolar disorder and/or suicidal ideation, and inform parents or guardian of this risk so they can help observe child or adolescent patients

 Pregnancy
- Risk Category C [some animal studies show adverse effects, no controlled studies in humans]
- Not generally recommended for use during pregnancy, especially during first trimester
- Possible increased incidence of fetal malformations if phenelzine is taken during the first trimester
- Should evaluate patient for treatment with an antidepressant with a better risk/benefit ratio

Breast Feeding
- Some drug is found in mother's breast milk

- If child becomes irritable or sedated, breast feeding or drug may need to be discontinued
- Immediate postpartum period is a high-risk time for depression, especially in women who have had prior depressive episodes, so drug may need to be reinstituted late in the third trimester or shortly after childbirth to prevent a recurrence during the postpartum period
- Should evaluate patient for treatment with an antidepressant with a better risk/benefit ratio

THE ART OF PSYCHOPHARMACOLOGY

Potential Advantages
- Atypical depression
- Severe depression
- Treatment-resistant depression or anxiety disorders

Potential Disadvantages
- Requires compliance to dietary restrictions, concomitant drug restrictions
- Patients with cardiac problems or hypertension
- Multiple daily doses

Primary Target Symptoms
- Depressed mood
- Somatic symptoms
- Sleep and eating disturbances
- Psychomotor retardation
- Morbid preoccupation

Pearls
- MAOIs are generally reserved for second-line use after SSRIs, SNRIs, and combinations of newer antidepressants have failed
- Patient should be advised not to take any prescription or over-the-counter drugs without consulting their doctor because of possible drug interactions with the MAOI
- Headache is often the first symptom of hypertensive crisis
- Foods generally to avoid as they are usually high in tyramine content: dry sausage, pickled herring, liver, broad bean pods, sauerkraut, cheese, yogurt, alcoholic beverages, nonalcoholic beer and wine, chocolate, caffeine, meat and fish

- The rigid dietary restrictions may reduce compliance
- Mood disorders can be associated with eating disorders (especially in adolescent females), and phenelzine can be used to treat both depression and bulimia
- MAOIs are a viable second-line treatment option in depression, but are not frequently used
- ✳ Myths about the danger of dietary tyramine can be exaggerated, but prohibitions against concomitant drugs often not followed closely enough
- Orthostatic hypotension, insomnia, and sexual dysfunction are often the most troublesome common side effects
- ✳ MAOIs should be for the expert, especially if combining with agents of potential risk (e.g., stimulants, trazodone, TCAs)
- ✳ MAOIs should not be neglected as therapeutic agents for the treatment-resistant
- Although generally prohibited, a heroic but potentially dangerous treatment for severely treatment-resistant patients is for an expert to give a tricyclic/tetracyclic antidepressant other than clomipramine simultaneously with an MAO inhibitor for patients who fail to respond to numerous other antidepressants
- Use of MAOIs with clomipramine is always prohibited because of the risk of serotonin syndrome and death
- Amoxapine may be the preferred trycyclic/tetracyclic antidepressant to combine with an MAOI in heroic cases due to its theoretically protective 5HT2A antagonist properties
- If this option is elected, start the MAOI with the tricyclic/tetracyclic antidepressant simultaneously at low doses after appropriate drug washout, then alternately increase doses of these agents every few days to a week as tolerated
- Although very strict dietary and concomitant drug restrictions must be observed to prevent hypertensive crises and serotonin syndrome, the most common side effects of MAOI and tricyclic/tetracyclic combinations may be weight gain and orthostatic hypotension

Suggested Reading

Kennedy SH. Continuation and maintenance treatments in major depression: the neglected role of monoamine oxidase inhibitors. J Psychiatry Neurosci 1997;22:127–31.

Lippman SB, Nash K. Monoamine oxidase inhibitor update. Potential adverse food and drug interactions. Drug Saf 1990;5:195–204.

Parsons B, Quitkin FM, McGrath PJ, Stewart JW, Tricamo E, Ocepek-Welikson K, Harrison W, Rabkin JG, Wager SG, Nunes E. Phenelzine, imipramine, and placebo in borderline patients meeting criteria for atypical depression. Psychopharmacol Bull 1989; 25:524–34.

PROTRIPTYLINE

Brands • Triptil
• Vivactil
see index for additional brand names

Generic? Yes

Class
• Tricyclic antidepressant (TCA)
• Predominantly a norepinephrine/noradrenaline reuptake inhibitor

Commonly Prescribed For
(bold for FDA approved)
• **Mental depression**
• Treatment-resistant depression

How The Drug Works
• Boosts neurotransmitter norepinephrine/noradrenaline
• Blocks norepinephrine reuptake pump (norepinephrine transporter), presumably increasing noradrenergic neurotransmission
• Since dopamine is inactivated by norepinephrine reuptake in frontal cortex, which largely lacks dopamine transporters, protriptyline can increase dopamine neurotransmission in this part of the brain
• A more potent inhibitor of norepinephrine reuptake pump than serotonin reuptake pump (serotonin transporter)
• At high doses may also boost neurotransmitter serotonin and presumably increase serotonergic neurotransmission

How Long Until It Works
✳ Some evidence it may have an early onset of action with improvement in activity and energy as early as 1 week
• Onset of therapeutic actions usually not immediate, but often delayed 2 to 4 weeks
• If it is not working within 6 to 8 weeks for depression, it may require a dosage increase or it may not work at all
• May continue to work for many years to prevent relapse of symptoms

If It Works
• The goal of treatment is complete remission of current symptoms as well as prevention of future relapses
• Treatment most often reduces or even eliminates symptoms, but not a cure since symptoms can recur after medicine stopped
• Continue treatment until all symptoms are gone (remission)
• Once symptoms gone, continue treating for 1 year for the first episode of depression
• For second and subsequent episodes of depression, treatment may need to be indefinite
• Use in anxiety disorders may also need to be indefinite

If It Doesn't Work
• Many patients only have a partial response where some symptoms are improved but others persist (especially insomnia, fatigue, and problems concentrating)
• Other patients may be nonresponders, sometimes called treatment-resistant or treatment-refractory
• Consider increasing dose, switching to another agent or adding an appropriate augmenting agent
• Consider psychotherapy
• Consider evaluation for another diagnosis or for a comorbid condition (e.g., medical illness, substance abuse, etc.)
• Some patients may experience apparent lack of consistent efficacy due to activation of latent or underlying bipolar disorder, and require antidepressant discontinuation and a switch to a mood stabilizer

Best Augmenting Combos for Partial Response or Treatment-Resistance
• Lithium, buspirone, thyroid hormone

Tests
• None for healthy individuals
✳ Since tricyclic and tetracyclic antidepressants are frequently associated with weight gain, before starting treatment, weigh all patients and determine if the patient is already overweight (BMI 25.0–29.9) or obese (BMI ≥30)
• Before giving a drug that can cause weight gain to an overweight or obese patient, consider determining whether the patient

already has pre-diabetes (fasting plasma glucose 100–125 mg/dl), diabetes (fasting plasma glucose >126 mg/dl), or dyslipidemia (increased total cholesterol, LDL cholesterol and triglycerides; decreased HDL cholesterol), and treat or refer such patients for treatment, including nutrition and weight management, physical activity counseling, smoking cessation, and medical management

✳ Monitor weight and BMI during treatment

✳ While giving a drug to a patient who has gained >5% of initial weight, consider evaluating for the presence of pre-diabetes, diabetes, or dyslipidemia, or consider switching to a different antidepressant

• EKGs may be useful for selected patients (e.g., those with personal or family history of QTc prolongation; cardiac arrhythmia; recent myocardial infarction; uncompensated heart failure; or taking agents that prolong QTc interval such as pimozide, thioridazine, selected antiarrhythmics, moxifloxacin, sparfloxacin, etc.)

• Patients at risk for electrolyte disturbances (e.g., patients on diuretic therapy) should have baseline and periodic serum potassium and magnesium measurements

SIDE EFFECTS

How Drug Causes Side Effects

✳ Anticholinergic activity for protriptyline may be more potent than for some other TCAs and may explain sedative effects, dry mouth, constipation, blurred vision, tachycardia, and hypotension

• Sedative effects and weight gain may be due to antihistamine properties

• Blockade of alpha adrenergic 1 receptors may explain dizziness, sedation, and hypotension

• Cardiac arrhythmias, especially in overdose, may be caused by blockade of ion channels

Notable Side Effects

• Blurred vision, constipation, urinary retention, increased appetite, dry mouth, nausea, diarrhea, heartburn, unusual taste in mouth, weight gain

• Fatigue, weakness, dizziness, sedation, headache, anxiety, nervousness, restlessness

• Sexual dysfunction (impotence, change in libido)

• Sweating, rash, itching

 Life Threatening or Dangerous Side Effects

• Paralytic ileus, hyperthermia (TCAs + anticholinergic agents)

• Lowered seizure threshold and rare seizures

• Orthostatic hypotension, sudden death, arrhythmias, tachycardia

• QTc prolongation

• Hepatic failure, extrapyramidal symptoms

• Increased intraocular pressure

• Rare induction of mania

• Rare activation of suicidal ideation and behavior (suidicality)

Weight Gain

unusual   not unusual   common   problematic

• Many experience and/or can be significant in amount

• Can increase appetite and carbohydrate craving

Sedation

unusual   not unusual   common   problematic

• Many experience and/or can be significant in amount

✳ Not as sedating as other TCAs; more likely to be activating than other TCAs

What To Do About Side Effects

• Wait

• Wait

• Wait

• Lower the dose

• Switch to an SSRI or newer antidepressant

Best Augmenting Agents for Side Effects

• Trazodone or a hypnotic for insomnia

• Benzodiazepines for agitation and anxiety

• Many side effects cannot be improved with an augmenting agent

DOSING AND USE

Usual Dosage Range
- 15–40 mg/day in 3–4 divided doses

Dosage Forms
- Tablets 5 mg, 10 mg

How to Dose
- Initial 15 mg/day in divided doses; increase morning dose as needed; maximum dose 60 mg/day

 Dosing Tips

❋ Be aware that among this class of agents (tricyclic/tetracyclic antidepressants), protriptyline has uniquely low dosing (15–40 mg/day for protriptyline compared to 75–300 mg/day for most other tricyclic/tetracyclic antidepressants)

❋ Be aware that among this class of agents (tricyclic/tetracyclic antidepressants), protriptyline has uniquely frequent dosing (3–4 times a day compared to once daily for most other tricyclic/tetracyclic antidepressants)

- If intolerable anxiety, insomnia, agitation, akathisia, or activation occur either upon dosing initiation or discontinuation, consider the possibility of activated bipolar disorder, and switch to a mood stabilizer or an atypical antipsychotic

Overdose
- Death may occur; CNS depression, convulsions, cardiac dysrhythmias, severe hypotension, ECG changes, coma

Long-Term Use
- Safe

Habit Forming
- No

How to Stop
- Taper to avoid withdrawal effects
- Even with gradual dose reduction some withdrawal symptoms may appear within the first 2 weeks
- Many patients tolerate 50% dose reduction for 3 days, then another 50% reduction for 3 days, then discontinuation
- If withdrawal symptoms emerge during discontinuation, raise dose to stop

symptoms and then restart withdrawal much more slowly

Pharmacokinetics
- Substrate for CYP450 2D6
- Half-life approximately 74 hours

 Drug Interactions

- Tramadol increases the risk of seizures in patients taking TCAs
- Use of TCAs with anticholinergic drugs may result in paralytic ileus or hyperthermia
- Fluoxetine, paroxetine, bupropion, duloxetine, and other 2D6 inhibitors may increase TCA concentrations
- Cimetidine may increase plasma concentrations of TCAs and cause anticholinergic symptoms
- Phenothiazines or haloperidol may raise TCA blood concentrations
- May alter effects of antihypertensive drugs; may inhibit hypotensive effects of clonidine
- Use with sympathomimetic agents may increase sympathetic activity
- Methylphenidate may inhibit metabolism of TCAs
- Activation and agitation, especially following switching or adding antidepressants, may represent the induction of a bipolar state, especially a mixed dysphoric bipolar II condition sometimes associated with suicidal ideation, and require the addition of lithium, a mood stabilizer or an atypical antipsychotic, and/or discontinuation of protriptyline

 Other Warnings/ Precautions

- Add or initiate other antidepressants with caution for up to 2 weeks after discontinuing protriptyline
- Generally, do not use with MAO inhibitors, including 14 days after MAOIs are stopped; do not start an MAOI until 2 weeks after discontinuing protriptyline
- Use with caution in patients with history of seizures, urinary retention, narrow angle-closure glaucoma, hyperthyroidism
- TCAs can increase QTc interval, especially at toxic doses, which can be attained not only by overdose but also by combining

with drugs that inhibit TCA metabolism via CYP450 2D6, potentially causing torsade de pointes-type arrhythmia or sudden death
- Because TCAs can prolong QTc interval, use with caution in patients who have bradycardia or who are taking drugs that can induce bradycardia (e.g., beta blockers, calcium channel blockers, clonidine, digitalis)
- Because TCAs can prolong QTc interval, use with caution in patients who have hypokalemia and/or hypomagnesemia or who are taking drugs that can induce hypokalemia and/or magnesemia (e.g., diuretics, stimulant laxatives, intravenous amphotericin B, glucocorticoids, tetracosactide)
- When treating children, carefully weigh the risks and benefits of pharmacological treatment against the risks and benefits of nontreatment with antidepressants and make sure to document this in the patient's chart
- Distribute the brochures provided by the FDA and the drug companies
- Warn patients and their caregivers about the possibility of activating side effects and advise them to report such symptoms immediately
- Monitor patients for activation of suicidal ideation, especially children and adolescents

Do Not Use
- If patient is recovering from myocardial infarction
- If patient is taking agents capable of significantly prolonging QTc interval (e.g., pimozide, thioridazine, selected antiarrhythmics, moxifloxacin, sparfloxacin)
- If there is a history of QTc prolongation or cardiac arrhythmia, recent acute myocardial infarction, uncompensated heart failure
- If patient is taking drugs that inhibit TCA metabolism, including CYP450 2D6 inhibitors, except by an expert
- If there is reduced CYP450 2D6 function, such as patients who are poor 2D6 metabolizers, except by an expert and at low doses
- If there is a proven allergy to protriptyline

Renal Impairment
- Use with caution; may need to lower dose
- Patient may need to be monitored closely

Hepatic Impairment
- Use with caution; may need to lower dose
- Patient may need to be monitored closely

Cardiac Impairment
- TCAs have been reported to cause arrhythmias, prolongation of conduction time, orthostatic hypotension, sinus tachycardia, and heart failure, especially in the diseased heart
- Myocardial infarction and stroke have been reported with TCAs
- TCAs produce QTc prolongation, which may be enhanced by the existence of bradycardia, hypokalemia, congenital or acquired long QTc interval, which should be evaluated prior to administering protriptyline
- Use with caution if treating concomitantly with a medication likely to produce prolonged bradycardia, hypokalemia, slowing of intracardiac conduction, or prolongation of the QTc interval
- Avoid TCAs in patients with a known history of QTc prolongation, recent acute myocardial infarction, and uncompensated heart failure
- TCAs may cause a sustained increase in heart rate in patients with ischemic heart disease and may worsen (decrease) heart rate variability, an independent risk of mortality in cardiac populations
- Since SSRIs may improve (increase) heart rate variability in patients following a myocardial infarct and may improve survival as well as mood in patients with acute angina or following a myocardial infarction, these are more appropriate agents for cardiac population than tricyclic/tetracyclic antidepressants
- ✳ Risk/benefit ratio may not justify use of TCAs in cardiac impairment

Elderly
- May be more sensitive to anticholinergic, cardiovascular, hypotensive, and sedative effects

- Recommended dose is between 15–20 mg/day; doses >20 mg/day require close monitoring of patient

Children and Adolescents

- Carefully weigh the risks and benefits of pharmacological treatment against the risks and benefits of nontreatment with antidepressants and make sure to document this in the patient's chart
- Monitor patients face-to-face regularly, particularly during the first several weeks of treatment
- Use with caution, observing for activation of known or unknown bipolar disorder and/or suicidal ideation, and inform parents or guardian of this risk so they can help observe child or adolescent patients
- Not recommended for use under age 12
- Not intended for use under age 6
- Several studies show lack of efficacy of TCAs for depression
- Some cases of sudden death have occurred in children taking TCAs
- Recommended dose: 15–20 mg/day

Pregnancy

- Risk Category C [some animal studies show adverse effects, no controlled studies in humans]
- Crosses the placenta
- Adverse effects have been reported in infants whose mothers took a TCA (lethargy, withdrawal symptoms, fetal malformations)
- Must weigh the risk of treatment (first trimester fetal development, third trimester newborn delivery) to the child against the risk of no treatment (recurrence of depression, maternal health, infant bonding) to the mother and child
- For many patients this may mean continuing treatment during pregnancy

Breast Feeding

- Some drug is found in mother's breast milk
- ✳ Recommended either to discontinue drug or bottle feed
- Immediate postpartum period is a high-risk time for depression, especially in women who have had prior depressive episodes, so drug may need to be reinstituted late in the third trimester or shortly after childbirth to prevent a recurrence during the postpartum period
- Must weigh benefits of breast feeding with risks and benefits of antidepressant treatment versus non-treatment to both the infant and the mother
- For many patients this may mean continuing treatment during breast feeding

THE ART OF PSYCHOPHARMACOLOGY

Potential Advantages
- Severe or treatment-resistant depression
- Withdrawn, anergic patients

Potential Disadvantages
- Pediatric, geriatric, and cardiac patients
- Patients concerned with weight gain
- Patients noncompliant with 3–4 times daily dosing

Primary Target Symptoms
- Depressed mood

Pearls

- Tricyclic antidepressants are no longer generally considered a first-line treatment option for depression because of their side effect profile
- Tricyclic antidepressants continue to be useful for severe or treatment-resistant depression
- ✳ Has some potential advantages for withdrawn, anergic patients
- ✳ May have a more rapid onset of action than some other TCAs
- ✳ May aggravate agitation and anxiety more than some other TCAs
- ✳ May have more anticholinergic side effects, hypotension, and tachycardia than some other TCAs
- Noradrenergic reuptake inhibitors such as protriptyline can be used as a second-line treatment for smoking cessation, cocaine dependence, and attention deficit disorder
- TCAs may aggravate psychotic symptoms
- Alcohol should be avoided because of additive CNS effects
- Underweight patients may be more susceptible to adverse cardiovascular effects

- Children, patients with inadequate hydration, and patients with cardiac disease may be more susceptible to TCA-induced cardiotoxicity than healthy adults
- For the expert only: a heroic treatment (but potentially dangerous) for severely treatment-resistant patients is to give simultaneously with monoamine oxidase inhibitors for patients who fail to respond to numerous other antidepressants, but generally recommend a different TCA than protriptyline for this use
- If this option is elected, start the MAOI with the tricyclic/tetracyclic antidepressant simultaneously at low doses after appropriate drug washout, then alternately increase doses of these agents every few days to a week as tolerated
- Although very strict dietary and concomitant drug restrictions must be observed to prevent hypertensive crises and serotonin syndrome, the most common side effects of MAOI and tricyclic/tetracyclic antidepressant combinations may be weight gain and orthostatic hypotension

- Patients on TCAs should be aware that they may experience symptoms such as photosensitivity or blue-green urine
- SSRIs may be more effective than TCAs in women, and TCAs may be more effective than SSRIs in men
- Since tricyclic/tetracyclic antidepressants are substrates for CYP450 2D6, and 7% of the population (especially Caucasians) may have a genetic variant leading to reduced activity of 2D6, such patients may not safely tolerate normal doses of tricyclic/tetracyclic antidepressants and may require dose reduction
- Phenotypic testing may be necessary to detect this genetic variant prior to dosing with a tricyclic/tetracyclic antidepressant, especially in vulnerable populations such as children, elderly, cardiac populations, and those on concomitant medications
- Patients who seem to have extraordinarily severe side effects at normal or low doses may have this phenotypic CYP450 2D6 variant and require low doses or switching to another antidepressant not metabolized by 2D6

 Suggested Reading

Anderson IM. Meta-analytical studies on new antidepressants. Br Med Bull. 2001; 57: 161–178.

Anderson IM. Selective serotonin reuptake inhibitors versus tricyclic antidepressants: a meta-analysis of efficacy and tolerability. J Aff Disorders. 2000; 58: 19–36.

Rudorfer MV, Potter WZ. Metabolism of tricyclic antidepressants. Cell Mol Neurobiol. 1999; 19 (3): 373–409.

REBOXETINE

THERAPEUTICS

Brands • Norebox
• Edronax
see index for additional brand names

Generic? No

 Class
• Selective norepinephrine reuptake inhibitor (NRI); antidepressant

Commonly Prescribed For
(bold for FDA approved)
• Major depressive disorder
• Dysthymia
• Panic disorder
• Attention deficit hyperactivity disorder

 How The Drug Works
• Boost neurotransmitter norepinephrine/noradrenaline and may also increase dopamine in prefrontal cortex
• Blocks norepinephrine reuptake pump (norepinephrine transporter)
• Presumably, this increases noradrenergic neurotransmission
• Since dopamine is inactivated by norepinephrine reuptake in frontal cortex which largely lacks dopamine transporters, reboxetine can increase dopamine neurotransmission in this part of the brain

How Long Until It Works
• Onset of therapeutic actions usually not immediate, but often delayed 2 to 4 weeks
• If it is not working within 6 to 8 weeks for depression, it may require a dosage increase or it may not work at all
• May continue to work for many years to prevent relapse of symptoms

If It Works
• The goal of treatment is complete remission of current symptoms as well as prevention of future relapses
• Treatment most often reduces or even eliminates symptoms, but not a cure since symptoms can recur after medicine stopped
• Continue treatment until all symptoms are gone (remission)

• Once symptoms gone, continue treating for 1 year for the first episode of depression
• For second and subsequent episodes of depression, treatment may need to be indefinite

If It Doesn't Work
• Many patients only have a partial response where some symptoms are improved but others persist (especially insomnia, fatigue, and problems concentrating)
• Other patients may be nonresponders, sometimes called treatment-resistant or treatment-refractory
• Consider increasing dose, switching to another agent or adding an appropriate augmenting agent
• Consider psychotherapy
• Consider evaluation for another diagnosis or for a comorbid condition (e.g., medical illness, substance abuse, etc.)
• Some patients may experience apparent lack of consistent efficacy due to activation of latent or underlying bipolar disorder, and require antidepressant discontinuation and a switch to a mood stabilizer

 Best Augmenting Combos for Partial Response or Treatment-Resistance
• Trazodone, especially for insomnia
• SSRIs, SNRIs, mirtazapine (use combinations of antidepressants with caution as this may activate bipolar disorder and suicidal ideation)
• Modafinil, especially for fatigue, sleepiness, and lack of concentration
• Mood stabilizers or atypical antipsychotics for bipolar depression, psychotic depression or treatment-resistant depression
• Benzodiazepines for anxiety
• Hypnotics for insomnia
• Classically, lithium, buspirone, or thyroid hormone

Tests
• None for healthy individuals

SIDE EFFECTS

How Drug Causes Side Effects
• Norepinephrine increases in parts of the brain and body and at receptors other than

those that cause therapeutic actions (e.g., unwanted actions of norepinephrine on acetylcholine release causing constipation and dry mouth, etc.)
- Most side effects are immediate but often go away with time

Notable Side Effects
- Insomnia, dizziness, anxiety, agitation
- Dry mouth, constipation
- Urinary hesitancy, urinary retention
- Sexual dysfunction (impotence)
- Dose-dependent hypotension

 Life Threatening or Dangerous Side Effects
- Rare seizures
- Rare induction of mania
- Rare activation of suicidal ideation and behavior (suicidality)

Weight Gain
 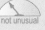
- Reported but not expected

Sedation

- Reported but not expected

What To Do About Side Effects
- Wait
- Wait
- Wait
- Lower the dose
- In a few weeks, switch or add other drugs

Best Augmenting Agents for Side Effects
- For urinary hesitancy, give an alpha 1 blocker such as tamsulosin
- Often best to try another antidepressant monotherapy prior to resorting to augmentation strategies to treat side effects
- Trazodone or a hypnotic for drug-induced insomnia
- Benzodiazepines for drug-induced anxiety and activation
- Mirtazapine for drug-induced insomnia or anxiety

- Many side effects are dose-dependent (i.e., they increase as dose increases, or they reemerge until tolerance re-develops)
- Many side effects are time-dependent (i.e., they start immediately upon dosing and upon each dose increase, but go away with time)
- Activation and agitation may represent the induction of a bipolar state, especially a mixed dysphoric bipolar II condition sometimes associated with suicidal ideation, and require the addition of lithium, a mood stabilizer or an atypical antipsychotic, and/or discontinuation of reboxetine

DOSING AND USE

Usual Dosage Range
- 8 mg/day in 2 doses (10 mg usual maximum daily dose)

Dosage Forms
- Tablet 2 mg, 4 mg scored

How to Dose
- Initial 2 mg/day twice a day for 1 week, 4 mg/day twice a day for second week

 Dosing Tips
- When switching from another antidepressant or adding to another antidepressant, dosing may need to be lower and titration slower to prevent activating side effects (e.g., 2 mg in the daytime for 2–3 days, then 2 mg bid for 1–2 weeks)
- Give second daily dose in late afternoon rather than at bedtime to avoid undesired activation or insomnia in the evening
- May not need full dose of 8 mg/day when given in conjunction with another antidepressant
- Some patients may need 10 mg/day or more if well-tolerated without orthostatic hypotension and if additional efficacy is seen at high doses in difficult cases
- Early dosing in patients with panic and anxiety may need to be lower and titration slower, perhaps with the use of concomitant short-term benzodiazepines to increase tolerability

Overdose
- Postural hypotension, anxiety, hypertension

Long-Term Use
- Safe

Habit Forming
- No

How to Stop
- Taper not necessary

Pharmacokinetics
- Metabolized by CYP450 3A4
- Inhibits CYP450 2D6 and 3A4 at high doses
- Elimination half-life approximately 13 hours

 Drug Interactions
- Tramadol increases the risk of seizures in patients taking an antidepressant
- May need to reduce reboxetine dose or avoid concomitant use with inhibitors of CYP450 3A4, such as azole and antifungals, macrolide antibiotics, fluvoxamine, nefazodone, fluoxetine, sertraline, etc.
- Via CYP450 2D6 inhibition, reboxetine could theoretically interfere with the analgesic actions of codeine, and increase the plasma levels of some beta blockers and of atomoxetine and TCAs
- Via CYP450 2D6 inhibition, reboxetine could theoretically increase concentrations of thioridazine and cause dangerous cardiac arrhythmias
- Via CYP450 3A4 inhibition, reboxetine may increase the levels of alprazolam, buspirone, and triazolam
- Via CYP450 3A4 inhibition, reboxetine could theoretically increase concentrations of certain cholesterol lowering HMG CoA reductase inhibitors, especially simvastatin, atorvastatin, and lovastatin, but not pravastatin or fluvastatin, which would increase the risk of rhabdomyolysis; thus, coadministration of reboxetine with certain HMG CoA reductase inhibitors should proceed with caution
- Via CYP450 3A4 inhibition, reboxetine could theoretically increase the concentrations of pimozide, and cause QTc prolongation and dangerous cardiac arrhythmias

- Use with ergotamine may increase blood pressure
- Hypokalemia may occur if reboxetine is used with diuretics
- Do not use with MAO inhibitors, including 14 days after MAOIs are stopped

 Other Warnings/ Precautions
- Use with caution in patients with bipolar disorder unless treated with concomitant mood stabilizing agent
- Use with caution in patients with urinary retention, benign prostatic hyperplasia, glaucoma, epilepsy
- Use with caution with drugs that lower blood pressure
- When treating children, carefully weigh the risks and benefits of pharmacological treatment against the risks and benefits of nontreatment with antidepressants and make sure to document this in the patient's chart
- Distribute the brochures provided by the FDA and the drug companies
- Warn patients and their caregivers about the possibility of activating side effects and advise them to report such symptoms immediately
- Monitor patients for activation of suicidal ideation, especially children and adolescents

Do Not Use
- If patient has narrow angle-closure glaucoma
- If patient is taking an MAO inhibitor
- If patient is taking pimozide or thioridazine
- If there is a proven allergy to reboxetine

SPECIAL POPULATIONS

Renal Impairment
- Plasma concentrations are increased
- May need to lower dose

Hepatic Impairment
- Plasma concentrations are increased
- May need to lower dose

Cardiac Impairment
- Use with caution

Elderly
• Lower dose is recommended (4–6 mg/day)

Children and Adolescents
• Carefully weigh the risks and benefits of pharmacological treatment against the risks and benefits of nontreatment with antidepressants and make sure to document this in the patient's chart
• Monitor patients face-to-face regularly, particularly during the first several weeks of treatment
• Use with caution, observing for activation of known or unknown bipolar disorder and/or suicidal ideation, and inform parents or guardian of this risk so they can help observe child or adolescent patients
• No guidelines for children; safety and efficacy have not been established

Pregnancy
• No controlled studies in humans
• Not generally recommended for use during pregnancy, especially during first trimester
• Must weigh the risk of treatment (first trimester fetal development, third trimester newborn delivery) to the child against the risk of no treatment (recurrence of depression, maternal health, infant bonding) to the mother and child
• For many patients this may mean continuing treatment during pregnancy

Breast Feeding
• Some drug is found in mother's breast milk
• Immediate postpartum period is a high-risk time for depression, especially in women who have had prior depressive episodes, so drug may need to be reinstituted late in the third trimester or shortly after childbirth to prevent a recurrence during the postpartum period
• Must weigh benefits of breast feeding with risks and benefits of antidepressant treatment versus non-treatment to both the infant and the mother
• For many patients, this may mean continuing treatment during breast feeding

THE ART OF PSYCHOPHARMACOLOGY

Potential Advantages
• Tired, unmotivated patients
• Patients with cognitive disturbances
• Patients with psychomotor retardation

Potential Disadvantages
• Patients unable to comply with twice-daily dosing
• Patients unable to tolerate activation

Primary Target Symptoms
• Depressed mood
• Energy, motivation, and interest
• Suicidal ideation
• Cognitive disturbance
• Psychomotor retardation

Pearls
• May be effective if SSRIs have failed or for SSRI "poop-out"
* May be more likely than SSRIs to improve social and work functioning
• Reboxetine is a mixture of an active and an inactive enantiomer, and the active enantiomer may be developed in future clinical testing
* Side effects may appear "anticholinergic", but reboxetine does not directly block muscarinic receptors
• Constipation, dry mouth, and urinary retention are noradrenergic, due in part to peripheral alpha 1 receptor stimulation causing decreased acetylcholine release
* Thus, antidotes for these side effects can be alpha 1 antagonists such as tamsulosin, especially for urinary retention in men over 50 with borderline urine flow
• Novel use of reboxetine may be for attention deficit disorder, analogous to the actions of another norepinephrine selective reuptake inhibitor, atomoxetine, but few controlled studies
• Another novel use may be for neuropathic pain, alone or in combination with other antidepressants, but few controlled studies
• Some studies suggest efficacy in panic disorder

Suggested Reading

Fleishaker JC. Clinical pharmacokinetics of reboxetine, a selective norepinephrine reuptake inhibitor for the treatment of patients with depression. Clin Pharmacokinet 2000;39(6):413–27.

Kasper S, el Giamal N, Hilger E. Reboxetine: the first selective noradrenaline re-uptake inhibitor. Expert Opin Pharmacother 2000;1(4):771–82.

Keller M. Role of serotonin and noradrenaline in social dysfunction: a review of data on reboxetine and the Social Adaptation Self-evaluation Scale (SASS). Gen Hosp Psychiatry 2001;23(1):15–9.

Tanum L. Reboxetine: tolerability and safety profile in patients with major depression. Acta Psychiatr Scand Suppl 2000;402:37–40.

SELEGILINE

THERAPEUTICS

Brands • EMSAM
• Eldepryl
see index for additional brand names

Generic? Yes (oral only)

Class
- Transdermal: tissue selective monoamine oxidase (MAO) inhibitor (MAO-A and MAO-B inhibitor in brain and relatively selective MAO-B inhibitor in gut)
- Oral: selective MAO-B inhibitor

Commonly Prescribed For
(bold for FDA approved)
- **Major depressive disorder (transdermal)**
- **Oral: Parkinson's disease or symptomatic Parkinsonism (adjunctive)**
- Treatment-resistant depression
- Panic disorder (transdermal)
- Social anxiety disorder (transdermal)
- Treatment-resistant anxiety disorders (transdermal)
- Alzheimer disease and other dementias (oral)

How The Drug Works
- Transdermal selegiline (recommended doses): in the brain, irreversibly inhibits both MAO-A and MAO-B from breaking down norepinephrine, serotonin, and dopamine, which presumably boosts noradrenergic, serotonergic, and dopaminergic neurotransmission
- Transdermal selegiline (recommended doses): in the gut, is a relatively selective irreversible inhibitor of MAO-B (intestine and liver), reducing the chances of dietary interactions with the MAO-A substrate tyramine
- Oral: at recommended doses, selectively and irreversibly blocks MAO-B, which presumably boosts dopaminergic neurotransmission
- Oral: above recommended doses, irreversibly blocks both MAO-A and MAO-B from breaking down norepinephrine, serotonin, and dopamine while simultaneously blocking metabolism of tyramine in the gut

- Thus, high dose oral administration is not tissue selective and is not MAO-A sparing in the gut, and may interact with tyramine-containing foods to cause hypertension

How Long Until It Works
- Onset of therapeutic actions in depression with transdermal administration is usually not immediate, but often delayed 2 to 4 weeks or longer
- If it is not working for depression within 6 to 8 weeks, it may require a dosage increase or it may not work at all
- May continue to work in depression for many years to prevent relapse of symptoms
- Can enhance the actions of levodopa in Parkinson's disease within a few weeks of initiating oral dosing
- Theoretical slowing of functional loss in both Parkinson's disease and Alzheimer disease is a provocative possibility under investigation and would take many months or more than a year to observe

If It Works
- The goal of treatment in depression is complete remission of current symptoms as well as prevention of future relapses
- Treatment of depression most often reduces or even eliminates symptoms, but not a cure since symptoms can recur after medicine stopped
- Continue treatment of depression until all symptoms of depression are gone (remission)
- Once symptoms of depression are gone, continue treating for 1 year for the first episode of depression
- For second and subsequent episodes of depression, treatment may need to be indefinite
- Continue use in Parkinson's disease as long as there is evidence that selegiline is favorably enhancing the actions of levodopa
- Use of selegiline to slow functional loss in Parkinson's disease or Alzheimer disease would be long-term if proven effective for this use

If It Doesn't Work
- Many depressed patients only have a partial response where some symptoms are improved but others persist (especially

insomnia, fatigue, and problems concentrating)
- Other depressed patients may be nonresponders, sometimes called treatment-resistant or treatment-refractory
- Some depressed patients who have an initial response may relapse even though they continue treatment, sometimes called "poop out"
- For depression, consider increasing dose, switching to another agent or adding an appropriate augmenting agent, psychotherapy, and evaluation for another diagnosis or for a comorbid condition (e.g., medical illness, substance abuse, etc.)
- Some patients may experience apparent lack of consistent efficacy due to activation of latent or underlying bipolar disorder, and require antidepressant discontinuation and a switch to a mood stabilizer
- Use alternate treatments for Parkinson's disease or Alzheimer's disease

 ### Best Augmenting Combos for Partial Response or Treatment-Resistance

✱ Augmentation of selegiline has not been systematically studied in depression, and this is something for the expert, to be done with caution and with careful monitoring
- A stimulant such as d-amphetamine or methylphenidate (with caution and by experts only as use of stimulants with selegiline is listed as a warning; may activate bipolar disorder and suicidal ideation; may elevate blood pressure)
- Lithium
- Mood stabilizing anticonvulsants
- Atypical antipsychotics (with special caution for those agents with monoamine reuptake blocking properties, such as ziprasidone and zotepine)
- Carbidopa-levodopa (for Parkinson's disease)

Tests
- Patients should be monitored for changes in blood pressure
- Although preliminary evidence from clinical trials suggests little or no weight gain, nonselective MAO inhibitors are frequently associated with weight gain. Thus, before starting treatment for depression with high doses of selegiline, weigh all patients and determine if the patient is already

overweight (BMI>25.0–29.9) or obese (BMI≥30)
- Before giving a drug that can cause weight gain to an overweight or obese patient, consider determining whether the patient already has pre-diabetes (fasting plasma glucose 100–125 mg/dl), diabetes (fasting plasma glucose >126 mg/dl), or dyslipidemia (increased total cholesterol, LDL cholesterol and triglycerides; decreased HDL cholesterol), and treat or refer such patients for treatment including nutrition and weight management, physical activity counseling, smoking cessation, and medical management
- ✱ Monitor weight and BMI during treatment
- ✱ While giving a drug to a patient who has gained >5% of initial weight, consider evaluating for the presence of pre-diabetes, diabetes, or dyslipidemia, or consider switching to a different antidepressant

SIDE EFFECTS

How Drug Causes Side Effects
- At recommended transdermal doses, norepinephrine, serotonin and dopamine increase in parts of the brain and at receptors other than those that cause therapeutic actions
- At high transdermal doses, loss of tissue selectivity and loss of MAO-A sparing actions in the gut may enhance the possibility of dietary tyramine interactions if MAO-B inhibition occurs in the gut
- At recommended oral doses, dopamine increases in parts of the brain and body and at receptors other than those that cause therapeutic actions
- Side effects are generally immediate, but immediate side effects often disappear in time

Notable Side Effects
- Transdermal: application site reactions, headache, insomnia, diarrhea, dry mouth
- Oral: exacerbation of levodopa side effects, especially nausea, dizziness, abdominal pain, dry mouth, headache, dyskinesia, confusion, hallucinations, vivid dreams

Life Threatening or Dangerous Side Effects

- Transdermal: hypertensive crisis was not observed with preliminary experience in clinical trials, even in patients who were not following a low tyramine diet
- Oral: hypertensive crisis (especially when MAOIs are used with certain tryamine-containing foods or prohibited drugs) – reduced risk at low oral doses compared to nonselective MAOIs
- Theoretically, when used at high doses may induce seizures and mania as do nonselective MAOIs
- Rare activation of suicidal ideation and behavior (suicidality)

Weight Gain

unusual   not unusual   common   problematic

- Transdermal: Reported but not expected; some patients may experience weight loss
- Oral: Occurs in significant minority

Sedation

unusual   not unusual   common   problematic

- Reported but not expected
- Can be activating in some patients

What To Do About Side Effects

- Wait
- Wait
- Wait
- Lower the dose
- Switch after appropriate washout to an SSRI or newer antidepressant (depression)
- Switch to other anti-parkinsonian therapies (Parkinson's Disease)

Best Augmenting Agents for Side Effects

- Trazodone (with caution) for insomnia in depression
- Benzodiazepines for insomnia in depression
- Single oral or sublingual dose of a calcium channel blocker (e.g., nifedipine) for urgent treatment of hypertension due to drug interaction or dietary tyramine
- Many side effects cannot be improved with an augmenting agent, especially at lower doses

DOSING AND USE

Usual Dosage Range

- Depression (transdermal): 6 mg/24 hours– 12 mg/24 hours
- Depression (oral): 30–60 mg/day
- Parkinson's disease/Alzheimer disease: 5–10 mg/day

Dosage Forms

- Transdermal patch 20 mg/20 cm² (6 mg/24 hours), 30 mg/30 cm² (9 mg/24 hours), 40 mg/40cm² (12 mg/24 hours)
- Capsule 5 mg
- Tablet 5 mg scored

How to Dose

- Depression (transdermal): Initial 6 mg/24 hours; can increase by 3 mg/24 hours every 2 weeks; maximum dose generally 12 mg/24 hours
- Parkinson's disease: Initial 2.5 mg/day twice daily; increase to 5 mg twice daily; reduce dose of levodopa after 2–3 days

Dosing Tips

- Transdermal patch contains 1 mg of selegiline per 1 cm² and delivers approximately 0.3 mg of selegiline per cm² over 24 hours
- Patch is available in three sizes – 20 mg/20 cm², 30 mg/30 cm², and 40 mg/40 cm² – that deliver doses of approximately 6 mg, 9 mg, and 12 mg, respectively, over 24 hours
- At 6 mg/24 hours (transdermal) dietary adjustments are not generally required
- Dietary modifications to restrict tyramine intake from foods are recommended for doses above 6 mg/24 hours (transdermal)
- Transdermal patch should only be applied to dry, intact skin on the upper torso, upper thigh, or outer surface of the upper arm
- New application site should be selected for each day; patch should be applied at approximately the same time every day; only one patch should be applied at a time; patches should not be cut
- Avoid touching the exposed (sticky) side of the patch, and after application, <u>wash hands</u> with soap and water; do not touch eyes until after hands have been washed

- Heat could theoretically increase the amount of selegiline absorbed from the transdermal patch, so patients should avoid exposing the application site to external sources of direct heat (e.g., heating pads, prolonged direct sunlight)
- Although there is theoretically a three day reservoir of drug in each patch, multiday administration from a single patch is generally not recommended and has not been tested; because of residual drug in the patch after 24 hours of administration, discard used patches in a manner that prevents accidental application or ingestion by children, pets, or others
- For Parkinson's disease, oral dosage above 10 mg/day generally not recommended
- Dosage of carbidopa-levodopa can at times be reduced by 10–30% after 2–3 days of administering oral selegiline 5–10 mg/day in Parkinson's disease
- At doses above 10 mg/day (oral), selegiline may become nonselective and inhibit both MAO-A and MAO-B
- At doses above 30 mg/day (oral), selegiline may have antidepressant properties
- Patients receiving high oral doses may need to be evaluated periodically for effects on the liver
- Doses above 10 mg/day (oral) may increase the risk of hypertensive crisis, tyramine interactions, and drug interactions similar to those of phenelzine and tranylcypromine

Overdose

- Overdose with the transdermal formulation is likely to produce substantial amounts of MAO-A inhibition as well as MAO-B inhibition, and should be treated the same as overdose with a nonselective oral MAO inhibitor
- Dizziness, anxiety, ataxia, insomnia, sedation, irritability, headache; cardiovascular effects, confusion, respiratory depression, coma

Long-Term Use

- Long-term use has not been systematically studied although generally recommended for chronic use as for other antidepressants

Habit Forming

- Lack of evidence for abuse potential with transdermal selegiline despite its metabolism to l-amphetamine and l-methamphetamine
- Some patients have developed dependence to other MAOIs

How to Stop

- Transdermal: MAO inhibition slowly recovers over 2–3 weeks after patch removed
- Oral: Generally no need to taper, as the drug wears off slowly over 2–3 weeks

Pharmacokinetics

- Clinical duration of action may be up to 21 days due to irreversible enzyme inhibition
- Major metabolite of selegiline is desmethylselegiline; other metabolites are L-methamphetamine and L-amphetamine
- Because first-pass metabolism is not extensive with transdermal dosing, this results in notably higher exposure to selegiline and lower exposure to metabolites as compared to oral dosing
- With transdermal selegiline, 25–30% of selegiline content is delivered systemically over 24 hours from each patch
- Mean half life of transdermal selegiline is approximately 18–25 hours
- Steady-state mean elimination half-life of oral selegiline is approximately 10 hours

Drug Interactions

- Many misunderstandings about what drugs can be combined with MAO inhibitors
- Theoretically and especially at high doses, selegiline could cause a fatal "serotonin syndrome" when combined with drugs that block serotonin reuptake (e.g., SSRIs, SNRIs, sibutramine, tramadol, clomipramine, etc), so do not use with a serotonin reuptake inhibitors for up to 5 half lives after stopping the serotonin reuptake inhibitor (i.e., "wash-in" of selegiline should be about 1 week after discontinuing most agents [except 5 weeks or more after discontinuing fluoxetine because of its long half-life and that of its active metabolite])
- When discontinuing selegiline ("wash-out" period), wait two weeks before starting

another antidepressant in order to allow enough time for the body to regenerate MAO enzyme
- Transdermal: no pharmacokinetic drug interactions present in studies with alprazolam, ibuprofen, levothyroxine, olanzapine, risperidone and warfarin
- Tramadol may increase the risk of seizures in patients taking an MAO inhibitor
- Selegiline may interact with opiate agonists to cause agitation, hallucination, or death
- Hypertensive crisis with headache, intracranial bleeding, and death may result from combining nonselective MAO inhibitors with sympathomimetic drugs (e.g., amphetamines, methylphenidate, cocaine, dopamine, epinephrine, nonepinephrine, and related compounds methyldopa, levodopa, L-tryptophan, L-tyrosine, and phenylalanine
- Excitation, seizures, delirium, hyperpyrexia, circulatory collapse, coma, and death may result from combining nonselective MAO inhibitors with mepiridine or dextromethorphan
- Do not combine with another MAO inhibitor, alcohol, buspirone, bupropion, or guanethidine
- Adverse drug reactions can result from combining MAO inhibitors with tricyclic/tetracyclic antidepressants and related compounds, including carbamazepine, cyclobenzaprine, and mirtazapine, and should be avoided except by experts to treat difficult cases
- Carbamazepine increases plasma levels of selegiline and is contraindicated with MAOIs
- MAO inhibitors in combination with spinal anesthesia may cause combined hypotensive effects
- Combination of MAOIs and CNS depressants may enhance sedation and hypotension

 Other Warnings/ Precautions
- Ingestion of a "high tyramine meal" is generally defined as 40 mg or more of tyramine in the fasted state
- Studies show that 200 to 400 mg of tyramine in the fasted state (and even more ingestion of tyramine in the fed state) may be required for a hypertensive response

with administration of the low dose transdermal patch (20 mg); thus, no dietary precautions are required at this dose
- Tyramine sensitivity of the low dose transdermal patch (20 mg) may be comparable to that of low dose oral selegiline (10 mg) with neither causing a hypertensive reaction to high tyramine meals
- Tyramine sensitivity and hypertensive responses to the high dose transdermal patch (40 mg) may occur with administration of 70–100 mg of tyramine in the fasted state, so dietary restrictions may also not be necessary at 30 mg or 40 mg of transdermal administration of selegiline
- However, insufficient studies have been performed to be sure of the safety of transdermal administration at 30 mg or 40 mg, so dietary restrictions of tyramine are still recommended at these higher doses
- Oral administration of nonselective irreversible MAO inhibitors generally requires adherence to a low tyramine diet
- Ingestion of a "high tyramine meal" defined as 40 mg or more of tyramine in the fasted state or as little as ingestion of 10 mg of tyramine in the fasted state can cause hypertensive reactions in patients taking a nonselective irreversible MAO inhibitor orally
- Foods to avoid for oral administration of nonselective irreversible MAO inhibitors include: dried, aged, smoked, fermented, spoiled, or improperly stored meat, poultry, and fish; broad bean pods; aged cheeses; tap and nonpasteurized beers; marmite; sauerkraut; soy products/tofu
- These restrictions are generally recommended for patients taking the higher doses of transdermal selegiline (30 mg and 40 mg transdermally) but not for the lower doses of transdermal selegiline (20 mg transdermally) or for the low dose orally (10 mg)
- Transdermal: studies of low dose transdermal administration of selegiline (20 mg) failed to show changes in systolic or diastolic blood pressure or pulse when administered to normal volunteers taking either pseudoephedrine 60 mg three times

a day for 2 days or 25 mg of phenylpropanolamine (no longer commercially available in the US) every 4 hours for 1 day

- However, sufficient safety information is not available to recommend administration of pseudoephedrine without a precaution; blood pressure should be monitored if low dose transdermal selegiline is given at all with pseudoephedrine
- Pseudoephedrine may need to be avoided when administering transdermal selegiline, particularly at higher doses of selegiline or in vulnerable patients with hypertension
- Although risk may be reduced with transdermal administration of selegiline, patient and prescriber must be vigilant to potential interactions with any drug, including antihypertensives and over-the-counter cough/cold preparations
- Over the counter medications to avoid or use with caution under the care of an expert include cough and cold preparations, including those containing dextromethorphan, nasal decongestants (tablets, drops, or spray), hay-fever medications, sinus medications, asthma inhalant medications, anti-appetite medications, weight reducing preparations, "pep" pills
- Hypoglycemia may occur in diabetic patients receiving insulin or oral antidiabetic agents
- Use cautiously in patients receiving reserpine, anesthetics, disulfiram, metrizamide, anticholinergic agents
- Selegiline is not recommended for use in patients who cannot be monitored closely
- Only use sympathomimetic agents or guanethidine with oral doses of selegiline below 10 mg/day
- When treating children, carefully weigh the risks and benefits of pharmacological treatment against the risks and benefits of nontreatment with antidepressants and make sure to document this in the patient's chart
- Distribute the brochures provide by the FDA and the drug companies
- Warn patients and their caregivers about the possibility of activating side effects and advise them to report such symptoms immediately

- Monitor patients for activation of suicidal ideation, especially children and adolescents

Do Not Use

- If patient is taking meperidine (pethidine)
- If patient is taking a sympathomimetic agent or taking guanethidine
- If patient is taking another MAOI
- If patient is taking any agent that can inhibit serotonin reuptake (e.g., SSRIs, sibutramine, tramadol, milnacipran, duloxetine, venlafaxine, clomipramine, etc.)
- If patient is taking diuretics, dextromethorphan, buspirone, bupropion
- If patient is taking St. John's wort, cyclobenzaprine, methadone, propoxyphene
- If patient has pheochromocytoma
- If patient is undergoing elective surgery and requires general anesthesia
- If there is a proven allergy to selegiline

SPECIAL POPULATIONS

Renal Impairment

- No dose adjustment necessary for transdermal administration in patients with mild to moderate renal impairment
- Use oral administration with caution – drug may accumulate in plasma in patients with renal impairment
- Oral administration may require lower than usual adult dose

Hepatic Impairment

- No dose adjustment necessary for transdermal administration in patients with mild to moderate hepatic impairment
- Oral administration may require lower than usual adult dose

Cardiac Impairment

- May require lower than usual adult dose
- Observe closely for orthostatic hypotension

Elderly

- Recommended dose for patients over 65 years old is 20 mg
- Dose increases in the elderly should be made with caution and patients should be observed for postural changes in blood pressure throughout treatment

Children and Adolescents

- Not recommended for use under 18
- Use with caution, observing for activation of known or unknown bipolar disorder and/or suicidal ideation, and inform parents or guardians of this risk so they can help observe child or adolescent patients
- Carefully weigh the risks and benefits of pharmacological treatment against the risks and benefits of nontreatment with antidepressants and make sure to document this in the patient's chart
- Monitor patients face-to-face regularly, particularly during the first several weeks of treatment

Pregnancy

- Risk Category C [some animal studies show adverse effects, no controlled studies in humans]
- Not generally recommended for use during pregnancy, especially during first trimester
- Should evaluate patient for treatment with an antidepressant with a better risk/benefit ratio

Breast Feeding

- Some drug is found in mother's breast milk
- Immediate postpartum period is a high-risk time for depression, especially in women who have had prior depressive episodes, so drug may need to be reinstituted late in the third trimester or shortly after childbirth to prevent a recurrence during the postpartum period
- Should evaluate patient for treatment with an antidepressant with a better risk/benefit ratio

THE ART OF PSYCHOPHARMACOLOGY

Potential Advantages

- Treatment-resistant depression
- Patients with atypical depression (hypersomnia, hyperphagia)
- Patients who wish to avoid weight gain and sexual dysfunction
- Parkinson's patients inadequately responsive to levodopa

Potential Disadvantages

- Non-compliant patients
- Patients with motor complications and fluctuations on levodopa treatment
- Patients with cardiac problems or hypertension

Primary Target Symptoms

- Depressed mood (depression)
- Somatic symptoms (depression)
- Sleep and eating disturbances (depression)
- Psychomotor disturbances (depression)
- Motor symptoms (Parkinson's disease)

Pearls

- Transdermal administration may allow freedom from dietary restrictions
- Transdermal selegiline theoretically appealing as a triple action agent (serotonin, norepinephrine and dopamine) for treatment-refractory and difficult cases of depression
- Transdermal selegiline may have low risk of weight gain and sexual dysfunction, and may be useful for cognitive dysfunction in attention deficit disorder and other cognitive disorders, as it increases dopamine and is metabolized to l-amphetamine and l-methamphetamine
- Low dose oral administration generally used as an adjunctive treatment for Parkinson's disease after other drugs have lost efficacy
- At oral doses used for Parkinson's disease, virtually no risk of interactions with food
- Neuroprotective effects are possible but unproved
- * Enhancement of levodopa action can occur for Parkinson's patients at low oral doses, but antidepressant actions probably require high oral doses that do not have the potential tissue selectivity and lack of dietary restrictions of the low dose transdermal formulation
- * High doses may lose safety features
- MAOIs are generally reserved for second-line use after SSRIs, SNRIs, and combinations of newer antidepressants have failed
- Patient should be advised not to take any prescription or over-the-counter drugs without consulting their doctor because of possible drug interactions

- Headache is often the first symptom of hypertensive crisis
- Myths about the danger of dietary tyramine can be exaggerated, but prohibitions against concomitant drugs often not followed closely enough
* Combining multiple psychotropic agents with MAOIs should be for the expert, especially if combining with agents of potential risk (e.g., stimulants, trazodone, TCAs)
* MAOIs should not be neglected as therapeutic agents for the treatment-resistant

Suggested Reading

Bodkin JA, Amsterdam JD. Transdermal selegiline in major depression: a double-blind, placebo-controlled, parallel-group study in outpatients. Am J Psychiatry 2002;159(11):1869-75.

Kennedy SH. Continuation and maintenance treatments in major depression: the neglected role of monoamine oxidase inhibitors. J Psychiatry Neurosci 1997;22:127-31.

Shulman KI, Walker SE. A reevaluation of dietary restrictions for irreversible monoamine oxidase inhibitors. Psychiatr Ann 2001;31:378-384.

SERTRALINE

THERAPEUTICS

Brands • Zoloft
see index for additional brand names

Generic? Not in U.S.

Class
- SSRI (selective serotonin reuptake inhibitor); often classified as an antidepressant, but it is not just an antidepressant

Commonly Prescribed For
(bold for FDA approved)
- **Major depressive disorder**
- **Premenstrual dysphoric disorder (PMDD)**
- **Panic disorder**
- **Posttraumatic stress disorder (PTSD)**
- **Social anxiety disorder (social phobia)**
- **Obsessive-compulsive disorder (OCD)**
- Generalized anxiety disorder (GAD)

How The Drug Works
- Boosts neurotransmitter serotonin
- Blocks serotonin reuptake pump (serotonin transporter)
- Desensitizes serotonin receptors, especially serotonin 1A receptors
- Presumably increases serotonergic neurotransmission
- ✳ Sertraline also has some ability to block dopamine reuptake pump (dopamine transporter), which could increase dopamine neurotransmission and contribute to its therapeutic actions
- Sertraline also has mild antagonist actions at sigma receptors

How Long Until It Works
- ✳ Some patients may experience increased energy or activation early after initiation of treatment
- Onset of therapeutic actions usually not immediate, but often delayed 2 to 4 weeks
- If it is not working within 6 to 8 weeks, it may require a dosage increase or it may not work at all
- May continue to work for many years to prevent relapse of symptoms

If It Works
- The goal of treatment is complete remission of current symptoms as well as prevention of future relapses
- Treatment most often reduces or even eliminates symptoms, but not a cure since symptoms can recur after medicine stopped
- Continue treatment until all symptoms are gone (remission) or significantly reduced (e.g., OCD, PTSD)
- Once symptoms gone, continue treating for 1 year for the first episode of depression
- For second and subsequent episodes of depression, treatment may need to be indefinite
- Use in anxiety disorders may also need to be indefinite

If It Doesn't Work
- Many patients only have a partial response where some symptoms are improved but others persist (especially insomnia, fatigue, and problems concentrating in depression)
- Other patients may be nonresponders, sometimes called treatment-resistant or treatment-refractory
- Some patients who have an initial response may relapse even though they continue treatment, sometimes called "poop-out"
- Consider increasing dose, switching to another agent or adding an appropriate augmenting agent
- Consider psychotherapy
- Consider evaluation for another diagnosis or for a comorbid condition (e.g., medical illness, substance abuse, etc.)
- Some patients may experience apparent lack of consistent efficacy due to activation of latent or underlying bipolar disorder, and require antidepressant discontinuation and a switch to a mood stabilizer

Best Augmenting Combos for Partial Response or Treatment-Resistance
- Trazodone, especially for insomnia ✓
- In the U.S., sertraline (Zoloft) is commonly augmented with bupropion (Wellbutrin) with good results in a combination anecdotally called "Well-loft" (use combinations of antidepressants with caution as this may activate bipolar disorder and suicidal ideation)

- Mirtazapine, reboxetine, or atomoxetine (add with caution and at lower doses since sertraline could theoretically raise atomoxetine levels); use combinations of antidepressants with caution as this may activate bipolar disorder and suicidal ideation
- Modafinil, especially for fatigue, sleepiness, and lack of concentration
- Mood stabilizers or atypical antipsychotics for bipolar depression, psychotic depression, treatment-resistant depression, or treatment-resistant anxiety disorders
- Benzodiazepines
- If all else fails for anxiety disorders, consider gabapentin or tiagabine
- Hypnotics for insomnia
- Classically, lithium, buspirone, or thyroid hormone

Tests
- None for healthy individuals

SIDE EFFECTS

How Drug Causes Side Effects
- Theoretically due to increases in serotonin concentrations at serotonin receptors in parts of the brain and body other than those that cause therapeutic actions (e.g., unwanted actions of serotonin in sleep centers causing insomnia, unwanted actions of serotonin in the gut causing diarrhea, etc.)
- * Increasing serotonin can cause diminished dopamine release and might contribute to emotional flattening, cognitive slowing, and apathy in some patients, although this could theoretically be diminished in some patients by sertraline's dopamine reuptake blocking properties
- Most side effects are immediate but often go away with time, in contrast to most therapeutic effects which are delayed and are enhanced over time
- Sertraline's possible dopamine reuptake blocking properties could contribute to agitation, anxiety, and undesirable activation, especially early in dosing

Notable Side Effects
- Sexual dysfunction (men: delayed ejaculation, erectile dysfunction; men and

women: decreased sexual desire, anorgasmia)
- Gastrointestinal (decreased appetite, nausea, diarrhea, constipation, dry mouth)
- Mostly central nervous system (insomnia but also sedation, agitation, tremors, headache, dizziness)
- Note: patients with diagnosed or undiagnosed bipolar or psychotic disorders may be more vulnerable to CNS-activating actions of SSRIs
- Autonomic (sweating)
- Bruising and rare bleeding
- Rare hyponatremia (mostly in elderly patients and generally reversible on discontinuation of sertraline)
- Rare hypotension

 Life Threatening or Dangerous Side Effects
- Rare seizures
- Rare induction of mania
- Rare activation of suicidal ideation and behavior (suicidality)

Weight Gain

unusual   not unusual   common   problematic

- Reported but not expected
- Some patients may actually experience weight loss

Sedation

unusual   not unusual   common   problematic

- Reported but not expected
- Possibly activating in some patients

What To Do About Side Effects
- Wait
- Wait
- Wait
- If sertraline is activating, take in the morning to help reduce insomnia
- Reduce dose to 25 mg or even 12.5 mg until side effects abate, then increase dose as tolerated, usually to at least 50 mg/day
- In a few weeks, switch or add other drugs

Best Augmenting Agents for Side Effects
- Often best to try another SSRI or another antidepressant monotherapy prior to

resorting to augmentation strategies to treat side effects
- Trazodone or a hypnotic for insomnia
- Bupropion, sildenafil, vardenafil or tadalafil for sexual dysfunction
- Bupropion for emotional flattening, cognitive slowing, or apathy
- Mirtazapine for insomnia, agitation, and gastrointestinal side effects
- Benzodiazepines for jitteriness and anxiety, especially at initiation of treatment and especially for anxious patients
- Many side effects are dose-dependent (i.e., they increase as dose increases, or they reemerge until tolerance re-develops)
- Many side effects are time-dependent (i.e., they start immediately upon dosing and upon each dose increase, but go away with time)
- Activation and agitation may represent the induction of a bipolar state, especially a mixed dysphoric bipolar II condition sometimes associated with suicidal ideation, and require the addition of lithium, a mood stabilizer or an atypical antipsychotic, and/or discontinuation of sertraline

DOSING AND USE

Usual Dosage Range
- 50–200 mg/day

Dosage Forms
- Tablets 25 mg scored, 50 mg scored, 100 mg

How to Dose
- Depression and OCD: initial 50 mg/day; usually wait a few weeks to assess drug effects before increasing dose, but can increase once a week; maximum generally 200 mg/day; single dose
- Panic and PTSD: initial 25 mg/day; increase to 50 mg/day after 1 week thereafter, usually wait a few weeks to assess drug effects before increasing dose; maximum generally 200 mg/day; single dose

 Dosing Tips
- All tablets are scored, so to save costs, give 50 mg as half of 100 mg tablet, since

100 mg and 50 mg tablets cost about the same in many markets
- Give once daily, often in the mornings to reduce chances of insomnia
- Many patients ultimately require more than 50 mg dose per day
- Some patients are dosed above 200 mg
- Evidence that some treatment-resistant OCD patients may respond safely to doses up to 400 mg/day, but this is for experts and use with caution
- The more anxious and agitated the patient, the lower the starting dose, the slower the titration, and the more likely the need for a concomitant agent such as trazodone or a benzodiazepine
- If intolerable anxiety, insomnia, agitation, akathisia, or activation occur either upon dosing initiation or discontinuation, consider the possibility of activated bipolar disorder and switch to a mood stabilizer or atypical antipsychotic
- Utilize half a 25 mg tablet (12.5 mg) when initiating treatment in patients with a history of intolerance to previous antidepressants

Overdose
- Rarely lethal in monotherapy overdose; vomiting, sedation, heart rhythm disturbances, dilated pupils, agitation; fatalities have been reported in sertraline overdose combined with other drugs or alcohol

Long-Term Use
- Safe

Habit Forming
- No

How to Stop
- Taper to avoid withdrawal effects (dizziness, nausea, stomach cramps, sweating, tingling, dysesthesias)
- Many patients tolerate 50% dose reduction for 3 days, then another 50% reduction for 3 days, then discontinuation
- If withdrawal symptoms emerge during discontinuation, raise dose to stop symptoms and then restart withdrawal much more slowly

Pharmacokinetics
- Parent drug has 22–36 hour half-life

- Metabolite half-life 62–104 hours
- Inhibits CYP450 2D6 (weakly at low doses)
- Inhibits CYP450 3A4 (weakly at low doses)

Drug Interactions

- Tramadol increases the risk of seizures in patients taking an antidepressant
- Can increase tricyclic antidepressant levels; use with caution with tricyclic antidepressants or when switching from a TCA to sertraline
- Can cause a fatal "serotonin syndrome" when combined with MAO inhibitors, so do not use with MAO inhibitors or for at least 14 days after MAOIs are stopped
- Do not start an MAO inhibitor for at least 2 weeks after discontinuing sertraline
- May displace highly protein bound drugs (e.g., warfarin)
- Can rarely cause weakness, hyperreflexia, and incoordination when combined with sumatriptan or possibly with other triptans, requiring careful monitoring of patient
- Via CYP450 2D6 inhibition, sertraline could theoretically interfere with the analgesic actions of codeine, and increase the plasma levels of some beta blockers and of atomoxetine
- Via CYP450 2D6 inhibition sertraline could theoretically increase concentrations of thioridazine and cause dangerous cardiac arrhythmias
- Via CYP450 3A4 inhibition, sertraline may increase the levels of alprazolam, buspirone, and triazolam
- Via CYP450 3A4 inhibition, sertraline could theoretically increase concentrations of certain cholesterol lowering HMG CoA reductase inhibitors, especially simvastatin, atorvastatin, and lovastatin, but not pravastatin or fluvastatin, which would increase the risk of rhabdomyolysis; thus, coadministration of sertraline with certain HMG CoA reductase inhibitors should proceed with caution
- Via CYP450 3A4 inhibition, sertraline could theoretically increase the concentrations of pimozide, and cause QTc prolongation and dangerous cardiac arrhythmias

Other Warnings/ Precautions

- Add or initiate other antidepressants with caution for up to 2 weeks after discontinuing sertraline
- Use with caution in patients with history of seizures
- Use with caution in patients with bipolar disorder unless treated with concomitant mood stabilizing agent
- When treating children, carefully weigh the risks and benefits of pharmacological treatment against the risks and benefits of nontreatment with antidepressants and make sure to document this in the patient's chart
- Distribute the brochures provided by the FDA and the drug companies
- Warn patients and their caregivers about the possibility of activating side effects and advise them to report such symptoms immediately
- Monitor patients for activation of suicidal ideation, especially children and adolescents

Do Not Use

- If patient is taking an MAO inhibitor
- If patient is taking pimozide
- If patient is taking thioridazine
- Use of sertraline oral concentrate is contraindicated with disulfiram due to the alcohol content of the concentrate
- If there is a proven allergy to sertraline

SPECIAL POPULATIONS

Renal Impairment

- No dose adjustment
- Not removed by hemodialysis

Hepatic Impairment

- Lower dose or give less frequently, perhaps by half

Cardiac Impairment

- Proven cardiovascular safety in depressed patients with recent myocardial infarction or angina
- Treating depression with SSRIs in patients with acute angina or following myocardial infarction may reduce cardiac events and improve survival as well as mood

Elderly
- Some patients may tolerate lower doses and/or slower titration better

 Children and Adolescents
- Carefully weigh the risks and benefits of pharmacological treatment against the risks and benefits of nontreatment with antidepressants and make sure to document this in the patient's chart
- Monitor patients face-to-face regularly, particularly during the first several weeks of treatment
- Use with caution, observing for activation of known or unknown bipolar disorder and/or suicidal ideation, and inform parents or guardian of this risk so they can help observe child or adolescent patients
- Approved for use in OCD
- Ages 6–12: initial dose 25 mg/day
- Ages 13 and up: adult dosing
- Long-term effects, particularly on growth, have not been studied

 Pregnancy
- Risk Category C [some animal studies show adverse effects, no controlled studies in humans]
- Not generally recommended for use during pregnancy, especially during first trimester
- Nonetheless, continuous treatment during pregnancy may be necessary and has not been proven to be harmful to the fetus
- At delivery there may be more bleeding in the mother and transient irritability or sedation in the newborn
- Must weigh the risk of treatment (first trimester fetal development, third trimester newborn delivery) to the child against the risk of no treatment (recurrence of depression, maternal health, infant bonding) to the mother and child
- For many patients this may mean continuing treatment during pregnancy
- Neonates exposed to SSRIs or SNRIs late in the third trimester have developed complications requiring prolonged hospitalization, respiratory support, and tube feeding; reported symptoms are consistent with either a direct toxic effect of SSRIs and SNRIs or, possibly, a drug discontinuation syndrome, and include respiratory distress, cyanosis, apnea, seizures, temperature instability, feeding difficulty, vomiting, hypoglycemia, hypotonia, hypertonia, hyperreflexia, tremor, jitteriness, irritability, and constant crying

Breast Feeding
- Some drug is found in mother's breast milk
- Trace amounts may be present in nursing children whose mothers are on sertraline
- Sertraline has shown efficacy in treating postpartum depression
- If child becomes irritable or sedated, breast feeding or drug may need to be discontinued
- Immediate postpartum period is a high-risk time for depression, especially in women who have had prior depressive episodes, so drug may need to be reinstituted late in the third trimester or shortly after childbirth to prevent a recurrence during the postpartum period
- Must weigh benefits of breast feeding with risks and benefits of antidepressant treatment versus nontreatment to both the infant and the mother
- For many patients, this may mean continuing treatment during breast feeding

THE ART OF PSYCHOPHARMACOLOGY

Potential Advantages
- Patients with atypical depression (hypersomnia, increased appetite)
- Patients with fatigue and low energy
- Patients who wish to avoid hyperprolactinemia (e.g., pubescent children, girls and women with galactorrhea, girls and women with unexplained amenorrhea, postmenopausal women who are not taking estrogen replacement therapy)
- Patients who are sensitive to the prolactin-elevating properties of other SSRIs (sertraline is the one SSRI that generally does not elevate prolactin)

Potential Disadvantages
- Initiating treatment in anxious patients with some insomnia
- Patients with comorbid irritable bowel syndrome
- Can require dosage titration

Primary Target Symptoms

- Depressed mood
- Anxiety
- Sleep disturbance, both insomnia and hypersomnia (eventually, but may actually cause insomnia, especially short-term)
- Panic attacks, avoidant behavior, re-experiencing, hyperarousal

 Pearls

- ✳ May be a type of "dual action" agent with both potent serotonin reuptake inhibition and less potent dopamine reuptake inhibition, but the clinical significance of this is unknown
- Cognitive and affective "flattening" may theoretically be diminished in some patients by sertraline's dopamine reuptake blocking properties
- ✳ May be a first-line choice for atypical depression (e.g., hypersomnia, hyperphagia, low energy, mood reactivity)
- Best documented cardiovascular safety of any antidepressant, proven safe for depressed patients with recent myocardial infarction or angina
- May block sigma 1 receptors, enhancing sertraline's anxiolytic actions
- Can have more gastrointestinal effects, particularly diarrhea, than some other antidepressants

- May be more effective treatment for women with PTSD or depression than for men with PTSD or depression, but the clinical significance of this is unknown
- SSRIs may be less effective in women over 50, especially if they are not taking estrogen
- SSRIs may be useful for hot flushes in perimenopausal women
- For sexual dysfunction, can augment with bupropion, sildenafil, vardenafil, tadalafil, or switch to a non-SSRI such as bupropion or mirtazapine
- Some postmenopausal women's depression will respond better to sertraline plus estrogen augmentation than to sertraline alone
- Nonresponse to sertraline in elderly may require consideration of mild cognitive impairment or Alzheimer disease
- Not as well tolerated as some SSRIs for panic, especially when dosing is initiated, unless given with co-therapies such as benzodiazepines or trazodone
- Relative lack of effect on prolactin may make it a preferred agent for some children, adolescents, and women
- Some evidence suggests that sertraline treatment during only the luteal phase may be more effective than continuous treatment for patients with PMDD

 Suggested Reading

DeVane CL, Liston HL, Markowitz JS. Clinical pharmacokinetics of sertraline. Clin Pharmacokinet. 2002;41:1247–66.

Flament MF, Lane RM, Zhu R, Ying Z. Predictors of an acute antidepressant response to fluoxetine and sertraline. International Clinical Psychopharmacology. 1999;14:259–275.

Khouzam HR, Emes R, Gill T, Raroque R. The antidepressant sertraline: a review of its uses in a range of psychiatric and medical conditions. Compr Ther. 2003;29:47–53.

McRae AL, Brady KT. Review of sertraline and its clinical applications in psychiatric disorders. Expert Opin Pharmacother. 2001;2:883–92.

TIANEPTINE

THERAPEUTICS

Brands • Coaxil
• Stablon
see index for additional brand names

Generic? No

Class

• Tricyclic antidepressant
• Serotonin reuptake enhancer

Commonly Prescribed For
(bold for FDA approved)
• Major depressive disorder
• Dysthymia
• Anxiety associated with depression, alcohol dependence

How The Drug Works

✳ Possibly increases serotonin uptake, but could also act similarly to agents that block serotonin reuptake

How Long Until It Works

• Onset of therapeutic actions usually not immediate, but often delayed 2 to 4 weeks
• If it is not working within 6 to 8 weeks for depression, it may require a dosage increase or it may not work at all
• May continue to work for many years to prevent relapse of symptoms

If It Works

• The goal of treatment is complete remission of current symptoms as well as prevention of future relapses
• Treatment most often reduces or even eliminates symptoms, but not a cure since symptoms can recur after medicine stopped
• Continue treatment until all symptoms are gone (remission)
• Once symptoms gone, continue treating for 1 year for the first episode of depression
• For second and subsequent episodes of depression, treatment may need to be indefinite

If It Doesn't Work

• Many patients only have a partial response where some symptoms are improved but others persist (especially insomnia, fatigue, and problems concentrating)
• Other patients may be nonresponders, sometimes called treatment-resistant or treatment-refractory
• Consider increasing dose, switching to another agent or adding an appropriate augmenting agent
• Consider psychotherapy
• Consider evaluation for another diagnosis or for a comorbid condition (e.g., medical illness, substance abuse, etc.)

Best Augmenting Combos for Partial Response or Treatment-Resistance

• Augmentation has not been systematically studied with tianeptine

Tests

• None for healthy individuals
✳ Since other tricyclic and tetracyclic antidepressants are frequently associated with weight gain, it is possible that this may also be the case for tianeptine; thus, before starting treatment, weigh all patients and determine if the patient is already overweight (BMI 25.0–29.9) or obese (BMI ≥30)
• Before giving a drug that can cause weight gain to an overweight or obese patient, consider determining whether the patient already has pre-diabetes (fasting plasma glucose 100–125 mg/dl), diabetes (fasting plasma glucose >126 mg/dl), or dyslipidemia (increased total cholesterol, LDL cholesterol and triglycerides; decreased HDL cholesterol), and treat or refer such patients for treatment, including nutrition and weight management, physical activity counseling, smoking cessation, and medical management
✳ Monitor weight and BMI during treatment
✳ While giving a drug to a patient who has gained >5% of initial weight, consider evaluating for the presence of pre-diabetes, diabetes, or dyslipidemia, or consider switching to a different antidepressant
• Theoretically, by analogy with other TCAs, EKGs may be useful for selected patients (e.g., those with personal or family history of QTc prolongation; cardiac arrhythmia; recent myocardial infarction; uncompensated heart failure; or taking agents that prolong QTc interval such as

TIANEPTINE (continued)

pimozide, thioridazine, selected antiarrhythmics, moxifloxacin, sparfloxacin, etc.)
- On a theoretical basis and by analogy with other TCAs, patients at risk for electrolyte disturbances (e.g., patients on diuretic therapy) should have baseline and periodic serum potassium and magnesium measurements

SIDE EFFECTS

How Drug Causes Side Effects
✳ Mild anticholinergic activity (less than some other tricyclic antidepressants) could possibly lead to sedative effects, dry mouth, constipation, and blurred vision
- Most side effects are immediate but often go away with time
✳ Pharmacologic studies indicate tianeptine may not be a potent alpha 1antagonist or H1 antihistamine
- Theoretically, cardiac arrhythmias and seizures, especially in overdose, may be caused by blockade of ion channels

Notable Side Effects
- Headache, dizziness, insomnia, sedation
- Nausea, constipation, abdominal pain, dry mouth
- Abnormal dreams
- Rare hepatotoxicity
- Tachycardia

 Life Threatening or Dangerous Side Effects
- Theoretically, lowered seizure threshold and rare seizures
- Theoretically, rare induction of mania and activation of suicidal ideation or behavior
- Theoretically, could prolong QTc interval, but not well-studied

Weight Gain

unusual | not unusual | common | problematic
- Not well studied

Sedation

unusual | not unusual | common | problematic
- Occurs in significant minority

What To Do About Side Effects
- Wait
- Wait
- Wait
- Lower the dose
- In a few weeks, switch or add other drugs

Best Augmenting Agents for Side Effects
- Augmentation for side effects of tianeptine has not been systematically studied

DOSING AND USE

Usual Dosage Range
- 25–50 mg/day

Dosage Forms
- Tablet 12.5 mg

How to Dose
- 12.5 mg 3 times/day

 Dosing Tips
- Tianeptine's rapid elimination necessitates strict adherence to the dosing schedule
✳ Short half-life means multiple daily doses
✳ Although tianeptine has a tricyclic structure, it is dosed lower than usual TCA dosing

Overdose
- Effects are generally mild and nonfatal; unlikely to cause cardiovascular effects

Long-Term Use
- Safe

Habit Forming
- No

How to Stop
- Taper to avoid withdrawal symptoms
- Many patients tolerate 50% dose reduction for 3 days, then another 50% reduction for 3 days, then discontinuation
- If withdrawal symptoms emerge during discontinuation, raise dose to stop symptoms and then restart withdrawal much more slowly

Pharmacokinetics
- Not primarily metabolized by CYP 450 enzyme system
- Tianeptine is rapidly eliminated
- Half-life approximately 3 hours

 Drug Interactions
- Tramadol increases the risk of seizures in patients taking TCAs
- Activation and agitation, especially following switching or adding antidepressants, may represent the induction of a bipolar state, especially a mixed dysphoric bipolar II condition sometimes associated with suicidal ideation, and require the addition of lithium, a mood stabilizer or an atypical antipsychotic, and/or discontinuation of tianeptine
- Other drug interactions not well-studied

 Other Warnings/ Precautions
- Add or initiate other antidepressants with caution for up to 2 weeks after discontinuing tianeptine
- For elective surgery, tianeptine should be stopped 24–48 hours before general anesthesia is administered
- Generally, do not use with MAO inhibitors, including 14 days after MAOIs are stopped; do not start an MAOI until 2 weeks after discontinuing tianeptine
- Although not well studied for tianeptine, other TCAs can prolong QTc interval, especially at toxic doses, potentially causing torsade de pointes-type arrhythmia or sudden death; this has not been reported specifically for tianeptine
- Because other TCAs can prolong QTc interval, use with caution in patients who have bradycardia or who are taking drugs that can induce bradycardia (e.g., beta blockers, calcium channel blockers, clonidine, digitalis)
- Because other TCAs can prolong QTc interval, use with caution in patients who have hypokalemia and/or hypomagnesemia or who are taking drugs that can induce hypokalemia and/or magnesemia (e.g., diuretics, stimulant laxatives, intravenous amphotericin B, glucocorticoids, tetracosactide)

- When treating children, carefully weigh the risks and benefits of pharmacological treatment against the risks and benefits of nontreatment with antidepressants and make sure to document this in the patient's chart
- Warn patients and their caregivers about the possibility of activating side effects and advise them to report such symptoms immediately
- Monitor patients for activation of suicidal ideation, especially children and adolescents

Do Not Use
- If patient is taking an MAO inhibitor
- If patient is pregnant or nursing
- On a theoretical basis, if patient is taking agents capable of significantly prolonging QTc interval (e.g., pimozide, thioridazine, selected antiarrhythmics, moxifloxacin, sparfloxacin)
- On a theoretical basis, if there is a history of QTc prolongation or cardiac arrhythmia, recent acute myocardial infarction, uncompensated heart failure
- If there is a proven allergy to tianeptine

SPECIAL POPULATIONS

Renal Impairment
- Dose should be reduced for severe impairment to 25 mg/day
- Dose reduction not necessary for patients on hemodialysis

Hepatic Impairment
- No dose adjustment necessary

Cardiac Impairment
- No dose adjustment necessary
- Safety of tianeptine in patients with cardiac impairment has not been specifically demonstrated
- TCAs have been reported to cause arrhythmias, prolongation of conduction time, orthostatic hypotension, sinus tachycardia, and heart failure, especially in the diseased heart
- Myocardial infarction and stroke have been reported with TCAs
- TCAs produce QTc prolongation, which may be enhanced by the existence of bradycardia, hypokalemia, congenital or

TIANEPTINE (continued)

acquired long QTc interval, which should be evaluated prior to administering tianeptine
- Avoid TCAs in patients with a known history of QTc prolongation, recent acute myocardial infarction, and uncompensated heart failure
- TCAs may cause a sustained increase in heart rate in patients with ischemic heart disease and may worsen (decrease) heart rate variability, an independent risk of mortality in cardiac populations
- ✳ Risk/benefit ratio may not justify use of TCAs in cardiac impairment

Elderly
- Dose should be reduced to 25 mg/day

 Children and Adolescents
- Carefully weigh the risks and benefits of pharmacological treatment against the risks and benefits of nontreatment with antidepressants and make sure to document this in the patient's chart
- Monitor patients face-to-face regularly, particularly during the first several weeks of treatment
- Use with caution, observing for activation of known or unknown bipolar disorder and/or suicidal ideation, and inform parents or guardian of this risk so they can help observe child or adolescent patients
- Has been used successfully to treat asthmatic symptoms in children
- Not recommended for use under age 15

 Pregnancy
- Risk Category not formally assessed by the US FDA
- Not recommended for use during pregnancy

Breast Feeding
- Some drug is found in mother's breast milk
- ✳ Not recommended for use during pregnancy
- Immediate postpartum period is a high-risk time for depression, especially in women who have had prior depressive episodes, so drug may need to be reinstituted late in the third trimester or shortly after childbirth to prevent a recurrence during the postpartum period
- Must weigh benefits of breast feeding with risks and benefits of antidepressant treatment versus non-treatment to both the infant and the mother
- For many patients, this may mean continuing treatment during breast feeding

THE ART OF PSYCHOPHARMACOLOGY

Potential Advantages
- Elderly patients
- Alcohol withdrawal

Potential Disadvantages
- Patients who have difficulty being compliant with multiple daily dosing

Primary Target Symptoms
- Depressed mood
- Symptoms of anxiety

 Pearls
- ✳ Possibly a unique mechanism of action
- However, mechanism of action not well understood
- Not marketed widely throughout the world, but mostly in France
- ✳ Effects on QTc prolongation not systematically studied

 Suggested Reading

Ginestet D. Efficacy of tianeptine in major depressive disorders with or without melancholia. Eur Neuropsychopharmacol 1997;7 Suppl 3:S341–5.

Wagstaff AJ, Ormrod D, Spencer CM. Tianeptine: a review of its use in depressive disorders. CNS Drugs 2001;15(3):231–59.

Wilde MI, Benfield P. Tianeptine. A review of its pharmacodynamic and pharmacokinetic properties, and therapeutic efficacy in depression and coexisting anxiety and depression. Drugs 1995;49(3):411–39.

PARNATE

TRANYLCYPROMINE

THERAPEUTICS

Brands • Parnate
see index for additional brand names

Generic? Not in U.S.

 Class
• Monoamine oxidase inhibitor (MAOI)

Commonly Prescribed For
(bold for FDA approved)
• **Major depressive episode without melancholia**
• Treatment-resistant depression
• Treatment-resistant panic disorder
• Treatment-resistant social anxiety disorder

 How The Drug Works
• Irreversibly blocks monoamine oxidase (MAO) from breaking down norepinephrine, serotonin, and dopamine
• This presumably boosts noradrenergic, serotonergic, and dopaminergic neurotransmission
✴ As the drug is structurally related to amphetamine, it may have some stimulant-like actions due to monoamine release and reuptake inhibition

How Long Until It Works
• Some patients may experience stimulant-like actions early in dosing
• Onset of therapeutic actions usually not immediate, but often delayed 2 to 4 weeks
• If it is not working within 6 to 8 weeks, it may require a dosage increase or it may not work at all
• May continue to work for many years to prevent relapse of symptoms

If It Works
• The goal of treatment is complete remission of current symptoms as well as prevention of future relapses
• Treatment most often reduces or even eliminates symptoms, but not a cure since symptoms can recur after medicine stopped
• Continue treatment until all symptoms are gone (remission)
• Once symptoms gone, continue treating for 1 year for the first episode of depression

• For second and subsequent episodes of depression, treatment may need to be indefinite
• Use in anxiety disorders may also need to be indefinite

If It Doesn't Work
• Many patients only have a partial response where some symptoms are improved but others persist (especially insomnia, fatigue, and problems concentrating)
• Other patients may be nonresponders, sometimes called treatment-resistant or treatment-refractory
• Some patients who have an initial response may relapse even though they continue treatment, sometimes called "poop-out"
• Consider increasing dose, switching to another agent or adding an appropriate augmenting agent
• Consider psychotherapy
• Consider evaluation for another diagnosis or for a comorbid condition (e.g., medical illness, substance abuse, etc.)
• Some patients may experience apparent lack of consistent efficacy due to activation of latent or underlying bipolar disorder, and require antidepressant discontinuation and a switch to a mood stabilizer

 Best Augmenting Combos for Partial Response or Treatment-Resistance
✴ Augmentation of MAOIs has not been systematically studied, and this is something for the expert, to be done with caution and with careful monitoring ✓
✴ A stimulant such as d-amphetamine or methylphenidate (with caution; may activate bipolar disorder and suicidal ideation; may elevate blood pressure)
• Lithium
• Mood stabilizing anticonvulsants
• Atypical antipsychotics (with special caution for those agents with monoamine reuptake blocking properties, such as ziprasidone and zotepine)

Tests
• Patients should be monitored for changes in blood pressure
• Patients receiving high doses or long-term treatment should have hepatic function evaluated periodically

SIDE EFFECTS

How Drug Causes Side Effects
- Theoretically due to increases in monoamines in parts of the brain and body and at receptors other than those that cause therapeutic actions (e.g., unwanted actions of serotonin in sleep centers causing insomnia, unwanted actions of norepinephrine on vascular smooth muscle causing hypertension, etc.)
- Side effects are generally immediate, but immediate side effects often disappear in time

Notable Side Effects
- Agitation, anxiety, insomnia, weakness, sedation, dizziness
- Constipation, dry mouth, nausea, diarrhea, change in appetite, weight gain
- Sexual dysfunction
- Orthostatic hypotension (dose-related); syncope may develop at high doses

Life Threatening or Dangerous Side Effects
- Hypertensive crisis (especially when MAOIs are used with certain tyramine-containing foods or prohibited drugs)
- Induction of mania
- Rare activation of suicidal ideation and behavior (suicidality)
- Seizures
- Hepatotoxicity

Weight Gain

- Occurs in significant minority

Sedation

- Many experience and/or can be significant in amount
- Can also cause activation

What To Do About Side Effects
- Wait
- Wait
- Wait
- Lower the dose
- Take at night if daytime sedation; take in daytime if overstimulated at night

- Switch after appropriate washout to an SSRI or newer antidepressant

Best Augmenting Agents for Side Effects
- Trazodone (with caution) for insomnia
- Benzodiazepines for insomnia
- ✳ Single oral or sublingual dose of a calcium channel blocker (e.g., nifedipine) for urgent treatment of hypertension due to drug interaction or dietary tyramine
- Many side effects cannot be improved with an augmenting agent

DOSING AND USE

Usual Dosage Range
- 30 mg/day in divided doses

Dosage Forms
- Tablet 10 mg

How to Dose
- Initial 30 mg/day in divided doses; after 2 weeks increase by 10 mg/day each 1–3 weeks; maximum 60 mg/day

 ### Dosing Tips
- Orthostatic hypotension, especially at high doses, may require splitting into 3–4 daily doses
- Patients receiving high doses may need to be evaluated periodically for effects on the liver

Overdose
- Dizziness, sedation, ataxia, headache, insomnia, restlessness, anxiety, irritability; cardiovascular effects, confusion, respiratory depression, or coma may also occur

Long-Term Use
- May require periodic evaluation of hepatic function
- MAOIs may lose efficacy long-term

Habit Forming
- Some patients have developed dependence to MAOIs

How to Stop
- Generally no need to taper, as the drug wears off slowly over 2–3 weeks

Pharmacokinetics
- Clinical duration of action may be up to 21 days due to irreversible enzyme inhibition

 Drug Interactions

- Tramadol may increase the risk of seizures in patients taking an MAO inhibitor
- Can cause a fatal "serotonin syndrome" when combined with drugs that block serotonin reuptake (e.g., SSRIs, SNRIs, sibutramine, tramadol, etc.), so do not use with a serotonin reuptake inhibitor or for up to 5 weeks after stopping the serotonin reuptake inhibitor
- Hypertensive crisis with headache, intracranial bleeding, and death may result from combining MAO inhibitors with sympathomimetic drugs (e.g., amphetamines, methylphenidate, cocaine, dopamine, epinephrine, norepinephrine, and related compounds methyldopa, levodopa, L-tryptophan, L-tyrosine, and phenylalanine
- Excitation, seizures, delirium, hyperpyrexia, circulatory collapse, coma, and death may result from combining MAO inhibitors with mepiridine or dextromethorphan
- Do not combine with another MAO inhibitor, alcohol, buspirone, bupropion, or guanethidine
- Adverse drug reactions can result from combining MAO inhibitors with tricyclic/tetracyclic antidepressants and related compounds, including carbamazepine, cyclobenzaprine, and mirtazapine, and should be avoided except by experts to treat difficult cases
- MAO inhibitors in combination with spinal anesthesia may cause combined hypotensive effects
- Combination of MAOIs and CNS depressants may enhance sedation and hypotension

 Other Warnings/ Precautions

- Use requires low tyramine diet
- Patients taking MAO inhibitors should avoid high protein food that has undergone protein breakdown by aging, fermentation, pickling, smoking, or bacterial contamination
- Patients taking MAO inhibitors should avoid cheeses (especially aged varieties), pickled herring, beer, wine, liver, yeast extract, dry sausage, hard salami, pepperoni, Lebanon bologna, pods of broad beans (fava beans), yogurt, and excessive use of caffeine and chocolate
- Patient and prescriber must be vigilant to potential interactions with any drug, including antihypertensives and over-the-counter cough/cold preparations
- Over-the-counter medications to avoid include cough and cold preparations, including those containing dextromethorphan, nasal decongestants (tablets, drops, or spray), hay-fever medications, sinus medications, asthma inhalant medications, anti-appetite medications, weight reducing preparations, "pep" pills
- Hypoglycemia may occur in diabetic patients receiving insulin or oral antidiabetic agents
- Use cautiously in patients receiving reserpine, anesthetics, disulfiram, metrizamide, anticholinergic agents
- Tranylcypromine is not recommended for use in patients who cannot be monitored closely
- When treating children, carefully weigh the risks and benefits of pharmacological treatment against the risks and benefits of nontreatment with antidepressants and make sure to document this in the patient's chart
- Distribute the brochures provided by the FDA and the drug companies
- Warn patients and their caregivers about the possibility of activating side effects and advise them to report such symptoms immediately
- Monitor patients for activation of suicidal ideation, especially children and adolescents

Do Not Use
- If patient is taking meperidine (pethidine)
- If patient is taking a sympathomimetic agent or taking guanethidine
- If patient is taking another MAOI
- If patient is taking any agent that can inhibit serotonin reuptake (e.g., SSRIs,

sibutramine, tramadol, milnacipran, duloxetine, venlafaxine, clomipramine, etc.)
- If patient is taking diuretics, dextromethorphan, buspirone, bupropion
- If patient has pheochromocytoma
- If patient has cardiovascular or cerebrovascular disease
- If patient has frequent or severe headaches
- If patient is undergoing elective surgery and requires general anesthesia
- If patient has a history of liver disease or abnormal liver function tests
- If patient is taking a prohibited drug
- If patient is not compliant with a low-tyramine diet
- If there is a proven allergy to tranylcypromine

SPECIAL POPULATIONS

Renal Impairment
- Use with caution – drug may accumulate in plasma
- May require lower than usual adult dose

Hepatic Impairment
- Tranylcypromine should not be used in patients with history of hepatic impairment or in patients with abnormal liver function tests

Cardiac Impairment
- Contraindicated in patients with any cardiac impairment

Elderly
- Initial dose lower than usual adult dose
- Elderly patients may have greater sensitivity to adverse effects

Children and Adolescents
- Not generally recommended for use under age 18
- Carefully weigh the risks and benefits of pharmacological treatment against the risks and benefits of nontreatment with antidepressants and make sure to document this in the patient's chart
- Monitor patients face-to-face regularly, particularly during the first several weeks of treatment

- Use with caution, observing for activation of known or unknown bipolar disorder and/or suicidal ideation, and inform parents or guardian of this risk so they can help observe child or adolescent patients

Pregnancy
- Risk Category C [some animal studies show adverse effects, no controlled studies in humans]
- Not generally recommended for use during pregnancy, especially during first trimester
- Should evaluate patient for treatment with an antidepressant with a better risk/benefit ratio

Breast Feeding
- Some drug is found in mother's breast milk
- Effects on infant unknown
- Immediate postpartum period is a high-risk time for depression, especially in women who have had prior depressive episodes, so drug may need to be reinstituted late in the third trimester or shortly after childbirth to prevent a recurrence during the postpartum period
- Should evaluate patient for treatment with an antidepressant with a better risk/benefit ratio

THE ART OF PSYCHOPHARMACOLOGY

Potential Advantages
- Atypical depression
- Severe depression
- Treatment-resistant depression or anxiety disorders

Potential Disadvantages
- Requires compliance to dietary restrictions, concomitant drug restrictions
- Patients with cardiac problems or hypertension
- Multiple daily doses

Primary Target Symptoms
- Depressed mood
- Somatic symptoms
- Sleep and eating disturbances
- Psychomotor retardation
- Morbid preoccupation

Pearls

- MAOIs are generally reserved for second-line use after SSRIs, SNRIs, and combinations of newer antidepressants have failed
- Patient should be advised not to take any prescription or over-the-counter drugs without consulting their doctor because of possible drug interactions with the MAOI
- Headache is often the first symptom of hypertensive crisis
- Foods generally to avoid as they are usually high in tyramine content: dry sausage, pickled herring, liver, broad bean pods, sauerkraut, cheese, yogurt, alcoholic beverages, nonalcoholic beer and wine, chocolate, caffeine, meat and fish
- The rigid dietary restrictions may reduce compliance
- Mood disorders can be associated with eating disorders (especially in adolescent females), and tranylcypromine can be used to treat both depression and bulimia
- MAOIs are a viable second-line treatment option in depression, but are not frequently used
- ✳ Myths about the danger of dietary tyramine can be exaggerated, but prohibitions against concomitant drugs often not followed closely enough
- Orthostatic hypotension, insomnia, and sexual dysfunction are often the most troublesome common side effects
- ✳ MAOIs should be for the expert, especially if combining with agents of potential risk (e.g., stimulants, trazodone, TCAs)
- ✳ MAOIs should not be neglected as therapeutic agents for the treatment-resistant
- Although generally prohibited, a heroic but potentially dangerous treatment for severely treatment-resistant patients is for an expert to give a tricyclic/tetracyclic antidepressant other than clomipramine simultaneously with an MAO inhibitor for patients who fail to respond to numerous other antidepressants
- Use of MAOIs with clomipramine is always prohibited because of the risk of serotonin syndrome and death
- Amoxapine may be the preferred trycyclic/tetracyclic antidepressant to combine with an MAOI in heroic cases due to its theoretically protective 5HT2A antagonist properties
- If this option is elected, start the MAOI with the tricyclic/tetracyclic antidepressant simultaneously at low doses after appropriate drug washout, then alternately increase doses of these agents every few days to a week as tolerated
- Although very strict dietary and concomitant drug restrictions must be observed to prevent hypertensive crises and serotonin syndrome, the most common side effects of MAOI and tricyclic/tetracyclic combinations may be weight gain and orthostatic hypotension

Suggested Reading

Baker GB, Coutts RT, McKenna KF, Sherry-McKenna RL. Insights into the mechanisms of action of the MAO inhibitors phenelzine and tranylcypromine: a review. J Psychiatry Neurosci 1992;17:206–14.

Kennedy SH. Continuation and maintenance treatments in major depression: the neglected role of monoamine oxidase inhibitors. J Psychiatry Neurosci 1997;22:127–31.

Lippman SB, Nash K. Monoamine oxidase inhibitor update. Potential adverse food and drug interactions. Drug Saf 1990;5:195–204.

Thase ME, Triyedi MH, Rush AJ. MAOIs in the contemporary treatment of depression. Neuropsychopharmacology 1995;12:185–219.

TRAZODONE

Brands • Desyrel
see index for additional brand names

Generic? Yes

Class
• SARI (serotonin 2 antagonist/reuptake inhibitor); antidepressant; hypnotic

Commonly Prescribed For
(bold for FDA approved)
• **Depression**
• Insomnia (primary and secondary)
• Anxiety

How The Drug Works
• Blocks serotonin 2A receptors potently
• Blocks serotonin reuptake pump (serotonin transporter) less potently

How Long Until It Works
✱ Onset of therapeutic actions in insomnia are immediate if dosing is correct
• Onset of therapeutic actions in depression usually not immediate, but often delayed 2 to 4 weeks whether given as an adjunct to another antidepressant or as a monotherapy
• If it is not working within 6 to 8 weeks for depression, it may require a dosage increase or it may not work at all
• May continue to work for many years to prevent relapse of symptoms in depression and to reduce symptoms of chronic insomnia

If It Works
✱ For insomnia, use possibly can be indefinite as there is no reliable evidence of tolerance, dependence, or withdrawal, but few long-term studies
• For secondary insomnia, if underlying condition (e.g., depression, anxiety disorder) is in remission, trazodone treatment may be discontinued if insomnia does not reemerge
• The goal of treatment for depression is complete remission of current symptoms of depression as well as prevention of future relapses

• Treatment most often reduces or even eliminates symptoms of depression, but is not a cure since symptoms can recur after medicine stopped
• Continue treatment until all symptoms of depression are gone (remission)
• Once symptoms of depression are gone, continue treating for 1 year for the first episode of depression
• For second and subsequent episodes of depression, treatment may need to be indefinite

If It Doesn't Work
• For insomnia, try escalating doses or switch to another agent
• Many patients only have a partial antidepressant response where some symptoms are improved but others persist (especially insomnia, fatigue, and problems concentrating)
• Other patients may be nonresponders, sometimes called treatment-resistant or treatment-refractory
• Consider increasing dose, switching to another agent or adding an appropriate augmenting agent for treatment of depression
• Consider psychotherapy
• Consider evaluation for another diagnosis or for a comorbid condition (e.g., medical illness, substance abuse, etc.)
• Some patients may experience apparent lack of consistent efficacy due to activation of latent or underlying bipolar disorder, and require antidepressant discontinuation and a switch to a mood stabilizer

Best Augmenting Combos for Partial Response or Treatment-Resistance

• Trazodone is not frequently used as a monotherapy for insomnia, but can be combined with sedative hypnotic benzodiazepines in difficult cases
• Trazodone is most frequently used in depression as an augmenting agent to numerous psychotropic drugs
• Trazodone can not only improve insomnia in depressed patients treated with antidepressants, but can also be an effective booster of antidepressant actions of other antidepressants (use combinations of antidepressants with caution as this may

activate bipolar disorder and suicidal ideation)
- Trazodone can also improve insomnia in numerous other psychiatric conditions (e.g., bipolar disorder, schizophrenia, alcohol withdrawal) and be added to numerous other psychotropic drugs (e.g., lithium, mood stabilizers, antipsychotics)

Tests
- None for healthy individuals

SIDE EFFECTS

How Drug Causes Side Effects
- Sedative effects may be due to antihistamine properties
- Blockade of alpha adrenergic 1 receptors may explain dizziness, sedation, and hypotension
- Most side effects are immediate but often go away with time

Notable Side Effects
- Nausea, vomiting, edema, blurred vision, constipation, dry mouth
- Dizziness, sedation, fatigue, headache, incoordination, tremor
- Hypotension, syncope
- Occasional sinus bradycardia (long-term)
- Rare rash

 Life Threatening or Dangerous Side Effects
- Rare priapism
- Rare seizures
- Rare induction of mania
- Rare activation of suicidal ideation and behavior (suicidality)

Weight Gain

unusual   not unusual   common   problematic
- Reported but not expected

Sedation

unusual   not unusual   common   problematic
- Many experience and/or can be significant in amount

What To Do About Side Effects
- Wait
- Wait
- Wait
- Take larger dose at night to prevent daytime sedation
- Switch to another agent

Best Augmenting Agents for Side Effects
- Most side effects cannot be improved with an augmenting agent
- Activation and agitation may represent the induction of a bipolar state, especially a mixed dysphoric bipolar II condition sometimes associated with suicidal ideation, and require the addition of lithium, a mood stabilizer or an atypical antipsychotic, and/or discontinuation of trazodone

DOSING AND USE

Usual Dosage Range
- 150–600 mg/day

Dosage Forms
- Tablet 50 mg scored, 100 mg scored, 150 mg, 150 mg with pividone scored, 300 mg with pividone scored

How to Dose
- For depression as a monotherapy, initial 150 mg/day in divided doses; can increase every 3–4 days by 50 mg/day as needed; maximum 400 mg/day (outpatient) or 600 mg/day (inpatient), split into 2 daily doses
- For insomnia, initial 25–50 mg at bedtime; increase as tolerated, usually to 50–100 mg/day, but some patients may require up to full antidepressant dose range
- For augmentation of other antidepressants in the treatment of depression, dose as recommended for insomnia

 Dosing Tips
- Start low and go slow
- ✱ Patients can have carryover sedation, ataxia, and intoxicated-like feeling if dosed

too aggressively, particularly when initiating dosing

* Do not discontinue trials if ineffective at low doses (<50 mg) as many patients with difficult cases may respond to higher doses (150–300 mg, even up to 600 mg in some cases)
* For relief of daytime anxiety, can give part of the dose in the daytime if not too sedating
* Although use as a monotherapy for depression is usually in divided doses due to its short half-life, use as an adjunct is often effective and best tolerated once daily at bedtime

Overdose
* Rarely lethal; sedation, vomiting, priapism, respiratory arrest, seizure, EKG changes

Long-Term Use
* Safe

Habit Forming
* No

How to Stop
* Taper is prudent to avoid withdrawal effects, but tolerance, dependence, and withdrawal effects have not been reliably demonstrated

Pharmacokinetics
* Metabolized by CYP450 3A4
* Half-life is biphasic; first phase is approximately 3–6 hours; second phase is approximately 5–9 hours

 Drug Interactions
* Tramadol increases the risk of seizures in patients taking an antidepressant
* Fluoxetine and other SSRIs may raise trazodone plasma levels
* Trazodone may block the hypotensive effects of some anti-hypertensive drugs
* Trazodone may increase digoxin or phenytoin concentrations
* Trazodone may interfere with the antihypertensive effects of clonidine
* Generally, do not use with MAO inhibitors, including 14 days after MAOIs are stopped
* Reports of increased and decreased prothrombin time in patients taking warfarin and trazodone

 Other Warnings/ Precautions
* Possibility of additive effects if trazodone is used with other CNS depressants
* Treatment should be discontinued if prolonged penile erection occurs because of the risk of permanent erectile dysfunction
* Advise patients to seek medical attention immediately if painful erections occur lasting more than one hour
* Generally, priapism reverses spontaneously, while penile blood flow and other signs being monitored, but in urgent cases, local phenylephrine injections or even surgery may be indicated
* Use with caution in patients with history of seizures
* Use with caution in patients with bipolar disorder unless treated with concomitant mood stabilizing agent
* When treating children, carefully weigh the risks and benefits of pharmacological treatment against the risks and benefits of nontreatment with antidepressants and make sure to document this in the patient's chart
* Distribute the brochures provided by the FDA and the drug companies
* Warn patients and their caregivers about the possibility of activating side effects and advise them to report such symptoms immediately
* Monitor patients for activation of suicidal ideation, especially children and adolescents

Do Not Use
* If patient is taking an MAO inhibitor, but see Pearls
* If there is a proven allergy to trazodone

SPECIAL POPULATIONS

Renal Impairment
* No dose adjustment necessary

Hepatic Impairment
* Drug should be used with caution

Cardiac Impairment
* Trazodone may be arrhythmogenic
* Monitor patients closely

- Not recommended for use during recovery from myocardial infarction

Elderly

- Elderly patients may be more sensitive to adverse effects and may require lower doses

Children and Adolescents

- Carefully weigh the risks and benefits of pharmacological treatment against the risks and benefits of nontreatment with antidepressants and make sure to document this in the patient's chart
- Monitor patients face-to-face regularly, particularly during the first several weeks of treatment
- Use with caution, observing for activation of known or unknown bipolar disorder and/or suicidal ideation, and inform parents or guardian of this risk so they can help observe child or adolescent patients
- Safety and efficacy have not been established, but trazodone has been used for behavioral disturbances, depression, and night terrors
- Children require lower initial dose and slow titration
- Boys may be even more sensitive to having prolonged erections than adult men

Pregnancy

- Risk Category C [some animal studies show adverse effects; no controlled studies in humans]
- Avoid use during first trimester
- Must weigh the risk of treatment (first trimester fetal development, third trimester newborn delivery) to the child against the risk of no treatment (recurrence of depression, maternal health, infant bonding) to the mother and child
- For many patients this may mean continuing treatment during pregnancy

Breast Feeding

- Some drug is found in mother's breast milk
- If child becomes irritable or sedated, breast feeding or drug may need to be discontinued
- Immediate postpartum period is a high-risk time for depression, especially in women

who have had prior depressive episodes, so drug may need to be reinstituted late in the third trimester or shortly after childbirth to prevent a recurrence during the postpartum period
- Must weigh benefits of breast feeding with risks and benefits of antidepressant treatment versus non-treatment to both the infant and the mother
- For many patients, this may mean continuing treatment during breast feeding

THE ART OF PSYCHOPHARMACOLOGY

Potential Advantages

- For insomnia when it is preferred to avoid the use of dependence-forming agents
- As an adjunct to the treatment of residual anxiety and insomnia with other antidepressants
- Depressed patients with anxiety
- Patients concerned about sexual side effects or weight gain

Potential Disadvantages

- For patients with fatigue, hypersomnia
- For patients intolerant to sedating effects

Primary Target Symptoms

- Depression
- Anxiety
- Sleep disturbances

Pearls

- May be less likely than some antidepressants to precipitate hypomania or mania
- Preliminary data suggest that trazodone may be effective treatment for drug-induced dyskinesias, perhaps in part because it reduces accompanying anxiety
- Trazodone may have some efficacy in treating agitation and aggression associated with dementia
- ✳ May cause sexual dysfunction only infrequently
- Can cause carryover sedation, sometimes severe, if dosed too high
- Often not tolerated as a monotherapy for moderate to severe cases of depression, as many patients cannot tolerate high doses (>150 mg)

- Do not forget to try at high doses, up to 600 mg/day, if lower doses well tolerated but ineffective
* For the expert psychopharmacologist, trazodone can be used cautiously for insomnia associated with MAO inhibitors, despite the warning – must be attempted only if patients closely monitored and by experts experienced in the use of MAOIs
- Priapism may occur in one in 8,000 men
- Early indications of impending priapism may be slow penile detumescence when awakening from REM sleep

- When using to treat insomnia, remember that insomnia may be a symptom of some other primary disorder, and not a primary disorder itself, and thus warrant evaluation for comorbid psychiatric and/or medical conditions
- Rarely, patients may complain of visual "trails" or after-images on trazodone

Suggested Reading

DeVane CL. Differential pharmacology of newer antidepressants. J Clin Psychiatry 1998;59 Suppl 20:85–93.

Haria M, Fitton A, McTavish D. Trazodone. A review of its pharmacology, therapeutic use in depression and therapeutic potential in other disorders. Drugs Aging 1994;4:331–55.

Rotzinger S, Bourin M, Akimoto Y, Coutts RT, Baker GB. Metabolism of some "second"- and "fourth"-generation antidepressants: iprindole, viloxazine, bupropion, mianserin, maprotiline, trazodone, nefazodone, and venlafaxine. Cell Mol Neurobiol 1999;19:427–42.

TRIMIPRAMINE

Brands • Surmontil
see index for additional brand names

Generic? Yes

Class

- Tricyclic antidepressant (TCA)
- Serotonin and norepinephrine/
  noradrenaline reuptake inhibitor

Commonly Prescribed For

(bold for FDA approved)
- **Depression**
- **Endogenous depression**
- Anxiety
- Insomnia
- Neuropathic pain/chronic pain
- Treatment-resistant depression

How The Drug Works

- Boosts neurotransmitters serotonin and
  norepinephrine/noradrenaline
- Blocks serotonin reuptake pump (serotonin
  transporter), presumably increasing
  serotonergic neurotransmission
- Blocks norepinephrine reuptake pump
  (norepinephrine transporter), presumably
  increasing noradrenergic
  neurotransmission
- Presumably desensitizes both serotonin 1A
  receptors and beta adrenergic receptors
- Since dopamine is inactivated by
  norepinephrine reuptake in frontal cortex,
  which largely lacks dopamine transporters,
  trimipramine can increase dopamine
  neurotransmission in this part of the brain

How Long Until It Works

- May have immediate effects in treating
  insomnia, agitation, or anxiety
- Onset of therapeutic actions usually not
  immediate, but often delayed 2 to 4 weeks
- If it is not working within 6 to 8 weeks for
  depression, it may require a dosage
  increase or it may not work at all
- May continue to work for many years to
  prevent relapse of symptoms

If It Works

- The goal of treatment of depression is
  complete remission of current symptoms
  as well as prevention of future relapses
- The goal of treatment of chronic
  neuropathic pain is to reduce symptoms as
  much as possible, especially in
  combination with other treatments
- Treatment of depression most often
  reduces or even eliminates symptoms, but
  not a cure since symptoms can recur after
  medicine stopped
- Treatment of chronic neuropathic pain may
  reduce symptoms, but rarely eliminates
  them completely, and is not a cure since
  symptoms can recur after medicine is
  stopped
- Continue treatment of depression until all
  symptoms are gone (remission)
- Once symptoms of depression are gone,
  continue treating for 1 year for the first
  episode of depression
- For second and subsequent episodes of
  depression, treatment may need to be
  indefinite
- Use in anxiety disorders and chronic pain
  may also need to be indefinite, but long-
  term treatment is not well studied in these
  conditions

If It Doesn't Work

- Many depressed patients only have a
  partial response where some symptoms
  are improved but others persist (especially
  insomnia, fatigue, and problems
  concentrating)
- Other depressed patients may be
  nonresponders, sometimes called
  treatment-resistant or treatment-refractory
- Consider increasing dose, switching to
  another agent or adding an appropriate
  augmenting agent
- Consider psychotherapy
- Consider evaluation for another diagnosis
  or for a comorbid condition (e.g., medical
  illness, substance abuse, etc.)
- Some patients may experience apparent
  lack of consistent efficacy due to activation
  of latent or underlying bipolar disorder, and
  require antidepressant discontinuation and
  a switch to a mood stabilizer

Best Augmenting Combos for Partial Response or Treatment-Resistance

- Lithium, buspirone, thyroid hormone (for depression)
- Gabapentin, tiagabine, other anticonvulsants, even opiates if done by experts while monitoring carefully in difficult cases (for chronic pain)

Tests

- None for healthy individuals
- ✳ Since tricyclic and tetracyclic antidepressants are frequently associated with weight gain, before starting treatment, weigh all patients and determine if the patient is already overweight (BMI 25.0–29.9) or obese (BMI ≥30)
- Before giving a drug that can cause weight gain to an overweight or obese patient, consider determining whether the patient already has pre-diabetes (fasting plasma glucose 100–125 mg/dl), diabetes (fasting plasma glucose >126 mg/dl), or dyslipidemia (increased total cholesterol, LDL cholesterol and triglycerides; decreased HDL cholesterol), and treat or refer such patients for treatment, including nutrition and weight management, physical activity counseling, smoking cessation, and medical management
- ✳ Monitor weight and BMI during treatment
- ✳ While giving a drug to a patient who has gained >5% of initial weight, consider evaluating for the presence of pre-diabetes, diabetes, or dyslipidemia, or consider switching to a different antipsychotic
- EKGs may be useful for selected patients (e.g., those with personal or family history of QTc prolongation; cardiac arrhythmia; recent myocardial infarction; uncompensated heart failure; or taking agents that prolong QTc interval such as pimozide, thioridazine, selected antiarrhythmics, moxifloxacin, sparfloxacin, etc.)
- Patients at risk for electrolyte disturbances (e.g., patients on diuretic therapy) should have baseline and periodic serum potassium and magnesium measurements

SIDE EFFECTS

How Drug Causes Side Effects

- Anticholinergic activity may explain sedative effects, dry mouth, constipation, and blurred vision
- Sedative effects and weight gain may be due to antihistamine properties
- Blockade of alpha adrenergic 1 receptors may explain dizziness, sedation, and hypotension
- Cardiac arrhythmias and seizures, especially in overdose, may be caused by blockade of ion channels

Notable Side Effects

- Blurred vision, constipation, urinary retention, increased appetite, dry mouth, nausea, diarrhea, heartburn, unusual taste in mouth, weight gain
- Fatigue, weakness, dizziness, sedation, headache, anxiety, nervousness, restlessness
- Sexual dysfunction (impotence, change in libido)
- Sweating, rash, itching

Life Threatening or Dangerous Side Effects

- Paralytic ileus, hyperthermia (TCAs + anticholinergic agents)
- Lowered seizure threshold and rare seizures
- Orthostatic hypotension, sudden death, arrhythmias, tachycardia
- QTc prolongation
- Hepatic failure, extrapyramidal symptoms
- Increased intraocular pressure
- Rare induction of mania
- Rare activation of suicidal ideation and behavior (suicidality)

Weight Gain

unusual / not unusual / **common** / problematic

- Many experience and/or can be significant in amount
- Can increase appetite and carbohydrate craving

Sedation

unusual / not unusual / **common** / problematic

- Many experience and/or can be significant in amount
- Tolerance to sedative effects may develop with long-term use

What To Do About Side Effects
- Wait
- Wait
- Wait
- Lower the dose
- Switch to an SSRI or newer antidepressant

Best Augmenting Agents for Side Effects
- Many side effects cannot be improved with an augmenting agent

DOSING AND USE

Usual Dosage Range
- 50–150 mg/day

Dosage Forms
- Capsule 25 mg, 50 mg, 100 mg

How to Dose
- Initial 25 mg/day at bedtime; increase by 75 mg every 3–7 days
- 75 mg/day in divided doses; increase to 150 mg/day; maximum 200 mg/day; hospitalized patients may receive doses up to 300 mg/day

 Dosing Tips
- If given in a single dose, should generally be administered at bedtime because of its sedative properties
- If given in split doses, largest dose should generally be given at bedtime because of its sedative properties
- If patients experience nightmares, split dose and do not give large dose at bedtime
- Patients treated for chronic pain may only require lower doses
- If intolerable anxiety, insomnia, agitation, akathisia, or activation occur either upon dosing initiation or discontinuation, consider the possibility of activated bipolar disorder, and switch to a mood stabilizer or an atypical antipsychotic

Overdose
- Death may occur; CNS depression, convulsions, cardiac dysrhythmias, severe hypotension, ECG changes, coma

Long-Term Use
- Safe

Habit Forming
- No

How to Stop
- Taper to avoid withdrawal effects
- Even with gradual dose reduction some withdrawal symptoms may appear within the first 2 weeks
- Many patients tolerate 50% dose reduction for 3 days, then another 50% reduction for 3 days, then discontinuation
- If withdrawal symptoms emerge during discontinuation, raise dose to stop symptoms and then restart withdrawal much more slowly

Pharmacokinetics
- Substrate for CYP450 2D6, 2C19, and 2C9
- Half-life approximately 7–23 hours

 Drug Interactions
- Tramadol increases the risk of seizures in patients taking TCAs
- Use of TCAs with anticholinergic drugs may result in paralytic ileus or hyperthermia
- Fluoxetine, paroxetine, bupropion, duloxetine, and other CYP450 2D6 inhibitors may increase TCA concentrations
- Cimetidine may increase plasma concentrations of TCAs and cause anticholinergic symptoms
- Phenothiazines or haloperidol may raise TCA blood concentrations
- May alter effects of antihypertensive drugs; may inhibit hypotensive effects of clonidine
- Use with sympathomimetic agents may increase sympathetic activity
- Methylphenidate may inhibit metabolism of TCAs
- Activation and agitation, especially following switching or adding antidepressants, may represent the induction of a bipolar state, especially a mixed dysphoric bipolar II condition sometimes associated with suicidal

ideation, and require the addition of lithium, a mood stabilizer or an atypical antipsychotic, and/or discontinuation of trimipramine

Other Warnings/ Precautions

- Add or initiate other antidepressants with caution for up to 2 weeks after discontinuing trimipramine
- Generally, do not use with MAO inhibitors, including 14 days after MAOIs are stopped; do not start an MAOI until 2 weeks after discontinuing trimipramine, but see Pearls
- Use with caution in patients with history of seizures, urinary retention, narrow angle-closure glaucoma, hyperthyroidism
- TCAs can increase QTc interval, especially at toxic doses which can be attained not only by overdose but also by combining with drugs that inhibit TCA metabolism via CYP450 2D6, potentially causing torsade de pointes-type arrhythmia or sudden death
- Because TCAs can prolong QTc interval, use with caution in patients who have bradycardia or who are taking drugs that can induce bradycardia (e.g., beta blockers, calcium channel blockers, clonidine, digitalis)
- Because TCAs can prolong QTc interval, use with caution in patients who have hypokalemia and/or hypomagnesemia or who are taking drugs that can induce hypokalemia and/or magnesemia (e.g., diuretics, stimulant laxatives, intravenous amphotericin B, glucocorticoids, tetracosactide)
- When treating children, carefully weigh the risks and benefits of pharmacological treatment against the risks and benefits of nontreatment with antidepressants and make sure to document this in the patient's chart
- Distribute the brochures provided by the FDA and the drug companies
- Warn patients and their caregivers about the possibility of activating side effects and advise them to report such symptoms immediately
- Monitor patients for activation of suicidal ideation, especially children and adolescents

Do Not Use

- If patient is recovering from myocardial infarction
- If patient is taking agents capable of significantly prolonging QTc interval (e.g., pimozide, thioridazine, selected antiarrhythmics, moxifloxacin, sparfloxacin)
- If there is a history of QTc prolongation or cardiac arrhythmia, recent acute myocardial infarction, uncompensated heart failure
- If patient is taking drugs that inhibit TCA metabolism, including CYP450 2D6 inhibitors, except by an expert
- If there is reduced CYP450 2D6 function, such as patients who are poor 2D6 metabolizers, except by an expert and at low doses
- If there is a proven allergy to trimipramine

SPECIAL POPULATIONS

Renal Impairment
- Use with caution; may need to lower dose

Hepatic Impairment
- Use with caution; may need to lower dose

Cardiac Impairment
- TCAs have been reported to cause arrhythmias, prolongation of conduction time, orthostatic hypotension, sinus tachycardia, and heart failure, especially in the diseased heart
- Myocardial infarction and stroke have been reported with TCAs
- TCAs produce QTc prolongation, which may be enhanced by the existence of bradycardia, hypokalemia, congenital or acquired long QTc interval, which should be evaluated prior to administering trimipramine
- Use with caution if treating concomitantly with a medication likely to produce prolonged bradycardia, hypokalemia, slowing of intracardiac conduction, or prolongation of the QTc interval
- Avoid TCAs in patients with a known history of QTc prolongation, recent acute myocardial infarction, and uncompensated heart failure
- TCAs may cause a sustained increase in heart rate in patients with ischemic heart

disease and may worsen (decrease) heart rate variability, an independent risk of mortality in cardiac populations
- Since SSRIs may improve (increase) heart rate variability in patients following a myocardial infarct and may improve survival as well as mood in patients with acute angina or following a myocardial infarction, these are more appropriate agents for cardiac population than tricyclic/tetracyclic antidepressants
* Risk/benefit ratio may not justify use of TCAs in cardiac impairment

Elderly
- May be more sensitive to anticholinergic, cardiovascular, hypotensive, and sedative effects
- Initial dose 50 mg/day; increase gradually up to 100 mg/day

Children and Adolescents
- Carefully weigh the risks and benefits of pharmacological treatment against the risks and benefits of nontreatment with antidepressants and make sure to document this in the patient's chart
- Monitor patients face-to-face regularly, particularly during the first several weeks of treatment
- Use with caution, observing for activation of known or unknown bipolar disorder and/or suicidal ideation, and inform parents or guardian of this risk so they can help observe child or adolescent patients
- Not recommended for use under age 12
- Several studies show lack of efficacy of TCAs for depression
- May be used to treat enuresis or hyperactive/impulsive behaviors
- Some cases of sudden death have occurred in children taking TCAs
- Adolescents: initial dose 50 mg/day; increase gradually up to 100 mg/day

Pregnancy
- Risk Category C [some animal studies show adverse effects, no controlled studies in humans]
- Crosses the placenta
- Adverse effects have been reported in infants whose mothers took a TCA

(lethargy, withdrawal symptoms, fetal malformations)
- Must weigh the risk of treatment (first trimester fetal development, third trimester newborn delivery) to the child against the risk of no treatment (recurrence of depression, maternal health, infant bonding) to the mother and child
- For many patients this may mean continuing treatment during pregnancy

Breast Feeding
- Some drug is found in mother's breast milk
* Recommended either to discontinue drug or bottle feed
- Immediate postpartum period is a high-risk time for depression, especially in women who have had prior depressive episodes, so drug may need to be reinstituted late in the third trimester or shortly after childbirth to prevent a recurrence during the postpartum period
- Must weigh the risk of treatment (first trimester fetal development, third trimester newborn delivery) to the child against the risk of no treatment (recurrence of depression, maternal health, infant bonding) to the mother and child
- For many patients this may mean continuing treatment during breast feeding

THE ART OF PSYCHOPHARMACOLOGY

Potential Advantages
- Patients with insomnia, anxiety
- Severe or treatment-resistant depression

Potential Disadvantages
- Pediatric and geriatric patients
- Patients concerned with weight gain and sedation

Primary Target Symptoms
- Depressed mood
- Symptoms of anxiety
- Somatic symptoms

Pearls
* May be more useful than some other TCAs for patients with anxiety, sleep disturbance, and depression with physical illness

✳ May be more sedating than some other TCAs

• Tricyclic antidepressants are often a first-line treatment option for chronic pain

• Tricyclic antidepressants are no longer generally considered a first-line option for depression because of their side effect profile

• Tricyclic antidepressants continue to be useful for severe or treatment-resistant depression

• TCAs may aggravate psychotic symptoms

• Alcohol should be avoided because of additive CNS effects

• Underweight patients may be more susceptible to adverse cardiovascular effects

• Children, patients with inadequate hydration, and patients with cardiac disease may be more susceptible to TCA-induced cardiotoxicity than healthy adults

• For the expert only: although generally prohibited, a heroic but potentially dangerous treatment for severely treatment-resistant patients is for an expert to give a tricyclic/tetracyclic antidepressant other than clomipramine simultaneously with an MAO inhibitor for patients who fail to respond to numerous other antidepressants

• If this option is elected, start the MAOI with the tricyclic/tetracyclic antidepressant simultaneously at low doses after appropriate drug washout, then alternately increase doses of these agents every few days to a week as tolerated

• Although very strict dietary and concomitant drug restrictions must be observed to prevent hypertensive crises and serotonin syndrome, the most common side effects of MAOI and tricyclic/tetracyclic antidepressant combinations may be weight gain and orthostatic hypotension

• Patients on tricyclics should be aware that they may experience symptoms such as photosensitivity or blue-green urine

• SSRIs may be more effective than TCAs in women, and TCAs may be more effective than SSRIs in men

• Since tricyclic/tetracyclic antidepressants are substrates for CYP450 2D6, and 7% of the population (especially Caucasians) may have a genetic variant leading to reduced activity of 2D6, such patients may not safely tolerate normal doses of tricyclic/tetracyclic antidepressants and may require dose reduction

• Phenotypic testing may be necessary to detect this genetic variant prior to dosing with a tricyclic/tetracyclic antidepressant, especially in vulnerable populations such as children, elderly, cardiac populations, and those on concomitant medications

• Patients who seem to have extraordinarily severe side effects at normal or low doses may have this phenotypic CYP450 2D6 variant and require low doses or switching to another antidepressant not metabolized by 2D6

Suggested Reading

Anderson IM. Meta-analytical studies on new antidepressants. Br Med Bull. 2001; 57:161–178.

Anderson IM. Selective serotonin reuptake inhibitors versus tricyclic antidepressants: a meta-analysis of efficacy and tolerability. J Aff Disorders. 2000;58:19–36.

Berger M, Gastpar M. Trimipramine: a challenge to current concepts on antidepressives. Eur Arch Psychiatry Clin Neurosci. 1996;246:235–9.

Lapierre YD. A review of trimipramine. 30 years of clinical use. Drugs. 1989;38 (Suppl 1):17–24;discussion 49–50.

VENLAFAXINE

THERAPEUTICS

Brands • Effexor
• Effexor XR
see index for additional brand names

Generic? No

 Class

- SNRI (dual serotonin and norepinephrine reuptake inhibitor); often classified as an antidepressant, but it is not just an antidepressant

Commonly Prescribed For
(bold for FDA approved)
- **Depression**
- **Generalized anxiety disorder (GAD)**
- **Social anxiety disorder (social phobia)**
- **Panic disorder**
- Posttraumatic stress disorder (PTSD)
- Premenstrual dysphoric disorder (PMDD)

 How The Drug Works

- Boosts neurotransmitters serotonin, norepinephrine/noradrenaline, and dopamine
- Blocks serotonin reuptake pump (serotonin transporter), presumably increasing serotonergic neurotransmission
- Blocks norepinephrine reuptake pump (norepinephrine transporter), presumably increasing noradrenergic neurotransmission
- Presumably desensitizes both serotonin 1A receptors and beta adrenergic receptors
- Since dopamine is inactivated by norepinephrine reuptake in frontal cortex, which largely lacks dopamine transporters, venlafaxine can increase dopamine neurotransmission in this part of the brain
- Weakly blocks dopamine reuptake pump (dopamine transporter), and may increase dopamine neurotransmission

How Long Until It Works
- Onset of therapeutic actions usually not immediate, but often delayed 2 to 4 weeks
- If it is not working within 6 to 8 weeks for depression, it may require a dosage increase or it may not work at all
- By contrast, for generalized anxiety, onset of response and increases in remission

rates may still occur after 8 weeks, and for up to 6 months after initiating dosing
- May continue to work for many years to prevent relapse of symptoms

If It Works
- The goal of treatment is complete remission of current symptoms as well as prevention of future relapses
- Treatment most often reduces or even eliminates symptoms, but not a cure since symptoms can recur after medicine stopped
- Continue treatment until all symptoms are gone (remission), especially in depression and whenever possible in anxiety disorders
- Once symptoms gone, continue treating for 1 year for the first episode of depression
- For second and subsequent episodes of depression, treatment may need to be indefinite
- Use in anxiety disorders may also need to be indefinite

If It Doesn't Work
- Many patients only have a partial response where some symptoms are improved but others persist (especially insomnia, fatigue, and problems concentrating)
- Other patients may be nonresponders, sometimes called treatment-resistant or treatment-refractory
- Some patients who have an initial response may relapse even though they continue treatment, sometimes called "poop-out"
- Consider increasing dose, switching to another agent or adding an appropriate augmenting agent
- Consider psychotherapy
- Consider evaluation for another diagnosis or for a comorbid condition (e.g., medical illness, substance abuse, etc.)
- Some patients may experience apparent lack of consistent efficacy due to activation of latent or underlying bipolar disorder, and require antidepressant discontinuation and a switch to a mood stabilizer

 Best Augmenting Combos for Partial Response or Treatment-Resistance

✳ Mirtazapine ("California rocket fuel"; a potentially powerful dual serotonin and norepinephrine combination, but observe

for activation of bipolar disorder and suicidal ideation)
- Bupropion, reboxetine, nortriptyline, desipramine, maprotiline, atomoxetine (all potentially powerful enhancers of noradrenergic action, but observe for activation of bipolar disorder and suicidal ideation)
- Modafinil, especially for fatigue, sleepiness, and lack of concentration
- Mood stabilizers or atypical antipsychotics for bipolar depression, psychotic depression or treatment-resistant depression
- Benzodiazepines
- If all else fails for anxiety disorders, consider gabapentin or tiagabine
- Hypnotics or trazodone for insomnia
- Classically, lithium, buspirone, or thyroid hormone

Tests
- Check blood pressure before initiating treatment and regularly during treatment

SIDE EFFECTS

How Drug Causes Side Effects
- Theoretically due to increases in serotonin and norepinephrine concentrations at receptors in parts of the brain and body other than those that cause therapeutic actions (e.g., unwanted actions of serotonin in sleep centers causing insomnia, unwanted actions of norepinephrine on acetylcholine release causing constipation and dry mouth, etc.)
- Most side effects are immediate but often go away with time

Notable Side Effects
- Most side effects increase with higher doses, at least transiently
- Headache, nervousness, insomnia, sedation
- Nausea, diarrhea, decreased appetite
- Sexual dysfunction (abnormal ejaculation/orgasm, impotence)
- Asthenia, sweating
- SIADH (syndrome of inappropriate antidiuretic hormone secretion)
- Hyponatremia
- Dose-dependent increase in blood pressure

Life Threatening or Dangerous Side Effects
- Rare seizures
- Rare induction of hypomania
- Rare activation of suicidal ideation and behavior (suicidality)

Weight Gain

unusual   not unusual   common   problematic

- Reported but not expected
- Possible weight loss, especially short-term

Sedation

unusual   not unusual   common   problematic

- Occurs in significant minority
- May also be activating in some patients

What To Do About Side Effects
- Wait
- Wait
- Wait
- Lower the dose
- In a few weeks, switch or add other drugs

Best Augmenting Agents for Side Effects
- Often best to try another antidepressant monotherapy prior to resorting to augmentation strategies to treat side effects
- Trazodone or a hypnotic for insomnia
- Bupropion, sildenafil, vardenafil, or tadalafil for sexual dysfunction
- Benzodiazepines for jitteriness and anxiety, especially at initiation of treatment and especially for anxious patients
- Mirtazapine for insomnia, agitation, and gastrointestinal side effects
- Many side effects are dose-dependent (i.e., they increase as dose increases, or they reemerge until tolerance re-develops)
- Many side effects are time-dependent (i.e., they start immediately upon dosing and upon each dose increase, but go away with time)
- Activation and agitation may represent the induction of a bipolar state, especially a mixed dysphoric bipolar II condition sometimes associated with suicidal ideation, and require the addition of lithium, a mood stabilizer or an atypical antipsychotic, and/or discontinuation of venlafaxine

DOSING AND USE

Usual Dosage Range
- Depression: 75–225 mg/day, once daily (extended release) or divided into 2–3 doses (immediate release)
- GAD: 150–225 mg/day

Dosage Forms
- Capsule (extended release) 37.5 mg, 75 mg, 150 mg
- Tablet 25 mg scored, 37.5 mg scored, 50 mg scored, 75 mg scored, 100 mg scored

How to Dose
- Initial dose 37.5 mg once daily (extended release) or 25–50 mg divided into 2–3 doses (immediate release) for a week, if tolerated; increase daily dose generally no faster than 75 mg every 4 days until desired efficacy is reached; maximum dose generally 375 mg/day
- Usually try doses at 75 mg increments for a few weeks prior to incrementing by an additional 75 mg

Dosing Tips
- At all doses, potent serotonin reuptake blockade
- 75–225 mg/day may be predominantly serotonergic in some patients, and dual serotonin and norepinephrine acting in other patients
- 225–375 mg/day is dual serotonin and norepinephrine acting in most patients
- ✳ Thus, nonresponders at lower doses should try higher doses to be assured of the benefits of dual SNRI action
- At very high doses (e.g., >375 mg/day), dopamine reuptake blocked as well in some patients
- Up to 600 mg/day has been given for heroic cases
- Venlafaxine has an active metabolite O-desmethylvenlafaxine (ODV), which is formed as the result of CYP450 2D6
- Thus, CYP450 2D6 inhibition reduces the formation of ODV, but this is of uncertain clinical significance
- ✳ Consider checking plasma levels of ODV and venlafaxine in nonresponders who tolerate high doses, and if plasma levels are low, experts can prudently prescribe doses above 375 mg/day while monitoring closely
- Do not break or chew venlafaxine XR capsules, as this will alter controlled release properties
- ✳ For patients with severe problems discontinuing venlafaxine, dosing may need to be tapered over many months (i.e., reduce dose by 1% every 3 days by crushing tablet and suspending or dissolving in 100 mL of fruit juice, and then disposing of 1 mL while drinking the rest; 3–7 days later, dispose of 2 mL, and so on). This is both a form of very slow biological tapering and a form of behavioral desensitization
- For some patients with severe problems discontinuing venlafaxine, it may be useful to add an SSRI with a long half-life, especially fluoxetine, prior to taper of venlafaxine; while maintaining fluoxetine dosing, first slowly taper venlafaxine and then taper fluoxetine
- Be sure to differentiate between re-emergence of symptoms requiring re-institution of treatment and withdrawal symptoms

Overdose
- Can be lethal; may cause no symptoms; possible symptoms include sedation, convulsions, rapid heartbeat
- Fatal toxicity index data from the U.K. suggest a higher rate of deaths from overdose with venlafaxine than with SSRIs
- Unknown whether this is related to differences in patients who receive venlafaxine or to potential cardiovascular toxicity of venlafaxine

Long-Term Use
- See doctor regularly to monitor blood pressure, especially at doses >225 mg/day

Habit Forming
- No

How to Stop
- Taper to avoid withdrawal effects (dizziness, nausea, stomach cramps, sweating, tingling, dysesthesias)
- Many patients tolerate 50% dose reduction for 3 days, then another 50% reduction for 3 days, then discontinuation

- If withdrawal symptoms emerge during discontinuation, raise dose to stop symptoms and then restart withdrawal much more slowly
- ✳ Withdrawal effects can be more common or more severe with venlafaxine than with some other antidepressants

Pharmacokinetics
- Parent drug has 3–7 hour half-life
- Active metabolite has 9–13 hour half-life

Drug Interactions
- Tramadol increases the risk of seizures in patients taking an antidepressant
- Can cause a fatal "serotonin syndrome" when combined with MAO inhibitors, so do not use with MAO inhibitors or for at least 14 days after MAOIs are stopped
- Do not start an MAO inhibitor for at least 2 weeks after discontinuing venlafaxine
- Concomitant use with cimetidine may reduce clearance of venlafaxine and raise venlafaxine levels
- Could theoretically interfere with the analgesic actions of codeine or possibly with other triptans
- Few known adverse drug interactions

⚠ Other Warnings/ Precautions
- Use with caution in patients with history of seizures
- Use with caution in patients with heart disease
- Use with caution in patients with bipolar disorder unless treated with concomitant mood stabilizing agent
- When treating children, carefully weigh the risks and benefits of pharmacological treatment against the risks and benefits of nontreatment with antidepressants and make sure to document this in the patient's chart
- Distribute the brochures provided by the FDA and the drug companies
- Warn patients and their caregivers about the possibility of activating side effects and advise them to report such symptoms immediately
- Monitor patients for activation of suicidal ideation, especially children and adolescents

Do Not Use
- If patient has uncontrolled narrow angle-closure glaucoma
- If patient is taking an MAO inhibitor
- If there is a proven allergy to venlafaxine

Renal Impairment
- Lower dose by 25–50%
- Patients on dialysis should not receive subsequent dose until dialysis is completed

Hepatic Impairment
- Lower dose by 50%

Cardiac Impairment
- Drug should be used with caution
- Venlafaxine has a dose-dependent effect on increasing blood pressure
- Venlafaxine is contraindicated in patients with heart disease in the U.K.
- Venlafaxine can block cardiac ion channels in vitro
- Venlafaxine worsens (i.e., reduces) heart rate variability in depression, perhaps due to norepinephrine reuptake inhibition

Elderly
- Some patients may tolerate lower doses better

Children and Adolescents
- Carefully weigh the risks and benefits of pharmacological treatment against the risks and benefits of nontreatment with antidepressants and make sure to document this in the patient's chart
- Monitor patients face-to-face regularly, particularly during the first several weeks of treatment
- Use with caution, observing for activation of known or unknown bipolar disorder and/or suicidal ideation, and inform parents or guardian of this risk so they can help observe child or adolescent patients
- Not specifically approved, but preliminary data suggest that venlafaxine is effective in children and adolescents with depression, anxiety disorders, and ADHD

Pregnancy

- Risk Category C [some animal studies show adverse effects, no controlled studies in humans]
- Not generally recommended for use during pregnancy, especially during first trimester
- Nonetheless, continuous treatment during pregnancy may be necessary and has not been proven to be harmful to the fetus
- Must weigh the risk of treatment (first trimester fetal development, third trimester newborn delivery) to the child against the risk of no treatment (recurrence of depression, maternal health, infant bonding) to the mother and child
- For many patients this may mean continuing treatment during pregnancy
- Neonates exposed to SSRIs or SNRIs late in the third trimester have developed complications requiring prolonged hospitalization, respiratory support, and tube feeding; reported symptoms are consistent with either a direct toxic effect of SSRIs and SNRIs or, possibly, a drug discontinuation syndrome, and include respiratory distress, cyanosis, apnea, seizures, temperature instability, feeding difficulty, vomiting, hypoglycemia, hypotonia, hypertonia, hyperreflexia, tremor, jitteriness, irritability, and constant crying

Breast Feeding

- Some drug is found in mother's breast milk
- Trace amounts may be present in nursing children whose mothers are on venlafaxine
- If child becomes irritable or sedated, breast feeding or drug may need to be discontinued
- Immediate postpartum period is a high-risk time for depression, especially in women who have had prior depressive episodes, so drug may need to be reinstituted late in the third trimester or shortly after childbirth to prevent a recurrence during the postpartum period
- Must weigh benefits of breast feeding with risks and benefits of antidepressant treatment versus non-treatment to both the infant and the mother
- For many patients, this may mean continuing treatment during breast feeding

THE ART OF PSYCHOPHARMACOLOGY

Potential Advantages

- Patients with retarded depression
- Patients with atypical depression
- Patients with comorbid anxiety
- Patients with depression may have higher remission rates on SNRIs than on SSRIs
- Depressed patients with somatic symptoms, fatigue, and pain
- Patients who do not respond or remit on treatment with SSRIs

Potential Disadvantages

- Patients sensitive to nausea
- Patients with borderline or uncontrolled hypertension
- Patients with cardiac disease

Primary Target Symptoms

- Depressed mood
- Energy, motivation, and interest
- Sleep disturbance
- Anxiety

Pearls

✳ May be effective in patients who fail to respond to SSRIs, and may be one of the preferred treatments for treatment-resistant depression

✳ May be used in combination with other antidepressants for treatment-refractory cases

- XR formulation improves tolerability, reduces nausea, and requires only once-daily dosing
- May be effective in a broad array of anxiety disorders
- May be effective in adult ADHD
- Not studied in stress urinary incontinence

✳ Has greater potency for serotonin reuptake blockade than for norepinephrine reuptake blockade, but this is of unclear clinical significance as a differentiating feature from other SNRIs

✳ In vitro binding studies tend to underestimate in vivo potency for reuptake blockade, as they do not factor in the presence of high concentrations of an active metabolite, higher oral mg dosing, or the lower protein binding which can increase functional drug levels at receptor sites

- Effective dose range is broad (i.e., 75 mg to 375 mg in many difficult cases, and up to 600 mg or more in heroic cases)
* Preliminary studies in neuropathic pain and fibromyalgia suggest potential efficacy
- Efficacy as well as side effects (especially nausea and increased blood pressure) are dose-dependent
- Blood pressure increases rare for XR formulation in doses up to 225 mg
- More withdrawal reactions reported upon discontinuation than for some other antidepressants
- May be helpful for hot flushes in perimenopausal women
- May be associated with higher depression remission rates than SSRIs

* Because of recent studies from the U.K. that suggest a higher rate of deaths from overdose with venlafaxine than with SSRIs, and because of its potential to affect heart function, venlafaxine can only be prescribed in the U.K. by specialist doctors and is contraindicated there in patients with heart disease
- Overdose data are from fatal toxicity index studies, which do not take into account patient characteristics or whether drug use was first- or second-line
- Venlafaxine's toxicity in overdose is less than that for tricyclic antidepressants

Suggested Reading

Buckley NA, McManus PR, Fatal toxicity of serotonergic and other antidepressant drugs: analysis of United Kingdom mortality data. BMJ 2002;325:1332–3.

Cheeta S, Schifano F, An Oyefeso A, Webb L, Ghodse AH. Antidepressant-related deaths and antidepressant prescriptions in England and Wales, 1998–2000. Br J Psychiatry 2004;184:41–7

Davidson J, Watkins L, Owens M, Krulewicz S, Connor K, Carpenter D et al. Effects of paroxetine and venlafaxine XR on heart rate variability in depression. J Clin Psychopharmacol 2005;25:480-4.

Hackett D. Venlafaxine XR in the treatment of anxiety. Acta Psychiatrica Scandinavica 2000; 406[suppl]:30–35.

Sheehan DV. Attaining remission in generalized anxiety disorder: venlafaxine extended release comparative data. J Clin Psychiatry 2001;62 Suppl 19:26–31.

Smith D, Dempster C, Glanville J, Freemantle N, Anderson I. Efficacy and tolerability of venlafaxine compared with selective serotonin reuptake inhibitors and other antidepressants: a meta-analysis. Br J Psychiatry 2002; 180:396–404.

Wellington K, Perry CM. Venlafaxine extended-release: a review of its use in the management of major depression. CNS Drugs 2001; 15:643–69.

Index by Drug Name

Acuilix (moclobemide), *125*
Adapin (doxepine), *57*
Adepil (amitriptyline), *1*
Adofen (fluoxetine), *77*
Allegron (nortriptyline), *137*
Alti-Desipramine (desipramine), *43*
Alti-Doxepin (doxepin), *57*
Alti-Trazodone (trazodone), *195*
Amboneural (selegiline), *171*
Ambo-neural (selegiline), *171*
Amilin (amitriptyline), *1*
Amilit (amitriptyline), *1*
Amindan (selegiline), *171*
Amineurin (amitriptyline), *1*
Aminuerin retard (amitriptyline), *1*
Amioxid (amitriptyline), *1*
Amitrip (amitriptyline), *1*
Amitriptilin (amitriptyline), *1*
Amitriptylin (amitriptyline), *1*
amitriptyline, *1*
Amitriptylinum (amitriptyline), *1*
Amitrol (amitriptyline), *1*
Amizol (amitriptyline), *1*
amoxapine, *9*
Anafranil (clomipramine), *35*
Anafranil 75 (clomipramine), *35*
Anafranil Retard (clomipramine), *35*
Aneural (maprotiline), *107*
Antideprin (imipramine), *89*
Antiparkin (selegiline), *171*
Apo-Amitriptyline (amitriptyline), *1*
Apo-Clomipramine (clomipramine), *35*
Apo-Desipramine (desipramine), *43*
Apo-Doxepin (doxepin), *57*
Apo-Fluoxetine (fluoxetine), *77*
Apo-Imipramine (imipramine), *89*
Aponal (doxepin), *57*
Apo-Selegiline (selegiline), *171*
Apo-Trazodone (trazodone), *195*
Apo-Trimip (trimipramine), *201*
Aremis (sertraline), *179*
Arima (moclobemide), *125*
Arol (moclobemide), *125*
Aropax (paroxetine), *145*
Asendin (amoxapine), *9*
Asendis (amoxapine), *9*
atomoxetine, *17*
Aurorix (moclobemide), *125*
Aventyl (nortriptyline), *137*
Avoxin (fluvoxamine), *83*
Azona (trazodone), *195*
Belpax (amitriptyline), *1*

Benpon (nortriptyline), *137*
Berk-Dothiepin (dothiepin), *51*
Besitran (sertraline), *179*
Bioxetin (fluoxetine), *77*
bupropion, *23*
bupropion SR, *23*
bupropion XL, *23*
Celexa (citalopram), *29*
Cidoxepin (doxepin), *57*
Cipram (citalopram), *29*
Cipramil (citalopram), *29*
citalopram, *29*
clomipramine, *35*
Clopress (clomipramine), *35*
Coaxil (tianeptine), *185*
Cognitiv (selegiline), *171*
Concordin (protriptyline), *159*
Concordine (protriptyline), *159*
Cosmopril (selegiline), *171*
Cymbalta (duloxetine), *65*
Dalcipran (milnacipran), *113*
Daprimen (amitriptyline), *1*
Defanyl (amoxapine), *9*
Deftan (lofepramine), *101*
Delgian (maprotiline), *107*
Demolox (amoxapine), *9*
Depramine (imipramine), *89*
Deprax (trazodone), *195*
Deprenon (fluoxetine), *77*
Deprenyl (selegiline), *171*
Depressase (maprotiline), *107*
Deprex (fluoxetine), *77*
Deprilan (selegiline), *171*
Deprilept (maprotiline), *107*
Deprimyl (lofepramine), *101*
Deprinol (imipramine), *89*
Deptran (doxepin), *57*
Deroxat (paroxetine), *145*
Desidox (doxepin), *57*
desipramine, *43*
Desitriptylin (amitriptyline), *1*
Desyrel (trazodone), *195*
Devidon (trazodone), *195*
Dinalexin (fluoxetine), *77*
Dobupal (venlafaxine), *207*
Domical (amitriptyline), *1*
Dominans (nortriptyline), *137*
DOM-trazodone (trazodone), *195*
Doneurin (doxepin), *57*
Dopress (dothiepin), *51*
Dothep (dothiepin), *51*
dothiepin, *51*

Doxal (doxepin), *57*
Doxedyn (doxepin), *57*
doxepin, *57*
duloxetine, *65*
Dumirox (fluvoxamine), *83*
Dumyrox (fluvoxamine), *83*
Dutonin (nefazodone), *131*
Edronax (reboxetine), *165*
Efectin (venlafaxine), *207*
Efexir (venlafaxine), *207*
Efexor (venlafaxine), *207*
Efexor XL (venlafaxine), *207*
Effexor (venlafaxine), *207*
Effexor XR (venlafaxine), *207*
Egibren (selegiline), *171*
Elavil (amitriptyline), *1*
Elavil Plus (amitriptyline), *1*
Eldepryl (selegiline), *171*
Eliwel (amitriptyline), *1*
Elopram (citalopram), *29*
Emdalen (lofepramine), *101*
Emsam (transdermal selegiline), *171*
Endep (amitriptyline), *1*
Erocap (fluoxetine), *77*
escitalopram, *71*
Eutimil (paroxetine), *145*
Exostrept (fluoxetine), *77*
Faverin (fluvoxamine), *83*
Felicium (fluoxetine), *77*
Fevarin (fluvoxamine), *83*
Flonital (fluoxetine), *77*
Floxyfral (fluvoxamine), *83*
Fluctin (fluoxetine), *77*
Fluctine (fluoxetine), *77*
Fluocim (fluoxetine), *77*
Fluoxeren (fluoxetine), *77*
fluoxetine, *77*
Fluoxifar (fluoxetine), *77*
Fluoxin (fluoxetine), *77*
Flutin (fluoxetine), *77*
Fluval (fluoxetine), *77*
fluvoxamine, *83*
Fluxadir (fluoxetine), *77*
Fluxonil (fluoxetine), *77*
Fondur (fluoxetine), *77*
Fontex (fluoxetine), *77*
Fonzac (fluoxetine), *77*
Frosinor (paroxetine), *145*
Frosnor (paroxetine), *145*
Gamanil (lofepramine), *101*
Gamonil (lofepramine), *101*
Gen-Clomipramine (clomipramine), *35*
Gladem (sertraline), *179*
Harmomed (dothiepin), *51*
Herphonal (trimipramine), *201*
Hydophen (clomipramine), *35*
Idom (dothiepin), *51*

Imavate (imipramine), *89*
Imipramiin (imipramine), *89*
Imipramin (imipramine), *89*
imipramine, *89*
isocarboxazid, *95*
Ixel (milnacipran), *113*
Janimine (imipramine), *89*
Jardin (dothiepin), *51*
Jatrosom (tranylcypromine), *189*
Jatrosom N (tranylcypromine), *189*
Julap (selegiline), *171*
Jumex (selegiline), *171*
Jumexal (selegiline), *171*
Kanopan 75 (maprotiline), *107*
Kinabide (selegiline), *171*
Ladose (fluoxetine), *77*
Laroxyl (amitriptyline), *1*
Lentizol (amitriptyline), *1*
Lexapro (escitalopram), *71*
Lilly Fluoxetine (fluoxetine), *77*
lofepramine, *101*
Lorien (fluoxetine), *77*
Lovan (fluoxetine), *77*
Ludiomil (maprotiline), *107*
Lustral (sertraline), *179*
Luvox (fluvoxamine), *83*
Maludil (maprotiline), *107*
Manerix (moclobemide), *125*
Mapro Gry (maprotiline), *107*
Mapro Tablinen (maprotiline), *107*
Maprolu (maprotiline), *107*
Maprolu-50 (maprotiline), *107*
Maprostad (maprotiline), *107*
Maprotibene (maprotiline), *107*
Maprotilin (maprotiline), *107*
maprotiline, *107*
Mareen 50 (doxepin), *57*
Marplan (isocarboxazid), *95*
Martimil (nortriptyline), *137*
Maveral (fluvoxamine), *83*
Maximed (protriptyline), *159*
Maxivalet (amitriptyline), *1*
Melipramin (imipramine), *89*
Melipramine (imipramine), *89*
Menfazona (nefazodone), *131*
Metylyl (desipramine), *43*
milnacipran, *113*
Mipralin (imipramine), *89*
Mirpan (maprotiline), *107*
mirtazapine, *119*
Mocloamine (moclobemide), *125*
moclobemide, *125*
Molipaxin (trazodone), *195*
Motipress (nortriptyline), *137*
Motival (nortriptyline), *137*
Motivan (paroxetine), *145*
Movergan (selegiline), *171*

Moverin (selegiline), *171*
Moxadil (amoxapine), *9*
Mutan (fluoxetine), *77*
Nailin (nortriptyline), *137*
Nalin (nortriptyline), *137*
Nardelzine (phenelzine), *153*
Nardil (phenelzine), *153*
Nefadar (nefazodone), *131*
nefazodone, *131*
Nefirel (nefazodone), *131*
Nicoflox (fluoxetine), *77*
Nopress (nortriptyline), *137*
Norebox (reboxetine), *165*
Norfenazin (nortriptyline), *137*
Noriline (nortriptyline), *137*
Noritren (nortriptyline), *137*
Norpramin (desipramine), *43*
Northiaden (dothiepin), *51*
Nortimil (desipramine), *43*
Nortix (nortriptyline), *137*
Nortrilen (nortriptyline), *137*
Nortriptilin (nortriptyline), *137*
nortriptyline, *137*
Novo-Clopamine (clomipramine), *35*
Novo-Doxepin (doxepin), *57*
Novo-fluoxetine (fluoxetine), *77*
Novo-Maprotiline (maprotiline), *107*
Novoprotect (amitriptyline), *1*
Novo-Selegine (selegiline), *171*
Novo-Trazodone (trazodone), *195*
Novo-Trimipramine (trimipramine), *201*
Nu-Trazodone (trazodone), *195*
Nu-Trimipramine (trimipramine), *201*
Nycoflox (fluoxetine), *77*
Omnipress (amoxapine), *9*
Orthon (fluoxetine), *77*
Pamelor (nortriptyline), *137*
Parkinyl (selegiline), *171*
Parmodalin (tranylcypromine), *189*
Parnate (tranylcypromine), *189*
paroxetine, *145*
paroxetine CR, *145*
Parstelin (tranylcypromine), *189*
Paxil (paroxetine), *145*
Paxil CR (paroxetine CR), *145*
Paxtibi (nortriptyline), *137*
Pertofrane (desipramine), *43*
Pertofrin (desipramine), *43*
phenelzine, *153*
Placil (clomipramine), *35*
Plurimen (selegiline), *171*
PMS-Desipramine (desipramine), *43*
PMS-Fluoxetine (fluoxetine), *77*
PMS-Trazodone (trazodone), *195*
Poldoxin (doxepin), *57*
Polysal (amitriptyline), *1*
Portal (fluoxetine), *77*

Pragmarel (trazodone), *195*
Prisdal (citalopram), *29*
Procythol (selegiline), *171*
Prothiaden (dothiepin), *51*
Protiaden (dothiepin), *51*
protriptyline, *159*
Prozac (fluoxetine), *77*
Prozyn (fluoxetine), *77*
Pryleugan (imipramine), *89*
Psymoin (maprotiline), *107*
Quitaxon (doxepin), *57*
reboxetine, *165*
Redomex (amitriptyline), *1*
RedomexDiffucaps (amitriptyline), *1*
Regepar (selegiline), *171*
Remergil (mirtazapine), *119*
Remeron (mirtazapine), *119*
Reneuron (fluoxetine), *77*
Reseril (nefazodone), *131*
Retinyl (maprotiline), *107*
Rexer (mirtazapine), *119*
Rho-Doxepin (doxepin), *57*
Rho-Trimine (trimipramine), *201*
Rimarix (moclobemide), *125*
Rulivan (nefazodone), *131*
Sanzur (fluoxetine), *77*
Sapilent (trimipramine), *201*
Sarafem (fluoxetine), *77*
Saroten (amitriptyline), *1*
Saroten Retard (amitriptyline), *1*
Sarotex (amitriptyline), *1*
Sartuzin (fluoxetine), *77*
Sedacoroxen (imipramine), *89*
Seledat (selegiline), *171*
Selegam (selegiline), *171*
selegiline, *171*
Selepar (selegiline), *171*
Selepark (selegiline), *171*
Seletop 5 (selegiline), *171*
Selgene (selegiline), *171*
Selpar (selegiline), *171*
Sensaval (nortriptyline), *137*
Sensival (nortriptyline), *137*
Sepatrem (selegiline), *171*
Serad (sertraline), *179*
Serafem (fluoxetine), *77*
Seralgan (citalopram), *29*
Sereupin (paroxetine), *145*
Serlain (sertraline), *179*
Serol (fluoxetine), *77*
Seronil (fluoxetine), *77*
Seropram (citalopram), *29*
Seroxal (paroxetine), *145*
Seroxat (paroxetine), *145*
Sertofren (desipramine), *43*
sertraline, *179*
Serzone (nefazodone), *131*

Sinequan (doxepin), *57*
Sinquan (doxepin), *57*
Sinquane (doxepin), *57*
SK-Pramine (imipramine), *89*
Solarix (moclobemide), *125*
Stablon (tianeptine), *185*
Stelminal (amitriptyline), *1*
Stephadilat (fluoxetine), *77*
Strattera (atomoxetine), *17*
Surmontil (trimipramine), *201*
Syneudon 50 (amitriptyline), *1*
Tagonis (paroxetine), *145*
Tatig (sertraline), *179*
Teledomin (milnacipran), *113*
Teperin (amitriptyline), *1*
Thaden (dothiepin), *51*
Thombran (trazodone), *195*
tianeptine, *185*
Timelit (lofepramine), *101*
Tingus (fluoxetine), *77*
Tofranil (imipramine), *89*
Tofranil pamoata (imipramine), *89*
Tofranil-PM (imipramine), *89*
Toledomin (milnacipran), *113*
Tramensan (trazodone), *195*
tranylcypromine, *189*
trazodone, *195*
Trazolan (trazodone), *195*
Tremorex (selegiline), *171*
Trepiline (amitriptyline), *1*
Tresleen (sertraline), *179*
Trevilor (venlafaxine), *207*

Trewilor (venlafaxine), *207*
trimipramine, *201*
Tripamine Surmontil (trimipramine), *201*
Triptil (protriptyline), *159*
Triptyl (amitriptyline), *1*
Triptyl Depot (amitriptyline), *1*
Trittico (trazodone), *195*
Tropargal (nortriptyline), *137*
Tryptanol (amitriptyline), *1*
Tryptine (amitriptyline), *1*
Tryptizol (amitriptyline), *1*
Tydamine (trimipramine), *201*
Tymelyt (lofepramine), *101*
Vandral (venlafaxine), *207*
Venefon (imipramine), *89*
venlafaxine, *207*
venlafaxine XR, *207*
Vivacti (protriptyline), *159*
Vivapryl (selegiline), *171*
Vividyl (nortriptyline), *137*
Wellbatrin (bupropion), *23*
Wellbutrin (bupropion), *23*
Wellbutrin SR (bupropion SR), *23*
Wellbutrin XL (bupropion XL), *23*
Xepin (doxepin), *57*
Zactin (fluoxetine), *77*
zelapon (selegiline), *171*
Zerenal (dothiepin), *51*
Zispin (mirtazapine), *119*
Zoloft (sertraline), *179*
Zonalon (doxepin), *57*
Zyban (bupropion), *23*

Index by Use

Bold for FDA approved

Anxiety
  amitriptyline, *1*
  amoxapine, *9*
  citalopram, *29*
  clomipramine, *35*
  desipramine, *43*
  dothiepin, *51*
  doxepin, *57*
  duloxetine, *65*
  escitalopram, *71*
  fluoxetine, *77*
  fluvoxamine, *83*
  imipramine, *89*
  isocarboxazid, *95*
  lofepramine, *101*
  maprotiline, *107*
  mirtazapine, *119*
  moclobemide, *125*
  nefazodone, *131*
  nortriptyline, *137*
  paroxetine, *145*
  phenelzine, *153*
  reboxetine, *165*
  sertraline, *179*
  tianeptine, *185*
  tranylcypromine, *189*
  trazodone, *195*
  trimipramine, *201*
  venlafaxine, *207*

Attention deficit/hyperactivity disorder
  atomoxetine, *17*
  bupropion, *23*
  reboxetine, *165*

Bipolar depression
  amoxapine, *9*
  bupropion, *23*
  fluoxetine, *77*

Bipolar disorder
  amoxapine, *9*
  bupropion, *23*
  doxepin, *57*
  fluoxetine, *77*

Bulimia nervosa/binge eating
  fluoxetine, *77*

Cataplexy syndrome
  clomipramine, *35*
  imipramine, *89*

Depression
  amitriptyline, *1*
  amoxapine, *9*
  atomoxetine, *17*
  bupropion, *23*
  citalopram, *29*
  clomipramine, *35*
  desipramine, *43*
  dothiepin, *51*
  doxepin, *57*
  duloxetine, *65*
  escitalopram, *71*
  fluoxetine, *77*
  fluvoxamine, *83*
  imipramine, *89*
  isocarboxazid, *95*
  lofepramine, *101*
  maprotiline, *107*
  milnacipran, *113*
  mirtazapine, *119*
  moclobemide, *125*
  nefazodone, *131*
  nortriptyline, *137*
  paroxetine, *145*
  phenelzine, *153*
  protriptyline, *159*
  reboxetine, *165*
  selegiline, *171*
  sertraline, *179*
  tianeptine, *185*
  tranylcypromine, *189*
  trazodone, *195*
  trimipramine, *201*
  venlafaxine, *207*

Enuresis
  imipramine, *89*

Fibromyalgia
  amitriptyline, *1*
  duloxetine, *65*
  milnacipran, *113*

Generalized anxiety disorder
  citalopram, *29*
  duloxetine, *65*
  escitalopram, *71*
  fluoxetine, *77*
  fluvoxamine, *83*
  mirtazapine, *119*
  paroxetine, *145*

sertraline, *179*
venlafaxine, *207*

Insomnia
amitriptyline, *1*
amoxapine, *9*
clomipramine, *35*
desipramine, *43*
dothiepin, *51*
doxepin, *57*
imipramine, *89*
lofepramine, *101*
maprotiline, *107*
nortriptyline, *137*
trazodone, *195*
trimipramine, *201*

Neuropathic pain/chronic pain
amitriptyline, *1*
amoxapine, *9*
clomipramine, *35*
desipramine, *43*
dothiepin, *51*
doxepin, *57*
duloxetine (DPNP), *65*
imipramine, *89*
lofepramine, *101*
maprotiline, *107*
milnacipran, *113*
nortriptyline, *137*
trimipramine, *201*

Nicotine addiction
bupropion, *23*

Obsessive-compulsive disorder
citalopram, *29*
clomipramine, *35*
escitalopram, *71*
fluoxetine, *77*
fluvoxamine, *83*
paroxetine, *145*
sertraline, *179*
venlafaxine, *207*

Panic disorder
citalopram, *29*
escitalopram, *71*
fluoxetine, *77*
fluvoxamine, *83*

isocarboxazid, *95*
mirtazapine, *119*
nefazodone, *131*
paroxetine, *145*
phenelzine, *153*
reboxetine, *165*
sertraline, *179*
tranylcypromine, *189*
venlafaxine, *207*

Parkinson's disease
selegiline, *171*

Posttraumatic stress disorder
citalopram, *29*
escitalopram, *71*
fluoxetine, *77*
fluvoxamine, *83*
mirtazapine, *119*
nefazodone, *131*
paroxetine, *145*
sertraline, *179*
venlafaxine, *207*

Premenstrual dysphoric disorder
citalopram, *29*
escitalopram, *71*
fluoxetine, *77*
paroxetine, *145*
sertraline, *179*
venlafaxine, *207*

Sexual dysfunction
bupropion, *23*

Social anxiety disorder
citalopram, *29*
escitalopram, *71*
fluoxetine, *77*
fluvoxamine, *83*
isocarboxazid, *95*
moclobemide, *125*
paroxetine, *145*
phenelzine, *153*
sertraline, *179*
tranylcypromine, *189*
venlafaxine, *207*

Stress urinary incontinence
duloxetine, *65*

Abbreviations

5HT	serotonin
ACH	acetylcholine
ACHE	acetylcholinesterase
ADHD	attention deficit hyperactivity disorder
ALT	alanine aminotransferase
ALPT	total serum alkaline phosphatase
AST	aspartate aminotransferase
BID	twice a day
BMI	body mass index
BuChE	butyrylcholinesterase
CMI	clomipramine
CNS	central nervous system
CYP450	cytochrome P450
De-CMI	desmethyl-clomipramine
DA	dopamine
dl	deciliter
DLB	dementia with Lewy bodies
DPNP	diabetic peripheral neuropathic pain
ECG	electrocardiogram
EEG	electroencephalogram
EKG	electrocardiogram
EPS	extrapyramidal side effects
ERT	estrogen replacement therapy
FDA	Food and Drug Administration
FSH	follicle-stimulating hormone
GAD	generalized anxiety disorder
GI	gastrointestinal
HDL	high-density lipoprotein
HMG CoA	beta-hydroxy-beta-methylglutaryl Coenzyme A
HRT	hormone replacement therapy
IM	intramuscular
IV	intravenous
LDL	low-density lipoprotein
LH	luteinizing hormone
Lb	pound
MAO	monoamine oxidase
MAOI	monoamine oxidase inhibitor
mCPP	meta-chloro-phenyl-piperazine
mg	milligram
mL	milliliter
mm Hg	millimeters of mercury

MDD	major depressive disorder
NE	norepinephrine
NMDA	N-methyl-d-aspartate
OCD	obsessive-compulsive disorder
ODV	O-desmethylvenlafaxine
PET	positron emission tomography
PK	pharmacokinetic
PMDD	premenstrual dysphoric disorder
PMS	premenstrual syndrome
PTSD	posttraumatic stress disorder
QD	once a day
QHS	once a day at bedtime
QID	four times a day
RIMA	reversible inhibitor of monoamine oxidase A
SNRI	dual serotonin and norepinephrine reuptake inhibitor
SSRI	selective serotonin reuptake inhibitor
TCA	tricyclic antidepressant
TID	three times a day
TSH	thyroid stimulating hormone

FDA Use-In-Pregnancy Ratings

Category A: Controlled studies show no risk: adequate, well-controlled studies in pregnant women have failed to demonstrate risk to the fetus

Category B: No evidence of risk in humans: either animal findings show risk, but human findings do not; or, if no adequate human studies have been performed, animal findings are negative

Category C: Risk cannot be ruled out: human studies are lacking, and animal studies are either positive for fetal risk or lacking as well. However, potential benefits may outweigh risks

Category D: Positive evidence of risk: investigational or postmarketing data show risk to the fetus. Nevertheless, potential benefits may outweigh risks

Category X: Contraindicated in pregnancy: studies in animals or humans, or investigational or postmarketing reports, have shown fetal risk that clearly outweighs any possible benefit to the patient